Atlas of
Differential Diagnosis in
Neoplastic Hematopathology

Dedication

To my teachers and friends: Prof. Stanislaw Woyke MD (Szczecin, Poland), Prof. Zbigniew Darzynkiewicz MD (Valhalla, New York), Prof. Wlodzimierz Olszewski MD (Warsaw, Poland), and Prof. MR Melamed MD (Valhalla, New York).

W Gorczyca

Atlas of
Differential Diagnosis in
Neoplastic Hematopathology

Wojciech Gorczyca MD PhD
Genzyme Genetics, New York, USA

with

James Weisberger MD and **Foxwell N Emmons** MT (ASCP) SH

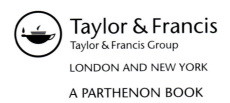

Taylor & Francis
Taylor & Francis Group

LONDON AND NEW YORK

A PARTHENON BOOK

First published in the United Kingdom in 2005
by Taylor & Francis,
an imprint of the Taylor & Francis Group,
2 Park Square, Milton Park
Abingdon, Oxon OX14 4RN, UK

Tel.:   +44 (0) 1235 828600
Fax.:   +44 (0) 1235 829000
Website: www.tandf.co.uk

British Library Cataloguing in Publication Data

Data available on application

Library of Congress Cataloging-in-Publication Data

Data available on application

ISBN 1-84214-247-X

Distributed in North and South America by

Taylor & Francis
2000 NW Corporate Blvd
Boca Raton, FL 33431, USA

Within Continental USA
Tel.: 800 272 7737; Fax.: 800 374 3401
Outside Continental USA
Tel.: 561 994 0555; Fax.: 561 361 6018
E-mail: orders@crcpress.com

Distributed in the rest of the world by
Thomson Publishing Services
Cheriton House
North Way
Andover, Hampshire SP10 5BE, UK
Tel.: +44 (0) 1264 332424
E-mail: salesorder.tandf@thomsonpublishingservices.co.uk

Composition by Siva Math Setters, Chennai, India
Printed and bound by T.G. Hostench, S.A., Spain

Contents

Contributors

Wojciech Gorczyca MD PhD
Director of Hematopathology/
    Oncology Services (New York)
Genzyme Genetics
521 West 57th Street
New York NY 10019, USA

Foxwell N Emmons MT (ASCP) SH
Bone Marrow Morphology Service
Genzyme Genetics
521 West 57th Street
New York, NY 10019, USA

James Weisberger MD
Vice-President and Director of Hematopathology
Bio-Reference Laboratories, Inc.
481 Edward H Ross Drive
Elmwood Park, NJ 07407, USA

Acknowledgments

The authors gratefully acknowledge the countless pathologists, hematologists and oncologists who entrusted their patient samples to our care at Genzyme Genetics, and enabled us to accrue the various cases depicted in this atlas. We would like to thank all hematopathologists at Genzyme Genetics, especially Drs Z Liu, H Dong, CD Wu, PS Lee, V Bhardwaj, P Cohen and HL Evans for their constructive remarks and for sharing interesting cases with us. We are grateful to Dr G Sun (Director of Cytogenetics at Genzyme Genetics) for his contribution of the cytogenetic and FISH images, and Prof. M Chosia (Medical School, Szczecin, Poland) for her contribution of cases.

We would like to thank M Gangi, immunohistochemistry laboratory manager and her team, whose devotion and hard work contributed so much to this project. We would also like to thank Dr S Tugulea and the Genzyme Genetics technologists from the immunohistochemistry, flow cytometry, bone marrow morphology and histology laboratories who prepared the samples depicted in this atlas, knowing that patient outcome depends on the expert handling of each specimen. We express our sincere appreciation to Dr Bruce C Horten, Medical Director, for his support and for creating a nurturing environment that allowed us to grow professionally.

Preface

The main purpose of this atlas is to provide the practicing pathologist, hematologist and oncologist, as well as physicians in training, with an overview of neoplastic hematopathology. The images, reflecting a multidisciplinary approach to the diagnosis of hematologic malignancies, include routine histology, cytology, immunohistochemistry and flow cytometry as well as cytogenetic, molecular and imaging studies. The emphasis of this atlas is on the differential diagnosis. The first chapter provides a general overview of the morphologic, cytologic, immunohistochemical and flow cytometric data useful in diagnostic hematopathology. It also includes normal hematopoiesis, cluster designation markers and algorithms to the diagnosis of lymphoma, chronic myelogenous leukemia, plasma cell neoplasia and anemia.

Chapters 2 through 12 present examples of the most useful diagnostic criteria in differentiating the various types of hematopoietic tumors, based on the WHO classification. The last three chapters are devoted entirely to the differential diagnosis based on cytohistologic features (Chapter 13), phenotypic markers (Chapter 14) and localization of the tumor (Chapter 15).

This atlas includes examples of the most common tumors as well as their variants. Illustrations are accompanied by tables, which present summary or statistical data of many entities based on the cases reviewed by the authors at Genzyme Genetics from 2000 to 2004. Brief discussions of each subject include relevant clinical presentation, prognosis and references.

Wojciech Gorczyca MD PhD
James Weisberger MD
Foxwell N Emmons MT (ASCP) SH
Genzyme Genetics, New York, 2004

CHAPTER 1

Introduction

GENERAL HISTOLOGIC AND CYTOLOGIC FEATURES

Lymph node – histology

Evaluation of the lymph node requires correlation of architectural characteristics (low power) with cytologic features (high-power evaluation). Evaluation of the lymph node at low power provides important information. Several major histologic patterns are recognized in the lymph node: nodular (follicular), diffuse, interfollicular, sinusoidal and mixed. A diffuse infiltrate composed of large cells (Figure 1.1A) can be present in diffuse large B-cell lymphoma (DLBCL), peripheral T-cell lymphoma and non-hematopoietic tumors. A diffuse lymphoid infiltrate with numerous histiocytes gives rise to a 'starry-sky' pattern (Figure 1.1B). This pattern is characteristic for Burkitt lymphoma and other high-grade lymphomas as well as precursor (lymphoblastic) tumors. The presence of clusters of paler-staining larger lymphocytes in the background of a small lymphocytic infiltrate gives rise to the 'pseudo-follicular' pattern (Figure 1.1C), characteristic of B-small lymphocytic lymphoma/chronic lymphocytic leukemia.

A nodular pattern is most characteristic for follicular lymphoma (Figure 1.1D). The nodular (follicular pattern) is typical also for several reactive conditions such as follicular hyperplasia, Kimura disease, Castleman's disease and rheumatoid lymphadenopathy. A nodular pattern with fibrous bands and scattered large multilobated cells (Figure 1.1E) is seen in the nodular sclerosis type of classical Hodgkin lymphoma (HL). A vague nodular pattern with rare large cells with vesicular nuclei (popcorn cells or L&H cells) is typical for nodular lymphocyte-predominant Hodgkin lymphoma (NLPHL; Figure 1.1F). The expanded nodules of NLPHL help to distinguish it from T-cell/histiocyte-rich large B-cell lymphoma.

A paracortical (interfollicular) infiltrate (Figure 1.1G) can be seen in peripheral T-cell lymphoma, 'not otherwise specified' (NOS). It can be also seen in extramedullary myeloid tumor (EMT; granulocytic sarcoma), blastic natural killer (NK)-cell lymphoma, classical Hodgkin lymphoma, anaplastic large cell lymphoma, occasional diffuse large B-cell lymphomas and metastatic tumors. Of those, EMT may be most difficult to identify on H&E examination alone (comparison of CD3 and CD43 staining will identify population of CD3$^-$/CD43$^+$ cells, which may stain for myeloperoxidase, CD34, CD117 and often TdT). The interfollicular pattern is seen also in some reactive conditions such as dermatopathic, post-vaccination lymphadenitis and viral lymphadenitis, and in some drug reactions.

Expansion of the marginal zone (Figure 1.1H) with prominent monocytoid B-cells is seen in marginal zone B-cell lymphoma and reactive hyperplasia. A mantle zone pattern (Figure 1.1I) can be seen in reactive processes and mantle cell lymphoma (MCL). MCL can present also diffuse and nodular patterns (see also Figures 2.75, 2.76 and 2.77; Chapter 2). A concentric arrangement of small lymphocytes ('onionskin', Figure 1.1J) with follicles composed of more than one germinal center is typical for Castleman's disease (hyaline-vascular type). Large expanded follicles composed of small lymphocytes with disruption of the follicular dendritic meshwork are termed 'progressively transformed germinal centers' (PTGC) (Figure 1.1K). They accompany reactive follicular hyperplasia and may be seen in patients with NLPHL (in prior or subsequent lymph node biopsies).

An intrasinusoidal pattern (Figure 1.1L) is typical for anaplastic large cell lymphoma, metastatic non-hematopoietic tumors, rare DLBCL and variants of peripheral T-cell lymphoma. T-cell lymphomas are additionally

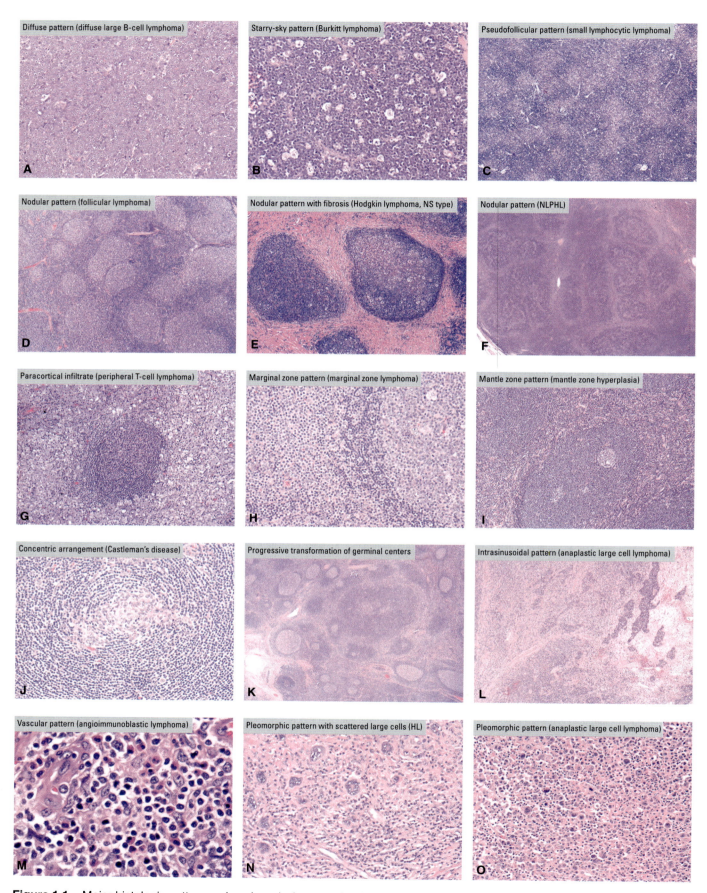

Figure 1.1   Major histologic patterns – lymph node (see text for details)

characterized by admixture of eosinophils and increased vascularity. The latter is especially prominent in angio-immunoblastic T-cell lymphoma (Figure 1.1M). A diffuse pleomorphic infiltrate composed of a mixed population of lymphocytes, eosinophils, plasma cells and histiocytes ('inflammatory background') and large multilobated cells is typical for classical Hodgkin lymphoma (Figure 1.1N). When large mononuclear highly atypical cells predominate, anaplastic large cell lymphoma should be considered (Figure 1.1O).

Differential diagnosis of lymph node patterns in malignant lymphoma is presented in Chapter 13 (Figures 13.2–13.13).

Bone marrow – histology

Histologic evaluation of the bone marrow core biopsy is an integral part of comprehensive marrow evaluation. It gives the information about marrow cellularity, M:E ratio and the architectural relationship between the various hematopoietic elements, number, distribution and cytomorphology of megakaryocytes, presence and distribution of lymphoid aggregates, presence of extrinsic elements, the status of the bony trabeculae, sinusoids and blood vessels[1–11].

A cellular marrow with an increased M:E ratio due to erythroid hypoplasia with scattered large cells containing prominent eosinophilic inclusions is characteristic for parvovirus infection (Figure 1.2A).

Reactive lymphoid aggregates (Figure 1.2B) are a common finding, especially in patients with chronic immune stimulation, and their likelihood and number(s) increase with age. They are composed of mixed population of small to intermediate lymphocytes, small blood vessels, and rare histiocytes. They are usually small and well demarcated. The immunohistochemistry (see Figures 13.13–13.16; Chapter 13) shows mixed B- and T-lymphocytes, intact follicular dendritic meshwork (CD21 staining) and bcl-2[-]/bcl6[+]/CD10[+] germinal center cells. Paratrabecular lymphoid aggregates (Figure 1.2C) are typical for follicular lymphoma, although occasional mantle cell lymphoma and other types of B-cell disorders can display a paratrabecular pattern.

A diffuse lymphoid infiltrate composed of small lymphocytes can be present in chronic lymphocytic leukemia/small lymphocytic lymphoma (B-CLL/SLL), mantle cell lymphoma, marginal zone B-cell lymphoma, lymphoplasmacytic lymphoma and some T-cell lymphoproliferative disorders. B-CLL/SLL shows predominance of small lymphocytes (Figure 1.2D) with groups of larger cells with nucleoli (prolymphocytes) giving rise to formation of proliferation centers (paler areas on HE preparations). A diffuse lymphoid infiltrate with blastic cytomorphology and occasional scattered histiocytes suggests precursor B-lymphoblastic leukemia (Figure 1.2E). The differential diagnosis includes T-ALL, metastatic tumors (neuroblastoma, rhabdomyosarcoma or carcinoma), large B-cell lymphoma, Langerhans cell histiocytosis, anaplastic myeloma and acute myeloid leukemia.

The presence of atypical lymphohistiocytic aggregates with scattered large multinucleated cells is highly suggestive of Hodgkin lymphoma (Figure 1.2F). A large cell infiltrate with nuclear outline irregularities and scattered eosinophils is seen in Langerhans cell histiocytosis (Figure 1.2G). The differential diagnosis of a spindle cell infiltrate (Figure 1.2H) includes metastases from malignant melanoma, sarcomatoid carcinoma, spindle cell sarcomas (leiomyosarcoma, gastrointestinal stromal tumors and vascular tumors) and anaplastic lymphomas.

An intrasinusoidal infiltrate (Figure 1.2I) may be seen in T-cell lymphomas, such as hepatosplenic gamma/delta T-cell lymphoma, anaplastic large cell lymphoma, enteropathy type T-cell lymphoma and B-cell lymphomas (e.g., splenic marginal zone lymphoma with villous lymphocytes or intravascular large B-cell lymphoma)[12,13]. A hypercellular marrow with increased M:E ratio and micromegakaryocytes suggests a chronic myeloproliferative disorder, such as chronic myelogenous leukemia (CML) (Figure 1.2J). The presence of diffuse fibrosis, megakaryocytosis and osteosclerosis is seen usually in chronic idiopathic myelofibrosis (Figure 1.2K). The differential diagnosis of marked megakaryocytosis with atypia and cluster formation includes acute megakaryoblastic leukemia (Figure 1.2L), polycythemia vera (Figure 1.2M), myelodysplastic syndrome and essential thrombocythemia.

Acute myeloid leukemias (Figure 1.2N) are characterized by a generally hypercellular marrow with sheets of immature cells replacing normal marrow elements.

Plasma cell infiltrates may be subtle (requiring immunohistochemical staining for identification) or very prominent (Figure 1.2O). Non-neoplastic plasma cell collections are often perivascular. Plasma cell neoplasia may be accompanied by other hematopoietic malignancies (AML, B-CLL/SLL, etc.).

Bone marrow mastocytosis (Figure 1.2P) is characterized by paratrabecular and/or interstitial aggregates of large cells with pale cytoplasm. Extrinsic tumors are usually easily discernible (Figure 1.2R). Some cases, however, require confirmatory immunohistochemistry staining

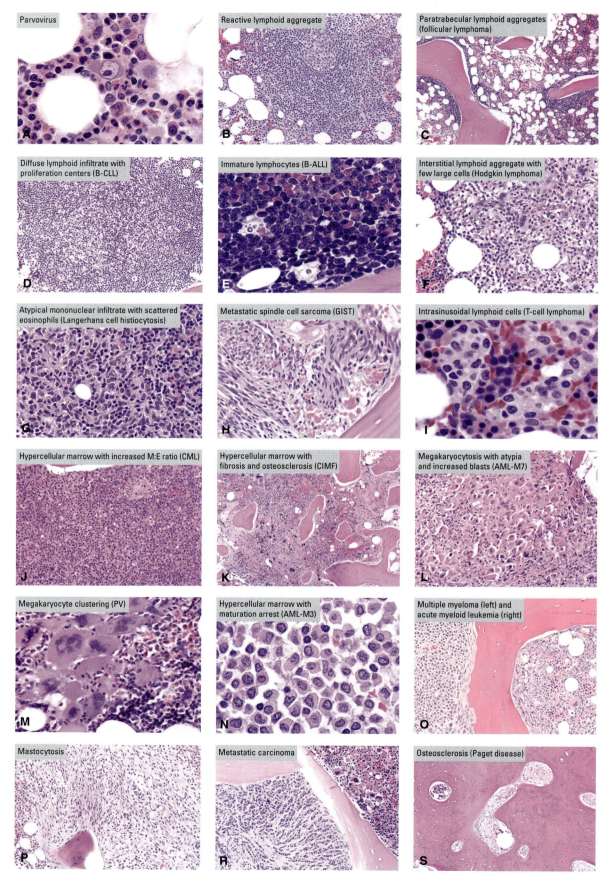

Figure 1.2   Histologic features – bone marrow (see text for details)

to identify metastatic disease (Figure 1.2Q). Evaluation of the core biopsy may determine the cause of other abnormal clinical/radiologic findings, such as Paget's disease (Figure 1.2R), bone remodeling after trauma, myxoid stromal changes after starvation or toxic insult to the marrow.

Differential diagnosis of lymphoid infiltrate in the bone marrow is presented in Chapter 13 (Figures 13.16–13.22).

Lymph node – cytology in histologic section

The morphologic diagnosis of hematolymphoid lesions requires correlation between histologic features (architecture; see above) and cytomorphology (cytologic features). The size of lymphoid cells is categorized by comparison with the nuclei of histiocytes or endothelial cells. Small lymphocytes are roughly the size of a histiocyte or endothelial cell nucleus (Figure 1.3A), and have scanty blue cytoplasm and small nuclei with dense (compact) chromatin. They are typically seen in chronic lymphocytic leukemia/small lymphocytic lymphoma (B-CLL/SLL), in which small lymphocytes are mixed with larger cells with prominent nucleoli – prolymphocytes or paraimmunoblasts (Figure 1.3B). Small lymphocytes with prominent nuclear irregularities in the form of indentation of the nuclear membrane (cleaved nuclei) are called centrocytes (Figure 1.3C). A mixture of small round lymphocytes and small cleaved lymphocytes is seen in mantle cell lymphoma. Small cleaved lymphocytes are also present in follicular lymphomas. Large B-lymphocytes are generally divided into centroblasts and immunoblasts. Centroblasts (Figure 1.3D) have large vesicular nuclei, and several nucleoli are often seen adjacent to the nuclear membrane. Immunoblasts (Figure 1.3E) are characterized by a prominent central eosinophilic macronucleolus.

Mast cells (Figure 1.3F) have small and often indented nuclei, inconspicuous nucleoli and abundant pale to clear cytoplasm (HE sections). Mast cells may be round, polygonal or spindle. Langerhans cells (Figure 1.3G) are usually large with pale eosinophilic cytoplasm. The nuclei have characteristic grooves (clefts) responsible for its 'coffee-bean' appearance. The chromatin is dispersed and nucleoli are inconspicuous, giving Langerhans cells bland cytologic features.

Prominent intracytoplasmic vacuoles may push the nucleus to the periphery with formation of 'signet-ring cells' (Figure 1.3H). This is usually a secondary phenomenon seen in a number of tumors, both hematolymphoid and non-hematopoietic, including follicular lymphoma, peripheral T-cell lymphoma, adenocarcinoma, etc. (see also Figure 13.9; Chapter 13). Plasma cells (Figure 1.3I),

the end product of the B-cell lineage, have abundant dense cytoplasm with a paler perinuclear area ('hof' or Golgi zone) and an eccentric nucleus. The chromatin is coarsely granular with formation of dark clumps at the periphery ('cartwheel' or 'clock-face' appearance). In a subset of plasma cell neoplasms, plasma cells may show significant anisopoikilocytosis with prominent nucleoli and immature, multinucleated or blastic forms (anaplastic plasma cells) (Figure 1.3J). Monocytoid B-cells (Figure 1.3K) are small to medium-sized lymphocytes with relatively abundant, pale or clear cytoplasm. They occur in reactive conditions, and are best appreciated in spleen follicles.

A tingible-body macrophage (Figure 1.3L) is a histiocytic cell with abundant cytoplasm containing numerous granules, which are the apoptotic debris of nearby proliferating cells. They occur inside the reactive follicles and in certain high-grade lymphomas (e.g., Burkitt lymphoma) and in precursor lymphoma/leukemia, giving the characteristic 'starry-sky' pattern. Small clusters of epithelioid cells (microgranulomas) (Figure 1.3M) are typical for reactive conditions (e.g., toxoplasmic lymphadenitis) and in some lymphomas. Sarcoidosis is characterized by granulomas in which some epithelioid cells contain crystalloid structures forming an 'asteroid body' (Figure 1.3N). Histiocytes with large vesicular nuclei, prominent nucleoli, abundant, pale, 'wispy' or frothy cytoplasm and engulfed lymphoid cells (emperipolesis or lymphocytophagocytosis) (Figure 1.3O), are typical for Rosai–Dorfman disease (sinus histiocytosis with massive lymphadenopathy). Histiocytes with melanin pigment (Figure 1.3P) are seen in dermatopathic lymphadenitis. Blastic features include a prominent nucleolus and fine, evenly distributed chromatin. Blastic/blastoid features may be present in mantle cell lymphoma (Figure 1.3Q), suggesting transformation into a more aggressive form of the disease. Differential diagnosis of blastoid infiltrate includes lymphoblastic lymphoma (Figure 1.3R), granulocytic sarcoma (Figure 1.3S) and blastic NK-cell lymphoma/leukemia (Figure 1.3T).

Multinucleated (or multilobated) cells with prominent nucleoli may be found in diffuse large B-cell lymphoma with anaplastic features (Figure 1.3U), Hodgkin lymphoma (Figure 1.3V–X), anaplastic large cell lymphoma (Figure 1.3Y–Z) and Kimura disease (Figure 1.3Z'). Reed–Sternberg cells are large multinucleated (Figure 1.3V), multilobated or bilobed cells with prominent eosinophilic nucleoli. Cells resembling Reed–Sternberg cells may be observed in diseases mimicking Hodgkin lymphoma, such as large B-cell lymphoma, anaplastic large cell lymphoma, etc. (see also

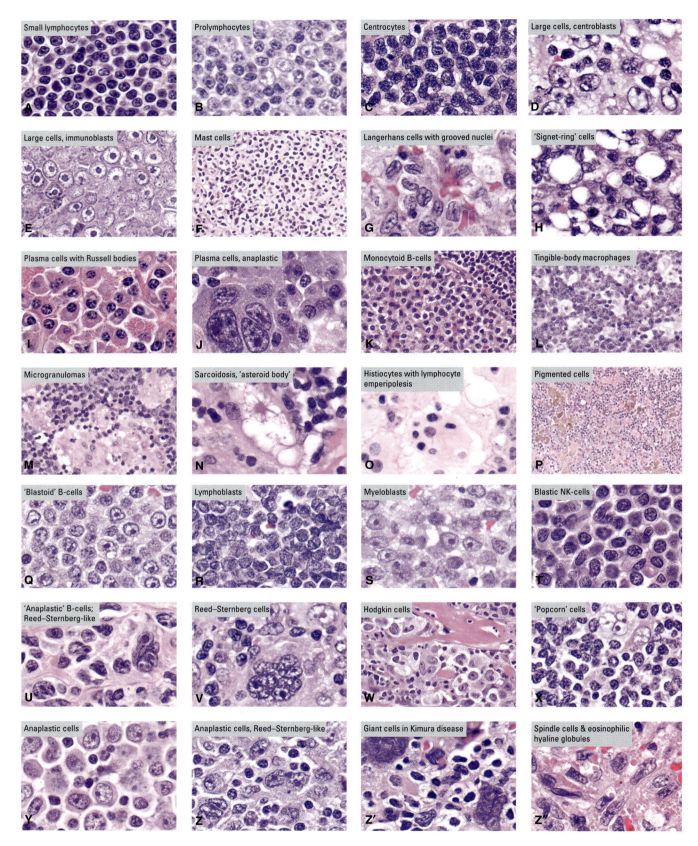

Figure 1.3   Cytologic features in histologic section from lymph nodes (see text for details)

Figure 13.11; Chapter 13). Popcorn cells (Figure 1.3X) or L&H cells are characteristic for nodular lymphocyte-predominant Hodgkin lymphoma (NLPHL). They are multilobated (multinucleated) cells which have scanty cytoplasm, highly irregular nuclear contours, pale, vesicular chromatin and prominent nucleoli. Popcorn cells differ from classic Reed–Sternberg cells by smaller size, less prominent nucleoli and paler chromatin with a thin delicate nuclear membrane. They are surrounded by a rim of small T-cells (CD57+ T/NK-rosettes) and are located within nodules of small B-cells, in contrast to Reed–Sternberg cells, which usually are present within the background of T-lymphocytes (see also Figure 4.5; Chapter 4).

Spindle cells with prominent eosinophilic cytoplasmic globules are typical for Kaposi's sarcoma (Figure 1.3Z″).

Lymph node – cytology in touch smear preparations

Touch smears stained with Wright–Giemsa (or H&E) are very useful in evaluation of the lymph nodes, especially during intraoperative consultations ('frozen' sections) and during flow cytometric analysis, when correlating immunophenotypic findings with cytomorphology. Reactive lymph nodes are characterized by a mixed population of small, medium-sized and, occasionally, large lymphocytes (Figure 1.4A) without overt atypia. Scattered tingible-body macrophages are often present. Histiocytes (Figure 1.4B) have abundant, pale and often vacuolated cytoplasm, ovoid or elongated nuclei with fine chromatin and inconspicuous nucleoli. They occur in reactive processes and in some high-grade lymphomas. Small lymphocytes (Figure 1.4C) have scanty cytoplasm and dark nuclei with compact or coarsely granular chromatin. The presence of a monotonous population of small lymphocytes with round nuclei suggests a low-grade lymphoma such as B-small lymphocytic lymphoma/chronic lymphocytic leukemia. Mantle cell lymphoma (Figure 1.4D) is characterized by round to angular lymphocytes with irregular nuclear contours, often in the form of indentations of the nuclear membrane. Cells with eccentric small mature round nuclei and mild to moderate amounts of cytoplasm, often accompanied by frank plasma cells, are seen in lymphoplasmacytic lymphoma. Plasma cells (usually IgA+) may contain eosinophilic material (immunoglobulins) in the cytoplasm, referred to as 'flame cells' (Figure 1.4E). Follicular lymphoma (Figure 1.4F) on touch smears may show a heterogeneous population of lymphocytes with atypical large cells with nucleoli (centroblasts). Large lymphocytes (Figure 1.4G–I) have a moderate amount of cytoplasm, a large nucleus and from one to several nucleoli. Centroblasts usually have two to three nucleoli located at the periphery of the nucleus, often adjacent to the nuclear membrane. Immunoblasts (Figure 1.4H) are characterized by a prominent, centrally located macronucleolus. Although T-cell lymphomas may have more irregular nuclear outlines, large T-cell lymphomas (Figure 1.4I) are often indistinguishable from their B-cell counterpart and phenotypic studies are needed for definite diagnosis.

Lymphoblasts (Figure 1.4J) are medium-sized with scanty cytoplasm, delicate chromatin and inconspicuous nucleoli. Neoplastic cells from blastic NK-cell lymphoma/leukemia (Figure 1.4K) resemble lymphoblasts and occasionally agranular myeloblasts. Large lymphocytes from anaplastic, large cell lymphomas have abundant cytoplasm, which is often vacuolated, and highly pleomorphic large nuclei with nucleoli (Figure 1.4L). The presence of cytoplasmic vacuoles is typically seen in Burkitt lymphoma (Figure 1.4M). The lymphoid cells are medium to large in size with blastoid nuclear characteristics.

Reed–Sternberg cells (Figure 1.4N) are characterized by large size, abundant cytoplasm and several nuclei, each with prominent nucleolus. Popcorn cells from nodular lymphocyte-predominant Hodgkin lymphoma (Figure 1.4O) are smaller than Reed–Sternberg cells, and have irregular nuclear borders and prominent nucleoli.

Bone marrow – cytology

The quality of the aspirate with adequate spicules and optimal Wright–Giemsa staining is crucial for proper analysis of the maturation sequence, cytomorphology, differential counts, assessment of the myeloid to erythroid ratio (M:E) and identification of any abnormalities such as dysplasia or the presence of extrinsic cells. The bone marrow aspirates are used also for evaluation of the bone marrow iron profile (amount and distribution of sideroblastic iron, including ringed sideroblasts) and for cytochemical stains such as myeloperoxidase (MPO) and alpha naphthyl butyrate esterase (NSE). Bone marrow fibrosis (e.g., chronic idiopathic myelofibrosis, myelodysplastic syndrome with fibrosis, metastatic tumor or acute megakaryocytic leukemia) may result in a non-representative hemodilute aspirate or a 'dry tap'. In that situation, a touch smear can be a valuable substitute. Normal bone marrow (Figure 1.5A) shows myeloid and erythroid cells at different stages of maturation (see also Figure 1.25).

Lymphoid cells are normally present in the bone marrow and account for approximately 10–20% of marrow cells in adults. The number of lymphocytes generally rises with age and/or the degree of chronic immune stimulation. The

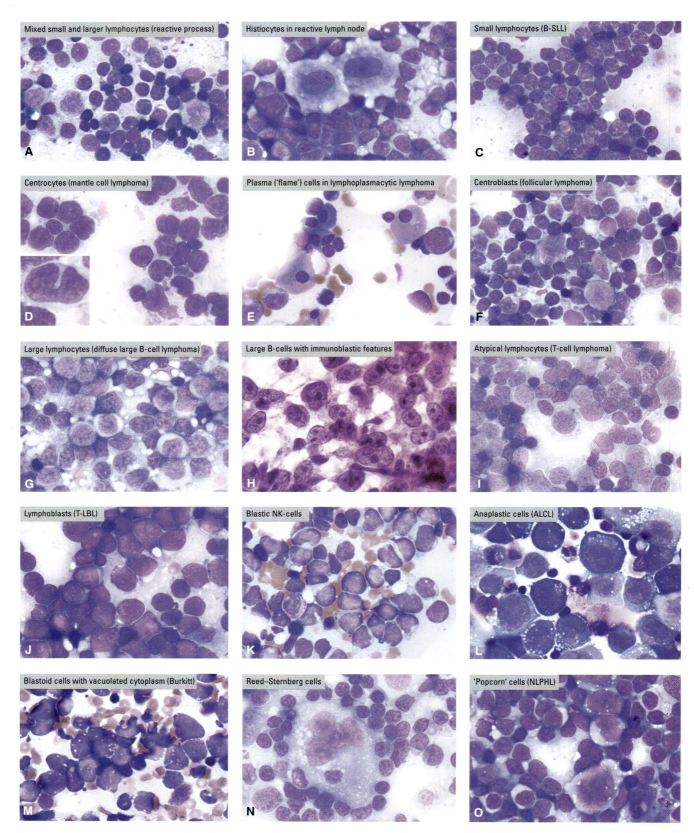

Figure 1.4   Cytologic features in touch smear preparations from lymph nodes (see text for details)

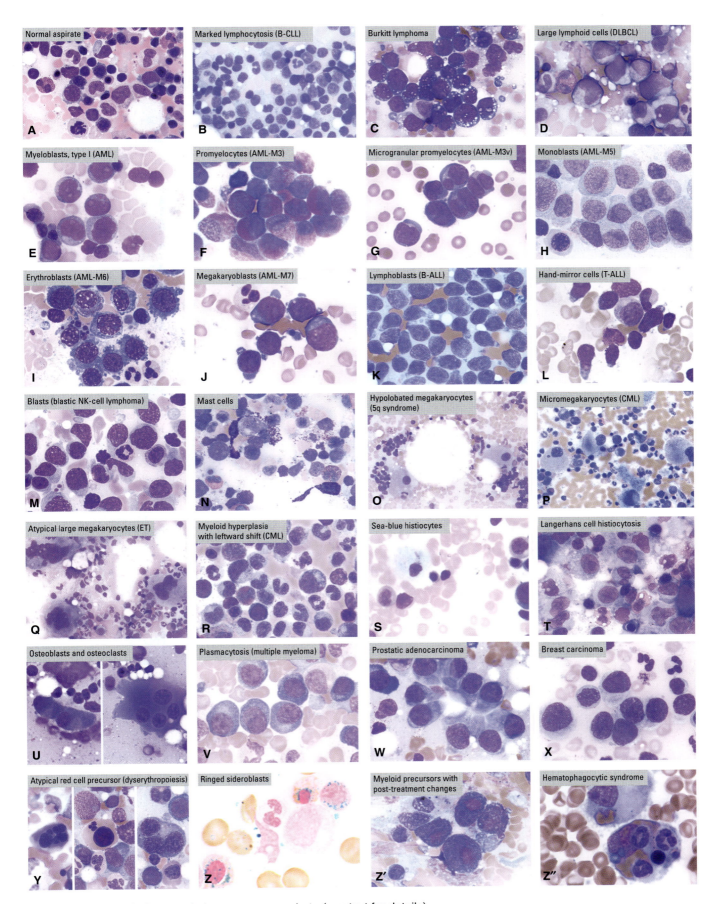

Figure 1.5 Cytologic features in bone marrow aspirate (see text for details)

presence of moderate to marked lymphocytosis of small lymphocytes is suggestive of a low-grade lymphoproliferative disorder, such as B-chronic lymphocytic leukemia (Figure 1.5B). Most of the lymphocytes of B-CLL have scanty cytoplasm, round (or rarely irregular) nuclei and condensed, dark chromatin. Lymphoid cells of Burkitt lymphoma (Figure 1.5C) are medium-sized with scanty, vacuolated cytoplasm, blastoid nuclei with finely dispersed chromatin and prominent nucleoli. Large cell lymphomas (Figure 1.5D) have large, often irregular nuclei, abundant cytoplasm and one to several nucleoli. The nuclear and cytoplasmic characteristics vary depending on the type of large cell lymphoma.

Myeloblasts (Figure 1.5E) have scanty cytoplasm, round or slightly irregular nuclei, fine chromatin and prominent nucleoli. The cytoplasm may be agranular or with rare granules (type I myeloblasts), paucigranular (<15 primary azurophilic granules; type II myeloblasts) or granular with no Golgi zone but >20 granules (type III myeloblasts). Atypical promyelocytes (Figure 1.5F) from acute promyelocytic leukemia (hypergranular variant) are characterized by the presence of numerous small, azurophilic cytoplasmic granules and Auer rods. In the microgranular variant of acute promyelocytic leukemia (APL), the atypical promyelocytes have characteristic bilobed or dumbbell-shaped nuclei with delicate chromatin, bearing some resemblance to monoblasts (Figure 1.5G). Promyelocytes are strongly positive for MPO and negative for NSE, which helps to differentiate them from monoblastic leukemia. Monoblasts (Figure 1.5H) have large nuclei that often are folded or convoluted, finely dispersed chromatin and abundant pale cytoplasm.

Early erythroid precursors from pure acute erythroid leukemia (Figure 1.5I) display prominent dyserythropoiesis, characteristic coarsely granular chromatin and irregular cytoplasmic borders. Often, there may be prominent cytoplasmic vacuolation. Megakaryoblasts are pleomorphic, may vary in cytologic appearance and may be indistinguishable from regular myeloblasts. The most characteristic feature of megakaryoblasts is prominent cytoplasmic budding (Figure 1.5J). Lymphoblasts (Figure 1.5K) have scanty cytoplasm, fine chromatin and inconspicuous nucleoli. Occasional cases of precursor T-lymphoblastic lymphoma/leukemia (and less often B-ALL) have elongated cytoplasm at one pole of the cell, giving a 'hand-mirror' appearance to the blast cells (Figure 1.5L). Blasts from blastic NK-cell lymphoma/leukemia (DC2 acute leukemia) (Figure 1.5M) resemble lymphoblasts or myeloblasts. They are negative for myeloperoxidase (MPO) and NSE and are positive for CD4 and CD56.

Mast cells (Figure 1.5N) may be round, polygonal or spindly shaped. They are characterized by purplish-black cytoplasmic granules.

Evaluation of megakaryocytes gives important clues in the diagnosis of thrombocytosis, thrombocytopenia, myeloproliferative disorders and myelodysplastic syndromes. At least 20 megakaryocytes should be analyzed. Hypolobated micromegakaryocytes may be found in del 5(q) syndrome (5q-minus syndrome) (Figure 1.5O) or chronic myeloid leukemia (CML) (Figure 1.5P). In the latter, they are often mixed with more pleomorphic and hyperchromatic megakaryocytes in the background of myeloid hyperplasia, eosinophilia and basophilia. The presence of increased numbers of enlarged atypical megakaryocytes with occasional clustering (best appreciated within spicules) is typical for non-CML chronic myeloproliferative disorders (Figure 1.5Q). Myeloid hyperplasia with a leftward shift, basophilia, eosinophilia and occasional sea-blue histiocytes raise the possibility of CML (Figure 1.5R–S).

Langerhans cells are large mononuclear cells with abundant vacuolated cytoplasm and large, round or oval nucleus with characteristic indentation (folding), giving a 'coffee-bean' appearance (Figure 1.5T). They are often accompanied by eosinophils. Osteoblasts (Figure 1.5U, left) are large cells with abundant dense basophilic (blue) cytoplasm with eccentric nuclei and perinuclear pale areas (halo). They are often present in small clusters and may be mistaken for plasma cells. Osteoclasts (Figure 1.5U, right) are large multinucleated cells with well-separated nuclei. Plasma cells (Figure 1.5V) have abundant cytoplasm with perinuclear 'halos' and eccentric nuclei with coarse chromatin. The chromatin may accumulate at the periphery of the nucleus with interspersed areas of parachromatin, giving rise to a clock-face or cartwheel appearance.

Extrinsic elements (Figure 1.5W–X) are easy to identify when they occur in clusters or cohesive sheets, as seen in well to moderately differentiated adenocarcinoma of prostate, breast or lung. On occasion, metastatic carcinomas may mimic immature myeloid cells (Figure 1.5X) or appear individually.

Dysplastic features of erythroid precursors (dyserythropoiesis) (Figure 1.5Y) include multinucleation (especially asymmetric), nuclear–cytoplasmic dyssynchrony, nuclear budding, basophilic stippling in the cytoplasm, and irregular (shaggy) cytoplasmic borders. The latter two features are non-specific. The presence of ringed sideroblasts (Figure 1.5Z) can be seen in myelodysplasia, as well as in many secondary causes (ethanol toxicity, chemotherapy with antituberculous agents, chloramphenicol or cycloserine, pyridoxine deficiency, and zinc toxicity). Ringed sideroblasts (>15% of erythroid precursors) are seen in refractory anemia with ringed sideroblasts (RARS), in refractory cytopenia with multilineage dysplasia and ringed sideroblasts (RCMD-RS) and in mixed myeloproliferative/myelodysplastic disease (refractory anemia with ringed sideroblasts and marked thrombocytosis). Features of dysmaturation can be seen in reactive processes and after treatment. Accumulation of azurophilic granules in the Golgi area of the maturing myeloid cells can be seen in regenerating marrows after chemotherapy (Figure 1.5Z′).

Reactive histiocytes which contain phagocytosed red cells and/or lymphocytes (Figure 1.5Z″) can be found in the bone marrow and other sites such as peripheral blood, spleen and lymph nodes. They are associated with reactive erythrophagocytic syndrome (RES or hemophagocytic syndrome) in certain viral infections and malignancies.

Peripheral blood – cytology

Prolymphocytes (Figure 1.6A) are larger than lymphocytes, with a moderate amount of cytoplasm, round (or occasionally irregular) nuclei and focally prominent nucleoli. Follicular lymphoma is characterized by cleaved cells or centrocytes (Figure 1.6B). Hairy cell leukemia (HCL) (Figure 1.6C) is characterized by medium-sized round lymphocytes with cytoplasmic 'hairy' projections and round or coffee-bean-shaped nuclei with evenly dispersed chromatin. Irregular or bipolar cytoplasmic projections may be seen also in splenic lymphoma with villous lymphocytes (Figure 1.6D). Large lymphoid cells (Figure 1.6E) have irregular nuclei, increased nuclear: cytoplasmic ratio and occasionally prominent nucleoli.

T-cell lymphoproliferations (Figure 1.6F–I) are characterized by prominent nuclear contour irregularities, with occasional flower-like cells. T-prolymphocytes have prominent nucleoli (Figure 1.6G), and large granular lymphocytes have coarse azurophilic granules in the cytoplasm (Figure 1.6H).

Lymphoblasts (Figure 1.6J) have scanty cytoplasm, a medium-sized nucleus with delicate, evenly distributed chromatin and one or more inconspicuous nucleoli.

Monocytosis in the peripheral blood may be associated with numerous reactive conditions and clonal disorders, including acute monocytic leukemia (Figure 1.6K) and chronic myelomonocytic leukemia (CMML). The presence of immature erythroid precursors (erythroblastosis) (Figure 1.6L) with prominent dyserythropoiesis may be seen in myelodysplastic syndromes or acute erythroid leukemia. In the pediatric age group, erythroblasts in peripheral blood

may be seen in erythroblastosis fetalis (Figure 1.6M) or transient myeloproliferative disorders. In the latter, circulating erythroblasts are accompanied by megakaryocytes and large platelets. A few erythroblasts may be present normally in newborn infants in the peripheral blood.

Circulating erythroid precursors mixed with leftward shifted myeloid cells (leukoerythroblastosis) (Figure 1.6N) is seen in a variety of reactive conditions as well as chronic myeloproliferative disorders and myelophthisic processes. Neutrophilia (Figure 1.6O) with a leftward shift accompanied by eosinophilia and basophilia is seen in CML.

Plasma cells in peripheral blood (Figure 1.6P) may indicate aggressive or advanced plasma cell myeloma; plasma cell leukemia is characterized by a leukocyte differential with >20% plasma cells. The presence of 'leukemic' carcinoma in peripheral blood is rare (Figure 1.6Q).

Erythrophagocytosis by immature cells is most often seen in acute monoblastic leukemia (Figure 1.6R) but can be also seen in other types of acute leukemias, including CD56-positive AML.

INTRODUCTION TO IMMUNOHISTOCHEMISTRY

Immunohistochemistry plays an important role in diagnostic hematopathology. It is helpful in the determination of (i) cell origin, (ii) degree of differentiation (maturation) and (iii) prognosis. The availability of monoclonal or polyclonal antibodies (Tables 1.1 and 1.2), automation, and protocols for antigen retrieval designed for formalin-fixed, paraffin-embedded tissues make immunohistochemical techniques a common practice in everyday diagnostic surgical pathology. Immunohistochemistry permits differentiation of epithelial tumors (cytokeratin positive) from hematolymphoid tumors (CD45 positive), but also allows for specific and detailed subclassification of tumors (melanoma versus sarcoma, T- versus B-cell, small lymphocytic versus mantle cell, myeloid versus lymphoblastic). It is also used to determine the prognosis and to optimize treatment strategies (estrogen/progesterone receptors in breast cancer, ZAP70 in B-CLL/SLL, Ki-67 proliferation fraction). Figure 1.7 presents the principles of immunohistochemical staining. In the indirect (two-step) method, antigen is detected by a primary antibody, which in turn is detected by a secondary antibody conjugated with an enzymatic complex. A colorimetric reaction of the substrate (e.g., DAB, alkaline phosphatase) identifies the presence of any given antigen under the microscope with its correlative morphologic parameters. In a direct (one-step) method, the primary antibody is conjugated with

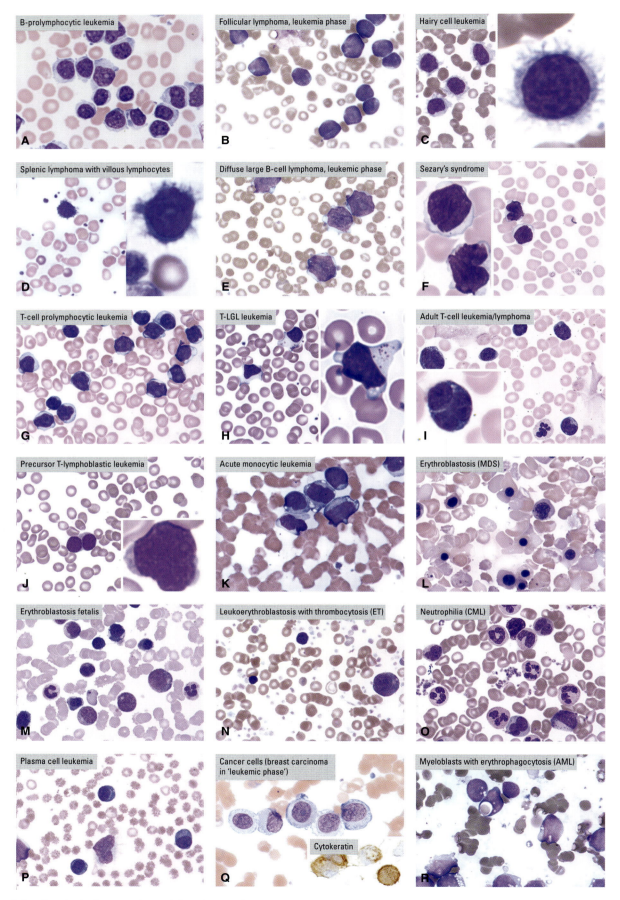

Figure 1.6   Cytologic features in peripheral blood (see text for details)

Table 1.1 Phenotypic markers in major types of hematopoietic cells

Target	Marker/antibody
Anaplastic large cell lymphoma	ALK-1, CD30, pan-T antigens, CD43, UCHL1, EMA
B-cell markers	CD19, CD20, CD79a, CD22, Pax-5, OCT-2, BOB-1
Blastic markers	CD34, CD117, TdT
Germinal center cells	CD10, bcl-6
Granulocytes	CD10, CD11b, CD15, CD16, MPO
Hodgkin lymphoma	CD30, CD15
Immature T-cells/thymocytes	CD1a, CD4, CD8, TdT, pan-T antigens, CD10
Mast cells	Mast cell tryptase, CD117, CD43, CD2
Megakaryocytes	CD41, CD61, (CD79a)
Monocytic markers	CD11b, CD11c, CD14, CD64, HLA-DR
Myeloid markers	CD13, CD15, CD33, CD68, MPO
NK-cell markers	CD16, CD56, CD57
Plasma cell markers	CD38, CD138, cytoplasmic light and heavy chains, CD56, CD117
Red cell markers	GPHA, hemoglobin A
T-cell markers (pan-T antigens)	CD2, CD3, CD5, CD7, UCHL1
T; helper/inducer	CD4
T; suppressor/cytotoxic	CD8

Table 1.2 CD antigens and other commonly used immunophenotypic markers

Antibody	Reactivity	IHC (paraffin)	Flow
AE1/AE3	Epithelial cells, mesothelial cells	+	−
Bcl-1	Mantle cell lymphoma, plasma cell myeloma, hairy cell leukemia (subset)	+	−
Bcl-2	Mature B-cells (except benign germinal center cells), T-cells, follicular lymphoma, epithelial tumors	+	+
Bcl-6	Germinal center cells, follicular lymphoma, some diffuse large B-cell lymphoma, subset of Hodgkin lymphoma	+	−
BOB-1	B-cells, multiple myeloma	+	−
CD1a	Thymocytes, immature T-cells	+	+
CD2	T-cells, large granular lymphocytes, NK-cells, some acute promyelocytic leukemias, mast cells (neoplastic)	+	+
CD3	T-cells, primary effusion lymphoma (PEL; subset)	+	+
CD4	T-cells (helper/inducer), monocytes, myeloblasts, blastic NK-cell lymphoma (DC2 leukemia)	+	+
CD5	T-cells, B-CLL/SLL, mantle cell lymphoma	+	+
CD7	T-cells, some myeloblasts	+	+
CD8	T-cells (cytotoxic), large granular lymphocytes	+	+
CD10	Follicle center cells, follicular lymphoma, some diffuse large B-cell lymphomas, precursor B-ALL, precursor T-ALL, thymocytes, Burkitt lymphoma, granulocytes	+	+
CD11b	Granulocytes, monocytes	−	+
CD11c	Monocytes, hairy cell leukemia, large granular lymphocytes, activated T-cells, marginal zone B-cell lymphoma	−	+
CD13	Myeloid cells, rare precursor B-ALL	−	+
CD14	Monocytes	−	+
CD15	Granulocytes, Hodgkin lymphoma (classical)	+	+
CD16	Granulocytes, NK-cells, large granular lymphocytes	−	+
CD19	B-cells, precursor B-ALL, subset of AML [*AML1/ETO* with t(8;21)]	−	+
CD20	B-cells, rare plasma cell myelomas	+	+
CD21	Follicular dendritic cells, AILD T-cell lymphoma	+	−
CD22	B-cells	+	+
CD23	B-SLL/CLL, plasma cells, follicular dendritic cells	+	+
CD25	Hairy cell leukemia, subset of B- and T-cell lymphomas	+	+
CD30	Hodgkin lymphoma, anaplastic large cell lymphoma, subset of diffuse large B-cell lymphoma, subset of T-cell lymphomas (NOS), primary mediastinal B-cell lymphoma, lymphomatoid papulosis	+	+
CD33	Myeloid cells, rare precursor B-ALL, rare blastic NK-cell lymphomas	+	+
CD34	Myeloblasts, lymphoblasts, endothelial cells, GIST	+	+
CD38	Plasma cells, activated B- and T-cells, subset B-CLL/SLL, epithelial cells	+	+
CD41	Megakaryocytes	−	+
CD43	Myeloid cells, T-cell lymphomas, precursor B- and T-cell leukemias, B-cell lymphoma (subset), plasma cells	+	+
CD45RB	B-cells, T-cells, myeloid cells, monocytes, L&H cells	+	+
CD56	NK-cells, large granular lymphocytes, subset of AML, subset of granulocytes in MDS, rare diffuse large B-cell lymphomas, T-cell lymphomas (subset), multiple myeloma, neuroendocrine carcinoma	+	+
CD57	NK-cells, large granular lymphocytes	+	+
CD61	Megakaryocytes	+	+

(Continued)

Table 1.2   (*Continued*)

Antibody	Reactivity	IHC (paraffin)	Flow
CD79a	B-cells, plasma cells, megakaryocytes	+	+
CD103	Hairy cell leukemia, rare T-cell lymphomas	–	+
CD117	AML, mast cells, stromal tumors (GIST), plasma cells	+	–
DBA-44	Hairy cell leukemia, subset of B-cell lymphomas	+	–
EBV	Hodgkin lymphoma, post-transplant lymphomas, immunoblasts in AILD T-cell lymphoma, some B-cell lymphomas in elderly	+	–
EBER	See EBV	+	–
EMA	Plasma cells, epithelial cells, nodular lymphocyte-predominant Hodgkin lymphoma (L&H cells), DLBCL with ALK expression, erythroblasts (M6 AML), anaplastic large cell lymphoma (ALCL)	+	–
Heavy chains	B-cells, plasma cells, DLBCL with ALK expression (IgA)	+	+
HLA-DR	AML (except acute promyelocytic leukemia), B-cells, monocytes	+	+
Light chains	B-cells (surface), plasma cells (cytoplasmic)	+	+
OCT-2	B-cells, multiple myeloma	+	–
Pax-5	B-cells, subset of multiple myeloma, Hodgkin lymphoma (R–S cells), L&H cells in NLPHL	+	–
S100	Melanoma, Rosai–Dorfman disease, eosinophilic granuloma, interdigitating reticulum cells (IDC)	+	–
TdT	Precursor B-ALL, precursor T-ALL, some AML, hematogones	+	+

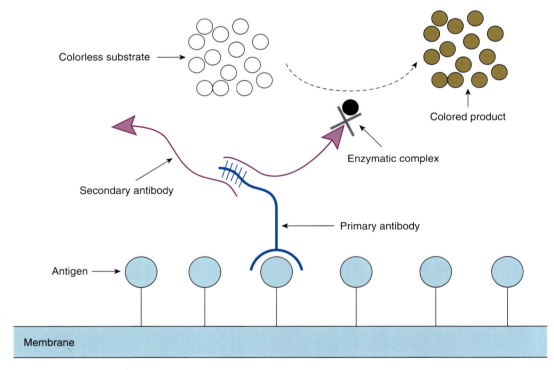

Figure 1.7   Immunohistochemical detection of antigen by indirect method (scheme) (see text for details)

an enzymatic complex. The two-step protocol is more sensitive. Depending on the location and distribution of the antigen(s), the color reaction may be visible in the nucleus, cytoplasm, cytoplasmic membrane and/or nucleolus (Figure 1.8). Nuclear staining (Figure 1.8A) is characteristic for bcl-1, bcl-6, BOB-1, EBER, HHV-8, Ki-67 (MIB-1), OCT-2, Pax-5 and TdT. Membrane staining (Figure 1.8B) occurs with CD20, CD30, CD45, CD138, EMA, and pan-T antigens. Cytoplasmic staining (Figure 1.8C) is seen with bcl-2, CD117, cytokeratins, myeloperoxidase and vimentin. Staining of the Golgi area (Figure 1.8D) as well as the membrane (dot-membrane pattern) is seen with CD15 and CD30. Cytoplasmic and nuclear staining is typical for ALK-1, ZAP70 and S100. ALK-1 may show only cytoplasmic staining or cytoplasmic, nuclear and nucleolar.

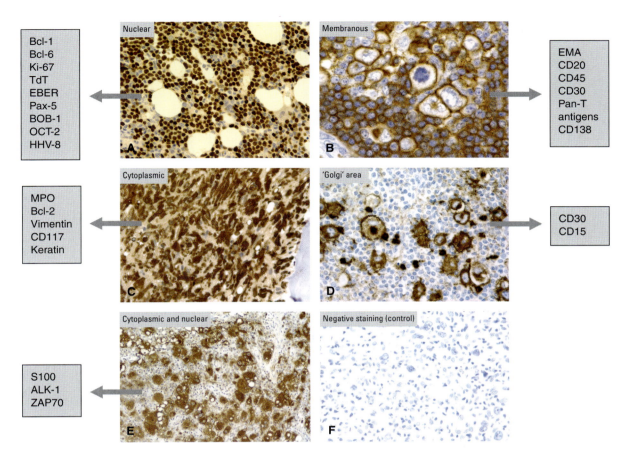

Figure 1.8 Major patterns of the immunohistochemical (IHC) staining in formalin-fixed and paraffin-embedded tissue sections. The pattern of IHC staining depends on the localization of the antigen: nuclear, cytoplasmic, cytoplasmic, and nuclear or membranous

Table 1.1 presents immunophenotypic markers useful in identifying major cell types and Table 1.2 presents the reactivity of most common antibodies used in diagnostic hematopathology.

INTRODUCTION TO FLOW CYTOMETRY

Flow cytometry (FC) uses the same principles in detection of antigens as described above for immunohistochemistry, except that it is performed on unfixed (fresh) cells suspended in a liquid medium. The antibodies are conjugated with fluorochromes, which are excited or stimulated by laser(s) in flow cytometers. Most of the antigens detected by FC are located on the cell surface. In order to stain intracellular components, cells have to be permeabilized (so that the antibody can enter cells through 'holes' in their membrane). FC is much faster than immunohistochemistry and can analyze thousands of cells within seconds. Another advantage of FC immunophenotyping is that it allows correlation of several markers on a single cell, and detects intensity of staining and aberrant expression of antigens. FC has high

sensitivity for B-cell lymphoproliferative disorders and acute leukemia, and high specificity for several categories of those neoplasms[14–34]. All these properties are used in diagnostic hematopathology for subclassification of neoplasms. The major disadvantage of FC is a need for liquid cell suspension and therefore lack of correlation with histomorphologic features (tissue architecture). FC requires viable fresh (unfixed) material. In a subset of neoplasms, especially high-grade lymphomas, decreased viability precludes FC analysis. FC analysis requires at least 10–20 000 cells/events acquired by tube, a fact which often limits its use in specimens from CSF, fine needle aspirates or paucicellular lesions. Dropout of neoplastic cells due to low viability or sample bias due to focal (partial) tissue involvement may lead to false-negative flow results.

In FC analysis, cells are tagged with fluorochrome-conjugated monoclonal antibodies directed toward specific surface, cytoplasmic or nuclear antigens. Intrinsic physical properties of the cells, especially their size and cytoplasmic granularity, are measured simultaneously with fluorescence emission as the fluorochrome-tagged cells pass through laser light. Forward angle light scatter

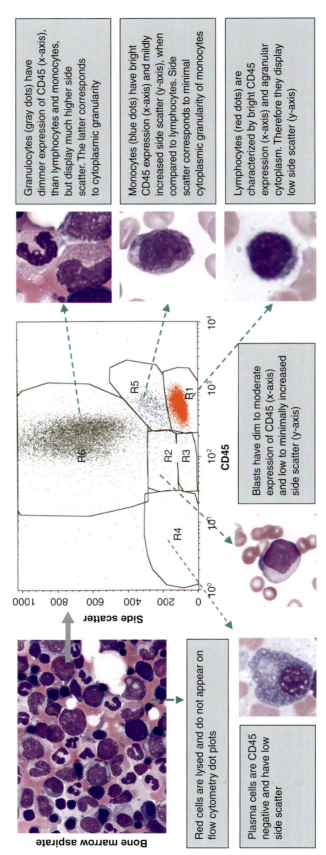

Figure 1.9   Flow cytometry immunophenotyping – gating strategy based on CD45 versus side (orthogonal) scatter (see text for details)

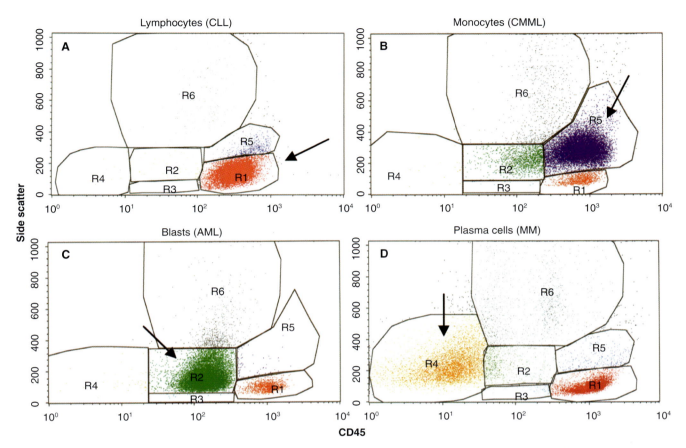

Figure 1.10 Flow cytometry immunophenotyping – localization of different types of hematopoietic tumors based on CD45 versus side scatter characteristics (see text for details)

(forward scatter; FSC) corresponds to cell size (i.e., the larger the cell, the higher the FSC) and right angle light scatter (side scatter; SSC) corresponds to the granularity of the cytoplasm (i.e., neutrophils with cytoplasmic granules have high SSC and lymphocytes have low SSC).

Flow cytometry of peripheral blood and bone marrow – gating strategy

Figure 1.9 illustrates gating strategy applied in the FC analysis of peripheral blood and bone marrow. Based on the intensity of CD45 staining (x-axis) and side scatter (SSC, y-axis), one can distinguish several major populations in normal bone marrow: lymphocytes (bright CD45 and low SCC; red), monocytes (bright CD45 and increased SSC; blue), and granulocytes (moderate CD45 and high SSC; gray). Red blood cells and their precursors are eliminated from FC analysis by lysis. Figure 1.10 presents examples of CD45 versus SSC in some neoplastic processes, to illustrate the properties mentioned above. B-CLL/SLL shows bright CD45 and low side scatter (Figure 1.10A). Other B- and T-cell lymphoproliferative disorders usually have a similar location. Neoplastic monocytes of chronic myelomonocytic leukemia (CMML)

(Figure 1.10B) have bright CD45, but SSC is higher than in lymphocytes. A similar distribution is often observed in hairy cell leukemia and T-LGL leukemia. Blasts usually have moderate CD45 and increased SSC (Figure 1.10C). Precursor B- and T-lymphoblastic leukemias, blastic NK-cell lymphoma/leukemia (DC2 acute leukemia) and occasional B- and T-cell lymphomas have a similar location in the blastic gate. Hematogones would have identical (moderate) CD45, but SSC would be very low. Plasma cells (Figure 1.10D) usually are CD45⁻ and have variable SSC. Small cell carcinoma also occurs in the CD45⁻ gate.

Intensity of staining and co-expression of antigens

Figure 1.11 presents the concept of intensity of staining and coexpression of antigen. The staining is negative when the results are the same as in negative (isotypic) control. In Figure 1.11A, blue dots representing hairy cell leukemia are negative for CD3. Dim staining is defined by the staining which is slightly brighter than the negative control. Moderate staining is defined as at least one log decade brighter than negative control without overlap. T-lymphocytes (red; * on Figure 1.11A) have

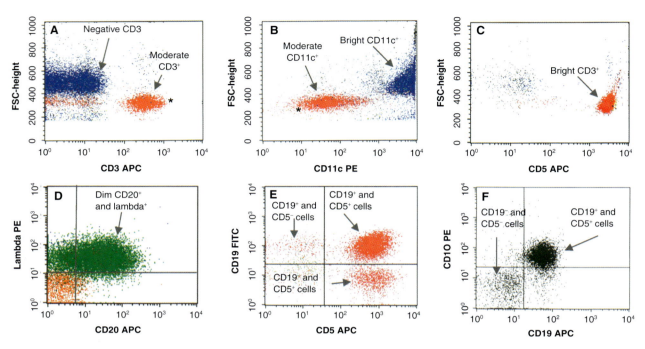

Figure 1.11   Flow cytometry immunophenotyping – concept of the intensity of staining and coexpression of antigens (see text for details)

moderate expression of CD3. Bright staining is at least two log decades brighter than negative control. Hairy cell leukemia (represented by blue; Figure 1.11B) and T-PLL cells (red; Figure 1.11C) display bright expression of CD11c and CD3, respectively. Figure 1.11D shows B-cell chronic lymphocytic leukemia/small lymphocytic lymphoma (B-CLL/SLL; green) with dim expression of CD20 (x-axis) and positive expression of lambda immunoglobulins (y-axis). As illustrated, FC gives information about the presence or absence of a given antigen as well as its intensity of expression. Dim expression of CD20 and surface light-chain immunoglobulin is characteristically seen in B-chronic lymphocytic leukemia/small lymphocytic lymphoma. Other low-grade lymphoproliferative disorders usually display moderate or bright expression of those markers. Figure 1.11E illustrates B-CLL/SLL co-expressing CD5 (x-axis) and CD19 (y-axis). The rare non-neoplastic B-cells (upper left quadrant) are CD19+/CD5− and residual T-cells (lower right quadrant) are CD19−/CD5+. Aberrant expression of CD5 by B-cells is typical for B-CLL/SLL and mantle cell lymphoma. Figure 1.11F illustrates moderate expression of CD10 by CD19+ B-cells (upper right quadrant).

Polyclonal versus monoclonal B-cell populations

Figure 1.12 presents the difference between polytypic and monoclonal expression of surface light-chain immunoglobulins. A reactive lymph node (Figure 1.12A) shows two distinct populations of cells, based on the expression of CD20 (B and C; x-axis): CD20+ cells (B-cells) and CD20− cells (T-cells). B-cells show kappa expression (B; upper right quadrant) and lambda expression (C; upper right quadrant); therefore, they are polytypic. Similar polytypic B-cells are present in follicular hyperplasia (Figure 1.12D). However, in follicular hyperplasia, a subset of B-cells has brighter expression of CD20 (germinal center cells; E and F). In contrast to a benign lymph node, B-cell lymphomas show monoclonal expression of surface immunoglobulins (either kappa or lambda). Figure 1.12G demonstrates follicular lymphoma with kappa-restricted expression of surface immunoglobulins (compare H and I).

Figure 1.13 shows FC findings in a case of partial lymph node involvement by malignant lymphoma. A histologic section shows a lymph node with reactive follicles (*) and a focus of follicular lymphoma (A; arrow). FC (B and C) shows two populations of B-cells: those with moderate expression of CD20 (*) and those with bright expression of CD20 (arrow). The latter are monoclonal lambda+ cells, representing follicular lymphoma. Residual benign B-cells with moderate CD20 expression are polytypic (compare B and C). The two populations differ not only in respect to the intensity of CD20 expression but also by forward scatter, which corresponds to cell size (D and E). Gating on cells with moderate CD20 and low forward scatter (D) yields polytypic cells

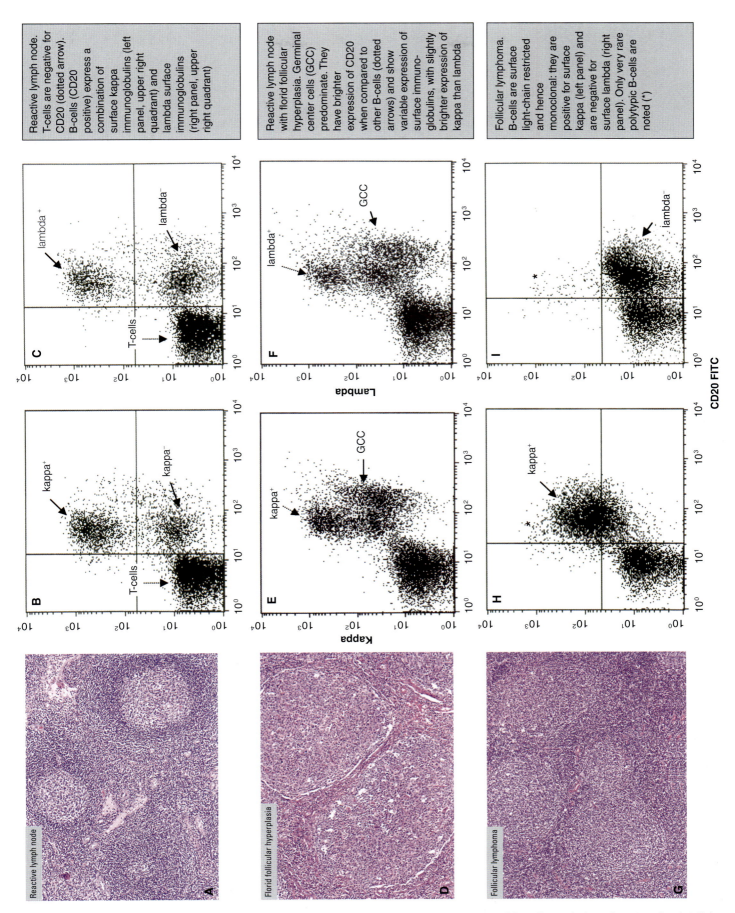

Figure 1.12   Flow cytometry immunophenotyping – concept of polytypic and monoclonal B-cell populations (see text for details)

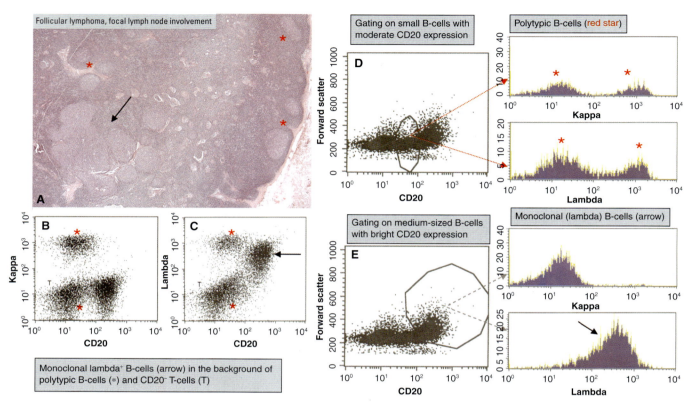

Figure 1.13   Flow cytometry immunophenotyping – gating strategy based on the intensity of CD20 expression (see text for details)

(see histograms on the right). Gating on cells with bright CD20 expression and slightly higher forward scatter (E) yields monoclonal lambda$^+$ population (arrow, histograms on the right).

Prognostic markers

Determination of the expression of ZAP70 and/or CD38 by FC can serve as a prognostic marker in patients with B-chronic lymphocytic leukemia (B-CLL). Naive-type CLL is more often positive for CD38 and/or ZAP70 and is associated with a poorer prognosis than the IgH-rearranged type of CLL, which is more often negative for these markers[35,36]. CD38 is a non-lineage-specific surface glycoprotein that in B-cells is expressed at times during B-cell development when cell-to-cell interactions are crucial to development. ZAP70 is a T-cell-specific signaling molecule (protein tyrosine kinase) which interacts with T-cell antigen receptors (TCR) during T-cell development. Figure 1.14 depicts B-CLL with positive expression of CD38 and ZAP70.

Aberrant expression of antigens

Benign B-cells are positive for B-cell markers (e.g., CD19, CD20, CD22 and CD79a) and negative for T-cell

markers (CD2, CD3, CD5 and CD7); conversely, normal T-cells are positive for T-antigens and are negative for B-cell markers. Other cell lineages have also characteristic immunophenotypic profiles; thus, monocytes have bright expression of CD11b, CD11c, CD14 and CD64 and are positive for HLA-DR. Positive expression of marker(s) not associated with the specific cell type (or the absence of an antigen which is normally positive) is termed aberrant antigen expression. Identification of an aberrant phenotype is used in FC evaluation of hematopoietic malignancies[14,20–23,29,31,32,37–39]. Figure 1.15 presents several examples of aberrant antigen expression. Figure 1.15A shows a peripheral T-cell lymphoma with aberrant expression of CD20 (arrow) on a subset of T-cells. Figure 1.15B shows a diffuse large B-cell lymphoma with aberrant expression of CD56. Figure 1.15C shows B-CLL/SLL with coexpression of CD8 (arrow). Figure 1.15D shows hairy cell leukemia (HCL) with aberrant expression of CD2 (T-cell marker) on a subset of leukemic cells (arrow). Figure 1.15E shows gamma/delta T-cell lymphoma with expression of B-cell-associated marker CD19 (arrow). Figure 1.15F shows acute monocytic leukemia with aberrant loss of HLA-DR expression. Figure 1.16 presents aberrant expression of bcl-6 and CD10 in mantle cell lymphoma.

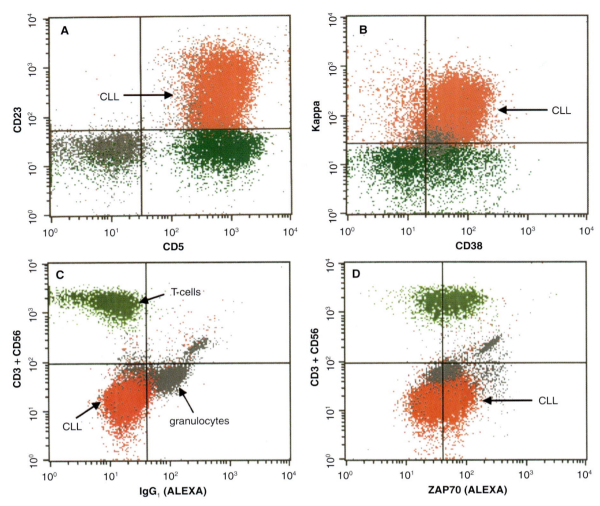

Figure 1.14   Evaluation of prognostic markers (CD38 and ZAP70) in B-chronic lymphocytic leukemia. Leukemic cells have typical phenotype with CD5 and CD23 coexpression (**A**). They are positive for CD38 (**B**) and ZAP70 (**D**). IgG$_1$ isotypic control for ZAP70 is presented in Panel **C**

Differential diagnosis of mature B-cell lymphoproliferative disorders

Table 1.3 presents the differential diagnosis of mature B-cell lymphoproliferative disorders. CD5 expression is typical for B-chronic lymphocytic leukemia/small lymphocytic lymphoma (B-CLL/SLL), mantle cell lymphoma (MCL) and a subset of diffuse large B-cell lymphoma with *de novo* CD5 expression. CD10 expression is most typical for follicular lymphoma (FL), Burkitt lymphoma and a subset of diffuse large B-cell lymphomas (DLBCL). Bright expression of CD11c is seen in HCL. Moderate expression of CD11c is observed in a subset of B-CLL/SLL, marginal zone B-cell lymphoma and occasional DLBCL. CD19 is positive in B-cell lymphomas and is negative in plasma cell neoplasms (~6% are CD19$^+$). Most B-cell lymphomas display moderate

expression of CD19, although FL may show dim CD19. Dim CD20 expression is typical for B-CLL/SLL, and bright CD20 is observed in HCL. Other B-cell lympho-proliferations show moderate CD20. Coexpression of CD5 and CD23 is most typical for B-CLL/SLL. CD25 is seen in all typical HCL, which are also positive for CD103 and CD11c. Other B-cell lymphomas are CD25$^+$, and therefore expression of this antigen is not specific for HCL. CD43 is useful in differentiating FL (CD43$^-$) from Burkitt lymphoma (CD43$^+$). These two lymphomas differ also in expression of bcl-2. Most FL are bcl-2$^+$ and Burkitt lymphomas are bcl-2$^-$. Bcl-2 is also helpful in differentiating follicular hyperplasia (CD10$^+$ germinal center cells are bcl-2$^-$) from FL (CD10$^+$ cells are most often bcl-2$^+$). Bcl-1 (cyclin D1) is positive in MCL and a subset of HCL and plasma cell myelomas. FL, Burkitt lymphoma and a subset of DLBCL are bcl-6$^+$.

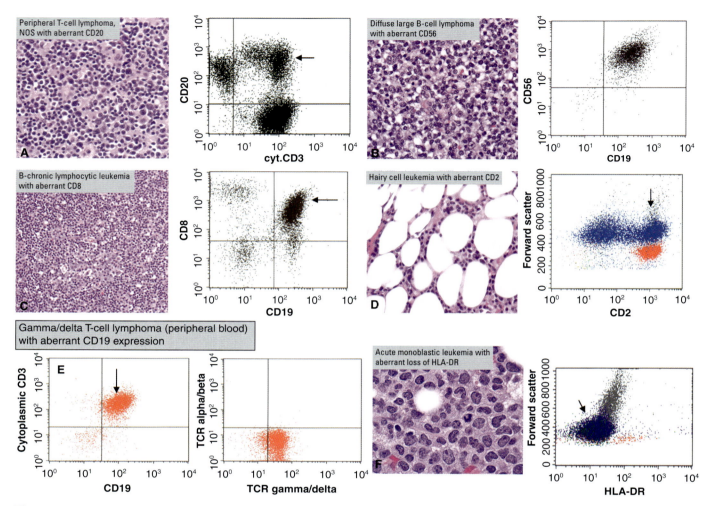

Figure 1.15   Flow cytometry immunophenotyping – concept of aberrant antigen expression (see text for details)

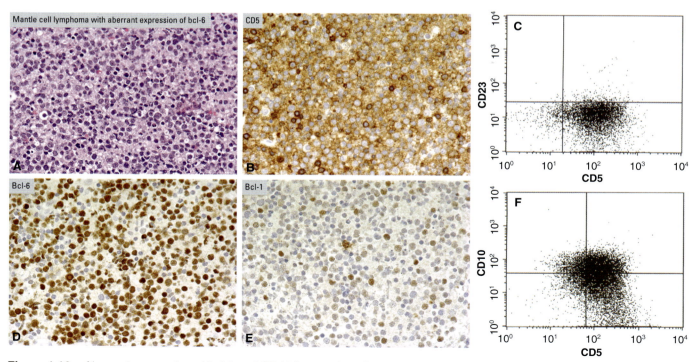

Figure 1.16   Aberrant expression of bcl-6 and CD10 by mantle cell lymphoma (**A**, histology; **B**, **D**, **E**, immunohistochemistry; **C**, **F**, flow cytometry). Tumor cells express CD5 (**B**, **C**), bcl-6 (**D**), bcl-1 (**E**) and CD10 (**F**). CD23 is negative (**C**)

Table 1.3 Immunophenotypic profiles of major types of B-cell disorders

Antibody	CLL/SLL	Mantle cell lymphoma	Marginal zone lymphoma	Follicular lymphoma	Hairy cell leukemia	Lymphoplasmacytic lymphoma	Diffuse large B-cell lymphoma	Burkitt lymphoma	Plasma cell myeloma
CD5	+	+/(rare −)	−	−	−	−	−/(rare +	−	−
CD10	−	−/(rare +)	−	+/(rare −)	−/(rare +)	−	+/−	+	−
CD11c	+ (dim)/−	−	+ (moderate)	−/+	+ (bright)	−	−/+	−	−
CD19	+	+	+	+ (dim)	+	+	+	+	−
CD20	+ (dim)	+	+	+	+ (bright)	+	+	+	+
CD23	++	−/(rare +)	−	−/+	−	−	−/+	−	+/−
CD25	−/+	−	−/+	−	+	−	−/+	−	−
CD43	+	+	+/−	−	−/+	−	−/+	+	++
Bcl-1	−	+	−	−	−/+	−	−	−	−/+
Bcl-2	+	+	+	+/rare −	+	+	+/−	+	−/(rare +)
Bcl-6	−	−	−	+	−	−	+/−	+	−
DBA44	−	−/(rare +)	−/+	−	+	−	−/(rare +)	−	−
Pax5	+	+	+	+	+	+	+	+	−/1/3 +

Table 1.4 Aberrant expression of antigens in B-cell neoplasms, as a percentage of each category

CD5-negative mantle cell lymphoma	11%
CD23-negative B-SLL/CLL	4%
CD10-positive hairy cell leukemia	12%
CD19-positive plasma cell myeloma	2%
CD56-positive diffuse large B-cell lymphoma	< 1%
CD10-negative follicular lymphoma	6%

There is an inverse correlation between bcl-6 expression and TdT (only very rare cases of TdT⁺ precursor B-lymphoblastic lymphomas are bcl-6⁺). DBA44 expression is similar to CD25. It is positive in HCL but is not specific for this entity. Pax-5 is a pan-B-cell marker present in a majority of B-cell neoplasms (both mature and immature). Approximately one-third of plasma cell neoplasms express Pax-5. Classical Hodgkin lymphoma is often Pax-5⁺, but the expression is dimmer than in B-cells. Popcorn cells (L&H cells) of nodular lymphocyte-predominant Hodgkin lymphoma are also Pax-5⁺. Sporadic cases of poorly differentiated carcinomas may express aberrantly Pax-5. Rare B-cell lymphomas co-express CD5 and CD10[40], most often DLBCL, followed by FL, MCL and others.

Table 1.4 presents the frequency of major B-cell lymphoproliferative disorders with aberrant phenotype.

Identification of abnormal T-cells by flow cytometry (FC)

An abnormal T-cell population may be identified by FC based on loss or diminished expression of one or more of the pan-T antigens (CD2, CD3, CD5, CD7), aberrant expression of CD4/CD8 (subset restriction, dual positive expression or lack of both markers), loss of expression of CD45, increased forward scatter, aberrant expression of TCR (dim expression of TCR alpha/beta, positive expression of TCR gamma/delta or lack of both TCR), and expression of additional markers, such as CD30, B-cell antigens (CD19, CD20), NK-cell markers (CD16, CD56, CD57), pan-myeloid antigens (CD13, CD33), CD117 and CD10[20,22,41]. Table 1.5 summarizes flow cytometric criteria to identify abnormal T-cell population.

Loss of one pan-T antigen is present in ~40% of peripheral (mature/post-thymic) T-cell neoplasms. CD7 is most commonly absent (~42%), followed by CD3 (~26%), CD5 (~22%) and CD2 (~11%). Lack of two pan-T antigens is present in ~16%, three pan-T antigens in ~7% and all four pan-T antigens in 2% of cases. Diminished expression of pan-T antigens is less specific

for T-cell neoplasms than complete lack of the expression. Diminished expression of one or even two pan-T antigens is often observed in reactive processes, such as viral infections, medication-associated changes or in the lymph nodes involved in non-T-cell disorders (e.g., diffuse large B-cell lymphoma, Hodgkin lymphoma). CD7 most often has aberrant dim expression in non-neoplastic lesions, followed by CD5. No reactive T-cell processes show aberrant (dim) expression of more than two markers. Therefore, the presence of dim expression of three or four pan-T antigens is considered highly suspicious for T-cell lymphoma/leukemia. Diminished expression of one or more antigens is suspicious for malignancy only if accompanied by other abnormalities (e.g., increased forward scatter). Figure 1.17 compares expression of pan-T antigens in benign lymph node (upper panels) and peripheral T-cell lymphoma (lower panels). Note increase in forward scatter and loss of CD5 and CD7 in T-cell lymphoma (residual benign T-cells are marked with *). Table 1.6 shows the frequency of loss or diminished expression of pan-T antigens in different types of peripheral T-cell lymphoproliferations.

Normal expression of all four pan-T antigens does not exclude T-cell lymphoma. Typical (moderate–bright) expression of all four antigens is present in 32% of peripheral (mature) T-cell lymphomas, most commonly in T-prolymphocytic leukemia (T-PLL; 57%), followed by AILD (25%), Sezary's syndrome (12%), anaplastic large cell lymphoma (11%), T-LGL (8%), and peripheral T-cell lymphoma, unspecified (7%). Therefore, lack of abnormal pan-T antigen expression does not exclude malignancy. Figure 1.18 presents T-PLL in the bone marrow (A) with clonal T-cells (PCR analysis; B), CD4 restriction (C) and normal expression of all four pan-T markers (D–G).

Restricted CD4 or CD8 expression, dual CD4/CD8 expression or lack of both CD4 and CD8 raises the possibility of lymphoma. Some non-T-cell disorders, such as Hodgkin lymphoma, may show marked predominance of CD4⁺ cells (Figure 1.19A). Lack of expression of CD4/CD8 is often seen in precursor T-lymphoblastic lymphoma (Figure 1.19B) and less commonly in peripheral (mature/post-thymic) T-cell disorders. Dual expression of CD4/CD8 is typical for thymocytes (Figure 1.19C) and therefore is not diagnostic for malignancy in lesions obtained from mediastinum. Occasional T-cell lymphoma may be CD8⁺ (Figure 1.19D). Predominance of CD8⁺ T-lymphocytes is often seen in viral infections.

Lack of CD45 is rarely observed in peripheral T-cell disorders (2.6%). When present, this is highly suggestive of malignancy. In contrast to precursor B-lymphoblastic

Table 1.5 Flow cytometric criteria to suspect T-cell neoplasm

Criteria	Comments
Loss of the expression of one or more pan-T antigens	Loss of one pan-T antigen is present in ~40% of peripheral T-cell neoplasms, most commonly CD7 (42%), followed by CD3 (~26%), CD5 (~22%) and CD2 (~11%). Lack of two pan-T antigens is present in ~16%, three pan-T antigens in ~7%, and all four pan-T antigens in 2% of cases. Positive expression of all four pan-T antigens does not exclude T-cell lymphoma. Positive expression of all four antigens is detected in 32% of peripheral T-cell lymphomas, most commonly in T-PLL (50%), followed by AILD lymphoma (25%) and others (see Table 1.6).
Diminished expression of more than two pan-T antigens	Diminished expression of one and even two pan-T antigens is often observed in reactive processes, such as viral infections (e.g., mononucleosis), medication-associated changes or in lymph nodes involved by non-T-cell disorders (e.g., diffuse large B-cell lymphoma or Hodgkin lymphoma). CD7 shows most often aberrant dim expression in non-neoplastic processes, followed by CD5. In many, CD5 expression is dim on a subset of cells (remaining T-cells show normal expression).
Aberrant CD4/CD8 expression (subset restriction, dual CD4/CD8 expression or lack of both antigens)	Restricted CD4 or CD8 expression, dual CD4/CD8 expression or lack of both antigens is suspicious for neoplasm. Reactive T-cells accompanying Hodgkin lymphoma and some other non-T-cell disorders may show marked predominance of CD4$^+$ cells. In some viral infections, CD4:CD8 ratio may be reversed. Dual expression of CD4/CD8 is typical for thymocytes (in both thymic hyperplasia and thymoma) and therefore is not diagnostic of malignancy in mediastinal lesions.
Loss of the expression of CD45	Lack of CD45 is rarely observed in peripheral T-cell disorders (2.6%). When present, it is highly suspicious for malignancy.
Increased forward scatter and diminished expression of one or more pan-T antigens	Increased forward scatter (FS) may be observed in rare reactive changes associated with treatment (e.g., in long-term phenytoin administration). Significantly increased FS coupled with diminished expression of pan-T antigens is highly suspicious for T-cell lymphoma. Note that a significant subset of high-grade large cell neoplasms (e.g., ALCL) may be missed by flow cytometry.
Dim expression of TCRαβ, lack of both TCRαβ and TCRγδ, or positive expression of TCRγδ	Dim expression of TCRαβ, lack of both TCR-associated antigens or positive expression of TCRγδ on significant numbers of T-cells indicates a malignant process.
Expression of additional markers: CD30, B-cell antigens (CD19, CD20), NK-cell associated antigens (CD16, CD56, CD57), pan-myeloid antigens (CD13, CD33), CD117 and CD10	CD30 is expressed by anaplastic large cell lymphoma and subset of other T-cell disorders. Rare cases of peripheral T-cell lymphomas show aberrant expression of B-cell antigens. Presence of NK-cell-associated antigens coupled with aberrant expression of pan-T antigens suggests T-cell disorders. Activated T-cells, however, often show dim expression of CD56 on subset of cells. Expression of pan-myeloid antigens and/or CD117 by T-cells is highly suspicious for malignancy. CD117 is rarely expressed by peripheral T-cell disorders (most often by T-PLL). Interestingly, CD117$^+$ peripheral T-cell disorders are always CD8$^+$. CD10, most often observed in AILD lymphoma, may be present in a minute subset of other mature T-cell neoplasms (see Table 1.4). Benign T-cells do not coexpress CD10.

lymphoma/leukemia, precursor T-cell neoplasms do not show loss of CD45. Dim expression of TCRαβ, lack of both TCR-associated antigens or positive expression of TCRγδ on a significant proportion of T-cells indicates a malignant process.

Of the additional (non-T-cell-associated) antigens useful in the diagnosis of T-cell lymphoproliferations, the most commonly applied are CD30, CD16, CD56, CD57, CD117 and CD10. CD30 is expressed by anaplastic large cell lymphoma and a subset of other T-cell disorders, including peripheral T-cell lymphoma, and unspecified and enteropathy-type T-cell lymphoma. T-cells in angioimmunoblastic T-cell lymphoma (AILD lymphoma) often express CD10 (50%) and bcl-6 (30%). CD10 is positive on a subset of benign thymocytes. CD117, a marker associated with acute myeloid leukemia and some spindle cell tumors (e.g., GIST), can be rarely expressed in both peripheral (mature) and precursor T-cell

lymphomas/leukemias (2.6% and 10%, respectively). Of interest, CD117 expression is restricted to CD8-positive lymphomas.

Pan-T antigens may be expressed in non-T-cell neoplasms (Table 1.7). CD2 may be positive in acute promyelocytic leukemia, blastic NK-cell lymphoma/leukemia (DC2 acute leukemia), and mast cell disorders. CD3 is often expressed by B-cells of primary effusion lymphoma. CD5 is aberrantly expressed in B-chronic lymphocytic leukemia/small lymphocytic lymphoma, mantle cell lymphoma, *de novo* diffuse large B-cell lymphoma and thymoma/thymic carcinoma. CD7 is often positive in acute myeloid leukemia, blastic NK-cell lymphoma/leukemia (DC2 acute leukemia) and acute monocytic leukemia.

Table 1.8 presents an immunophenotypic profile of major categories of peripheral (mature/post-thymic) T-cell disorders.

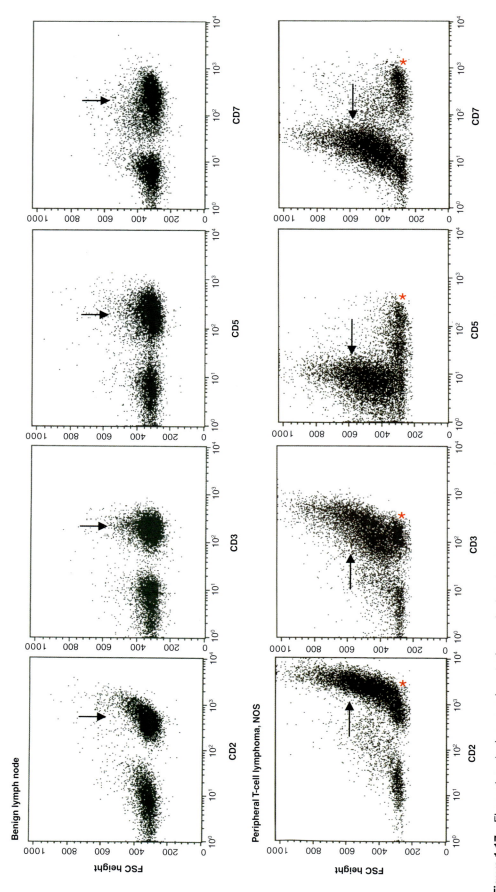

Figure 1.17   Flow cytometry immunophenotyping – criteria to identify abnormal T-cell population (see text for details). Upper panels represent a benign lymph node. Note moderate expression of all four pan-T antigens (arrow). Lower panels represent an example of T-cell lymphoma with aberrant expression of CD2 (brighter than normal T-cells marked with *), loss of CD5 and CD7, and increased forward scatter (arrow). Reactive conditions may be associated with loss or diminished expression of one of pan-T antigens (usually CD7) and coexpression of CD11c and CD38

Table 1.6   Frequency of aberrant expression of pan-T antigens in peripheral T-cell lymphomas

Pan-T antigen expression (CD2, CD3, CD5, CD7)	T-cell lymphoma, NOS	AILD lymphoma	Adult T-cell leukemia	T-PLL	Anaplastic large cell lymphoma	Hepatosplenic T-cell lymphoma	T-LGL leukemia	NK-LGL leukemia	Sezary's syndrome
1 antigen negative	49.2	58.3	66.7	20.8	16.7	55.5	30.5	0	62.5
2 antigens negative	25.4	16.7	16.7	8.3	27.8	33.3	0	100	12.5
3 antigens negative	7.5	0	16.7	0	22.2	0	0	0	0
4 antigens negative	0	0	0	0	22.2	0	0	0	0
All four antigens normal	**7.5**	**25**	**0**	**57.1**	**11.1**	**0**	**8.3**	**0**	**12.5**
1 antigen abnormal (negative or dim)	52.9	58.3	66.7	21.4	16.7	66.7	52.8	0	62.5
2 antigens abnormal (negative or dim)	41.8	33.3	16.7	10.8	27.8	33.3	30.5	69.7	25
3 antigens abnormal (negative or dim)	13.4	0	16.7	10.8	22.2	0	8.3	30.8	0
4 antigens abnormal (negative or dim)	1.5	0	0	0	22.2	0	0	0	0

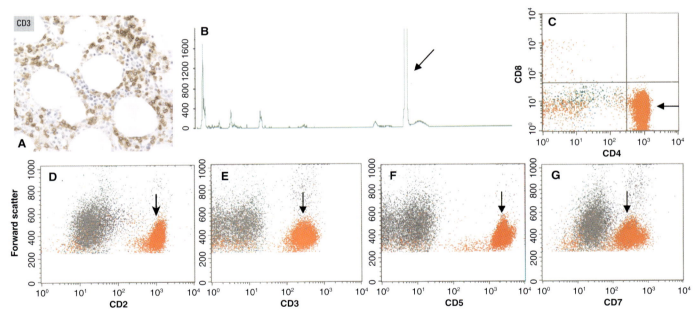

Figure 1.18   T-PLL (**A**, bone marrow staining for CD3; **B**, molecular test with clonal peak (arrow); **C–G**, flow cytometry). Flow cytometry immunophenotyping shows no loss of pan-T antigen expression (D–G). Lack of aberrant expression of pan-T antigens does no exclude malignancy. Other cricteria useful in flow cytometric diagnosis of T-cell proliferations include CD4 or CD8 subset restriction (**C**), increased forward or orthogonal side-scatter, presence of NK-cell associated antigens and aberrant expression of antigens, e.g. CD33 or CD117. Among peripheral T-cell disorders, T-cell prolymphocytic leukemia is a most common entity which lacks aberrant expression of pan-T markers (CD2, CD3, CD5 and CD7)

Table 1.7   Aberrant expression of pan-T antigens in non-T-cell neoplasms

CD2	APL, blastic NK-leukemia/lymphoma, mast cell disease
CD3	Primary effusion lymphoma
CD5	SLL/CLL, mantle cell lymphoma, *de novo* diffuse large B-cell lymphoma, thymoma/thymic carcinoma
CD7	AML, APL, blastic NK-cell leukemia/lymphoma, monocytic leukemia, AML with NK-cell differentiation

Mature T-cell disorders versus precursor T-lymphoblastic lymphoma/leukemia

Table 1.9 presents a comparison between the mature and precursor T-cell neoplasms. T-ALL/LBL more often shows dimmer expression of CD45, lack of CD2 and CD3 (surface), dual positive or dual negative CD4/CD8 expression, lack of TCR, and expression of CD10 and CD117 when compared to mature tumors[20,22]. Peripheral (mature/post-thymic) T-cell proliferations more often

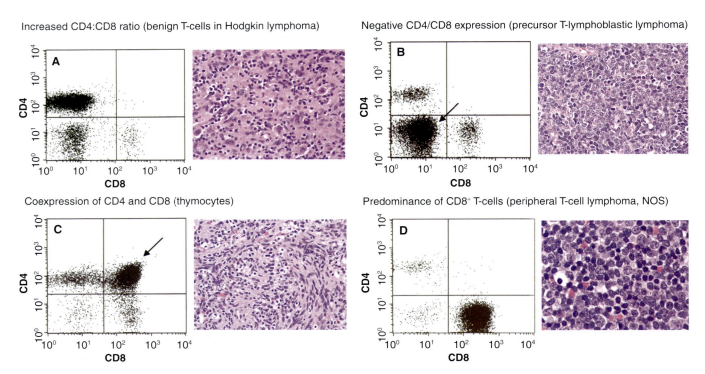

Figure 1.19 Flow cytometry immunophenotyping – CD4:CD8 ratio. Apart from evaluation of pan-T antigens, the CD4:CD8 ratio is a very useful parameter in flow cytometric analysis of hematolymphoid lesions (**A–D**). Predominance of either CD4⁺ or CD8⁺ cells, dual expression of CD4/CD8 or lack of both CD4/CD8, although not completely diagnostic, may indicate malignancy (including both mature/post-thymic and precursor lesions). Classical Hodgkin lymphoma and NLPHL are often associated with an increased CD4:CD8 ratio (**A**). Benign thymocytes (hyperplastic thymus or thymoma) typically coexpress CD4 and CD8 (**C**)

Table 1.8 Immunophenotypic profiles of major types of T-cell disorders (%)

Antibody	T-cell lymphoma, NOS	AILD lymphoma	Adult T-cell leukemia	T-PLL	Anaplastic large cell lymphoma	Hepatosplenic T-cell lymphoma	T-LGL leukemia	NK-LGL leukemia	Sezary's syndrome
CD2⁺	88	100	86	96	67	81	100	100	88
CD3⁺	60	67	71	89	33	100	100	0	100
CD5⁺	87	100	100	92	50	18	80	0	88
CD7⁺	45	42	0	89	22	90	89	100	37
CD4⁺	60	100	100	58	72	0	0	0	100
CD8⁺	12	0	0	13	17	10	89	23	0
CD4/8⁺	6	0	0	17	6	0	8	0	0
CD4/CD8⁻	22	0	0	12	5	90	3	77	0
TCRαβ⁺	76	100	71	91	67	10	78	8	100
TCRγδ⁺	0	0	0	0	0	90	22	0	0
TCR⁻	24	0	29	9	33	0	0	92	0
CD25⁺	15	Rare	100	Rare	25	0	0	0	14
CD30⁺	8	Rare	X	X	100	X	X	X	X
CD56⁺	13	0	0	4	Rare	100	33	70	0
CD57⁺	Rare	0	0	Rare	0	0	97	61	0
ALK-1⁺	0	0	X	X	66	X	X	X	X
EMA⁺	7	X	X	X	78	X	X	X	X
CD11b⁺	Rare	0	0	0	0	0	28	46	0
CD11c⁺	12	0	0	4	0	0	44	61	0
Other	CD10⁺ 7% CD117⁺ 1.5%	CD10⁺ 50% Bcl-6⁺ 30%		CD117⁺ 14.3%*	CD10⁺ 12%				

*All cases of CD117⁺ tumors were CD8⁺; X = not evaluated; CD10 expression in angioimmunoblastic lymphoma corresponds to cases in which majority of tumor cells were CD10⁺.

Table 1.9 Comparison of antigenic profile of peripheral T-cell lymphomas and precursor T-lymphoblastic lymphoma/leukemia

Antigen	Peripheral T-cell lymphoma/leukemia (%)	Precursor T-lymphoblastic lymphoma/leukemia (%)
CD45		
Moderate⁺	93.3	69.6
Dim⁺	4.1	30.4
Negative	2.6	0
Pan-T-cell antigens		
CD2⁺	89.1	65.2
CD3⁺	73.6	41.3
CD5⁺	77.7	87.0
CD7⁺	58.0	97.8
1 pan-T antigen negative	39.9	47.8
2 pan-T antigens negative	16.1	21.7
3 pan-T antigens negative	6.7	6.5
All pan-T antigens negative	2.0	0
All pan-T antigens positive	32.1	6.5
CD4/CD8		
CD4⁺	48.7	10.9
CD8⁺	29.0	8.7
CD4/CD8⁺	6.2	39.4
CD4/CD8⁻	16.1	41.3
TCR		
TCRαβ+	75.6	31.4
TCRγδ+	14.4	17.1
TCR⁻	10.0	51.4
CD1a⁺	0	32.0
CD10⁺	6.2	23.9
CD13⁺	0	17.4
CD33⁺	0	21.7
CD34⁺	0	36.9
CD56⁺	20.7	23.9
CD57⁺	24.3	4.3
CD117⁺	2.6	10.9
HLA-DR⁺	4.1	8.7
TdT⁺	0	87.0

show positive expression of all four pan-T antigens (32% vs 6.5%) and lack of CD7 (58% vs 98%) than T-ALL/LBL. The presence of CD1a, CD13, CD33, CD34, and TdT indicates T-ALL/LBL.

Differential diagnosis of acute leukemias

Table 1.10 summarizes FC phenotypic characteristics of different types of acute leukemias. The majority of acute leukemias have blasts with low orthogonal side scatter (SSC), whereas all cases of hypergranular variants of APL are characterized by high SSC (similar to maturing granulocytes). Occasional cases of non-APL leukemias may have blasts with high SSC. A majority of blasts display moderate expression of CD45. Acute monocytic leukemia usually shows bright CD45, and precursor B-lymphoblastic leukemia/lymphoma (B-ALL) usually shows dim expression of CD45 (many cases are CD45⁻). Negative expression of

CD45 apart from B-ALL is seen in acute erythroid leukemia. The most valuable markers to differentiate between acute myeloid leukemia (AML) and acute lymphoblastic leukemia (ALL) are CD13, CD33, CD117 (AML), CD10, CD19 and intracytoplasmic CD79a (B-ALL), and intracytoplasmic CD3 (T-ALL). Lack of expression of HLA-DR is seen in acute promyelocytic leukemia (APL) and in rare cases of other myeloid leukemias. Expression of HLA-DR differentiates acute monocytic leukemia from the microgranular variant of APL (only a minute subset of acute monocytic leukemias is HLA-DR⁻). HLA-DR in acute megakaryocytic leukemia is negative to dim. Positive expression of CD56 is seen most commonly in acute monocytic leukemia and blastic NK-cell lymphoma/leukemia. Other acute leukemias may be CD56⁺, especially AML with t(8;21), which often coexpress CD56 and CD19. AML with NK-cell differentiation is often positive for CD7. Expression of CD11b and CD11c is most typical for acute monocytic leukemia, where the expression tends to be bright or at least moderate. Other AMLs often have moderate CD11c, but CD11b is usually negative. Expression of pan-myeloid antigens (CD13, CD33) can be seen occasionally in precursor B- or T-lymphoblastic leukemias. Acute monocytic leukemia and acute megakaryoblastic leukemia show usually dim CD13 and bright CD33. The latter shows dim CD117 and negative CD34, which creates a characteristic FC pattern, prompting the addition of CD41 and CD61 during flow analysis. CD64 is more brightly expressed in acute monocytic leukemia than in megakaryoblastic or promyelocytic leukemias. CD23 can be expressed on a subset of acute monocytic leukemia and the microgranular variant of APL. CD34 expression is negative in hypergranular APL and megakaryocytic leukemia. CD117 is usually negative on monocytic cells, B-ALL and most cases of blastic NK-cell lymphoma/leukemia and T-ALL.

INTRODUCTION TO CYTOGENETICS/MOLECULAR PATHOLOGY

Cytogenetic/fluorescence *in situ* hybridization (FISH) and molecular tests, including polymerase chain reaction (PCR) and Southern blot are an integral part of evaluating hematopoietic tumors[36,42–71]. Detection of specific chromosomal changes is necessary for the diagnosis of chronic myeloid leukemia (Philadelphia chromosome leading to *bcr-abl* fusion gene), acute promyelocytic leukemia [t(15;17)], AML with t(8;21), T-prolymphocytic leukemia (chromosome 16 abnormalities), follicular lymphoma [t(14;18)] and Burkitt lymphoma (c-*myc*).

Table 1.10 Immunophenotypic profiles of major types of acute leukemias

Antibody	AML M0-2	AML-M2 t(8;21)	AML-M3 (APL)	AML-M4 Blasts	AML-M4 Monocytes	AML-M5	AML-M6	AML-M7	Blastic NK-cell leukemia	Precursor B-ALL	Precursor T-ALL
CD2	–	–	+/–	–	–	–	–	–	–	–	+
CD3	–	–	–	–	–	–	–	–	–	–	+
CD4	+/–	+/–	+/–	+/–	+	+	–	–/+	+	–	+/–
CD7	–/+	–/+	–/+	–/+	+/–	+/–	–	–/+	–/+	–	+/–
CD10	–	–	–	–	–	–	–	–	–	+/–	–/+
CD11b	–	–	–	–	+	+	–	–	–	–	–
CD11c	–/+	–/+	–/+	+/–	+	+	–	–	–	–	–
CD13	+	+	+	+	+	dim+	–	–/dim+	–	–/rare+	–
CD14	–	–	–	–	+	+/–	–	–	–	–	–
CD16	–	–	–	–	–	–/+	–	–	–	–	–
CD19	–	+	–	–	–	–	–	–	–	+	–
CD20	–	–	–	–	–	–	–	–	–	–/rare+	–
CD22	–	–	–	–	–	–	–	–	–	+/–	–
CD33	+	+	+	+	+	bright+	–	bright+	–/rare+	–/rare+	–/rare+
CD34	+	+	–	+	–	+/–	+/–	–/rare+	+/–	+	+/–
CD41	–	–	–	–	–	–	–	+	–	–	–
CD45	+	+	+	+	+	+	–/rare+	+/rare–	+	+/–	+
CD56	–/+	+/rare–	–/+	–	–/+	+/–	–/rare+	–/rare+	+	–	–/+
CD61	–	–	–	–	–	–	–	+	–	–	–
CD64	–/+	–/+	–/+	–/+	+	+/–	–	–	–	–	–
CD79a	–	–	–	–	–	–	–	–	–	+	–
CD117	+	+	+	+	–	–/+	dim+	dim+	–/rare+	–	–/rare+
HLA-DR	+/rare–	+/rare–	–	+	+	+/–	+	–/dim	+(dim)	+/–	–/+
TdT	–/+	–/+	–	–	–	–	–	–	–/+	+	+/–
GPHA	–	–	–	–	–	–	+	–	–	–	–
cIgM	–	–	–	–	–	–	–	–	–	+/–	–

Lymphomas most often display balanced translocations, whereas myelodysplastic syndromes often have deletion(s) or addition(s) of genetic material (e.g., monosomies and trisomies). Figure 1.20 and Table 1.11 present common chromosomal changes in hematopoietic tumors. Figure 1.21 shows examples of PCR studies.

NORMAL STRUCTURE OF HEMATOLYMPHOID ORGANS

The hematolymphoid system, in which leukemia and lymphoma arise, consists of lymph nodes, the bone marrow, the spleen and the thymus.

Lymph node

The lymph nodes act as a scaffolding system and home for lymphocytes and monocytes/histiocytes in the lymphatic system. Lymph nodes are ovoid, encapsulated structures composed of primary and secondary follicles, paracortex, medullary cords, vessels and sinuses (Figure 1.22A). Primary and secondary follicles are distributed within cortex (at the periphery of the lymph node). Primary follicles (unstimulated; resting) are composed of small and relatively monotonous B-cells. Special care must be made in interpretation of primary versus secondary follicles by

immunohistochemical studies, as the primary follicle B-cells are bcl-2[+] and can be confused with neoplastic follicles of follicular lymphoma. Secondary follicles are composed of two zones: central, pale-staining germinal centers and a darker-staining mantle zone composed of small lymphocytes. The germinal centers contain numerous larger lymphocytes with nucleoli (centroblasts) and tingible body macrophages. The secondary follicles often show polarization of their architecture (Figure 1.22B): one pole is composed of centrocytes and the other has an increased number of centroblasts and macrophages. Polarization helps to differentiate reactive follicles from follicular lymphoma. The polarization is best appreciated with Ki-67 (MIB-1) staining (see Figures 2.72 and 2.73; Chapter 2). Supporting the B-cells in the follicles are follicular dendritic cells, best visualized by staining with CD21 (Figure 1.22C) or CD23. Intact (compact) distributions of follicular dendritic cell meshwork favors a reactive process, whereas an expanded or disrupted meshwork is seen in lymphomas, such as marginal zone lymphoma, follicular lymphoma or nodular lymphocyte-predominant Hodgkin lymphoma. The lymphoid cells between follicles (paracortex or interfollicular region) are composed predominantly of small T-cells with rare centroblasts (depending on the degree of activation), scattered interdigitating

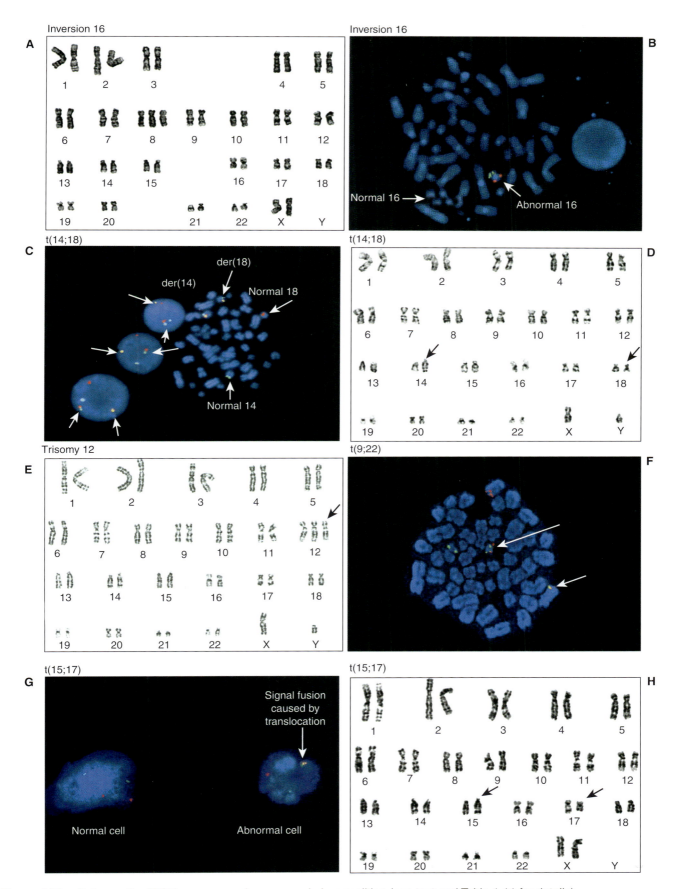

Figure 1.20   Cytogenetics/FISH – common chromosomal abnormalities (see text and Table 1.11 for details)

Table 1.11   Common chromosomal abnormalities in hematopoietic tumors

Lymphoma/leukemia	Chromosomal abnormality	Molecular basis	Clinical significance
CML	t(9;22)(q34;q11) Complex changes; i.e., extra Ph′, +8, i(17q)	BCR-ABL fusion gene	Response to imatinib (Gleevec©) Majority of patients in accelerated phase or blast phase
AML-M2	t(8;21)(q22;q22)	AML1-ETO	Good response to cytosine arabinoside
AML-M3 (APL)	t(15;17)(q22;q12)	PML-RARA	Responds to retinoic acid therapy
AML-M4eo	inv(16)(p13;q22)	MYH11-CBFB	Good response to cytosine arabinoside
AML-M5	Deletion or translocation of 11q23		
B-ALL	t(9;22)(q34;q11.2) t(12;21)(p13;q22)	BCR-ABL fusion gene	Poor prognosis
T-ALL	del(1p32) del(9p); others	TAL1 deletion	
Splenic marginal zone lymphoma	Allelic loss of 7q(21–32) Trisomy 3		
Follicular lymphoma	t(14;18)(q32;q21) t(2;18)(p12;q21)	BCL2-IGGH	
B-SLL/CLL	Trisomy 12		Atypical morphology and poor prognosis
Mantle cell lymphoma	t(11;14)	BCL1-IGGH	
Diffuse large B-cell lymphoma	t(3;14)	BCL6-IGGH	
Marginal zone B-cell lymphoma (MALT)	t(11;18)	API1-MALT1	
Burkitt's lymphoma	t(8;14,2, or 22)	MYC-IGH, IGK, or IGL	
Anaplastic large cell lymphoma	t(2;5)(p23;35) t(1;2)(a25;p23)	NPM-ALK	Good prognosis
Chronic myelomonocytic leukemia	+ 8, -7/del(7q), t(5;12)	TEL-PDGFβR	
Myelodysplastic syndrome (MDS)	del(20q), + 8, abnormalities of chromosome 5 and/or 7		
MDS with isolated del(5q)	del(5q) only		5q (−) syndrome

reticulum cells and the high endothelial venules. Sinuses contain macrophages and patency is best evaluated by the examination of the subcapsular region. The immunohistochemical staining of the lymph node with B-cell markers (e.g., CD20, CD79a), pan-T antigens (e.g., CD3, CD5), CD10, CD21 (to assess the dendritic cells) and bcl-2 helps to identify normal architecture and differentiate reactive process from lymphoma. Figure 1.22C–F shows a normal pattern of immunohistochemical staining with selected relevant markers.

Bone marrow

The bone marrow in the adult occupies the medullary spaces of large bones such as the femur, the hip, the sternum and the humerus. The marrow cellularity changes with age and can be roughly estimated as (100−age)% (100% at birth, 50% in a 50-year-old person and 10–20% in an 80-year-old person). The primary function of the bone marrow is the production of blood cells (hematopoiesis). The bone marrow (Figures 1.23 and 1.24) is composed of a matrix requisite for hematopoiesis as well as granulocytic precursors, erythroid precursors, megakaryocytes (platelet precursors), scattered monocytes, lymphocytes and plasma cells, adipocytes, blood vessels and other stromal elements (e.g., osteoblasts, osteoclasts, fibroblasts, etc.).

The bone marrow contains progenitor cells called stem cells. Stem cells have the pluripotent capacity for both self-renewal and differentiation. These cells give rise to all of the different cell series of lymphocytes and myeloid cells. The myeloid lineage is comprised of all nonlymphoid white cells, red cells, and platelets. The sequence of maturation stages on a bone marrow aspirate smear stained with Wright–Giemsa for different cell types is presented in Figure 1.25. The granulocytic series predominates

A   Polyclonal IgH gene rearrangement (PCR)

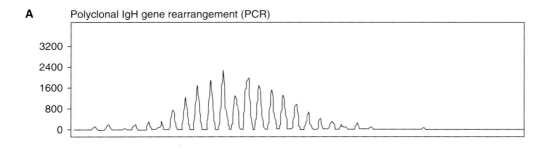

B   Monoclonal IgH gene rearrangement (PCR)

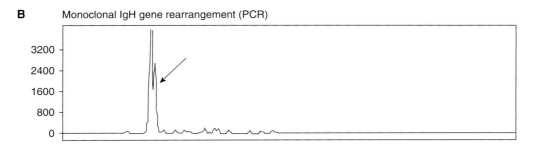

C   Monoclonal IgH gene rearrangement in the polyclonal background (PCR)

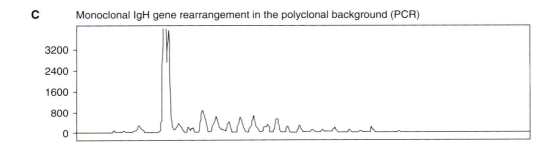

D   AML-ETO +

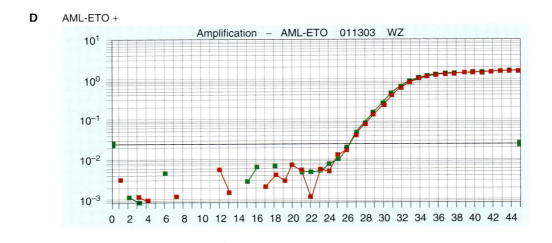

E   Monoclonal TCR gene rearrangement (PCR)

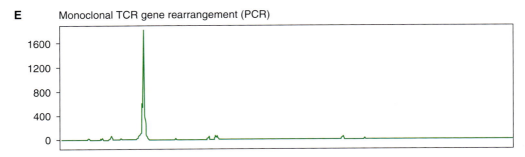

Figure 1.21   Molecular pathology – concept of clonal gene rearrangement (see text for details)

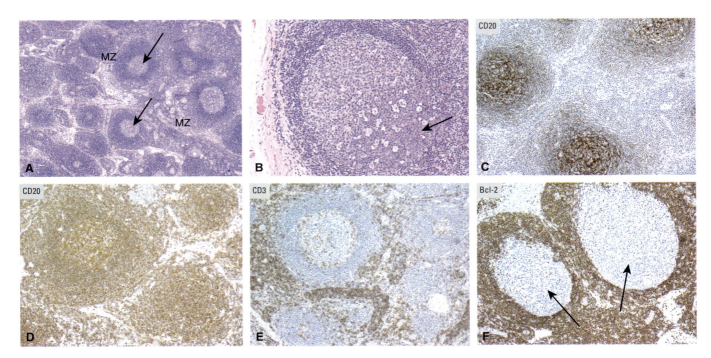

Figure 1.22 Benign lymph node – histology and immunohistochemistry. Low power (**A**) shows preserved architecture with follicles composed of germinal centers (arrow) and mantle zone (MZ). Higher magnification (**B**) shows germinal center with one pole composed of larger lymphocytes with macrophages (polarization, arrow). The follicular dendritic cell meshwork is preserved (**C**, CD21 staining). B-cells are visualized by staining with CD20 (**D**). T-cells are restricted to the perifollicular area (**E**, CD3 staining). Germinal center cells do not coexpress bcl-2, a useful parameter in distinguishing between follicular hyperplasia and follicular lymphoma (**F**)

over the erythroid series (the ratio is roughly 2:1). The recognized morphologic maturation stages in granulocytic lineage are blasts, promyelocytes, myelocytes, metamyelocytes, bands and polymorphonuclear leukocytes (neutrophils). In a normal marrow core biopsy, blasts (CD34⁺) comprise up to 3% of marrow cells (Figure 1.24B). Megakaryocytes (Figure 1.24C) are scattered individually, and usually do not exceed 4–5 per high-power field (objective × 40). Cytoplasmic fragments of megakaryocyte cells (platelets) are instrumental in primary hemostasis. The erythroid lineage matures from stem cell to red cells (which carry oxygen to peripheral tissues) through proerythroblast (pronormoblast), early normoblast (basophilic erythroblast), intermediate normoblast (polychromatic erythroblast), late normoblast (orthochromatic erythroblast) and reticulocyte. The lymphoid lineage also matures from stem cell to mature lymphocyte. A lymphocyte will become either a B-cell or a T-cell. T-cells are further subdivided into helper/inducer cells, suppressor/cytotoxic cells and NK-cells. T-cells regulate the B-cells, as well as kill infected cells in the body. The B-cells are programmed at birth to react against a specific glycoprotein sequence, or antigen. Each B-cell

has a surface immunoglobulin (antibody) which contains a specific kappa or lambda light-chain configuration. If the B-cell encounters its antigen match, the B-cell will undergo clonal expansion, making millions of copies of itself and differentiating into special types of B-cells eventually transforming into a plasma cell. Plasma cells secrete their immunoglobulin antibodies from their cytoplasm into the serum, thereby enabling the infection or intruder proteins to be eliminated. Programmed cell death (apoptosis), as well as suppressor T-cells, prevents the clonal cells from becoming autonomous, immortal and hence neoplastic.

Spleen

Spleen has a tripartite role, (i) acting as a sieve for the circulatory system (similar to that of lymph node for the lymphatic system), (ii) phagocytosis (elimination of senescent red blood cells, bacteria and other foreign material) and (iii) storing blood cell elements for possible future use. Figures 1.26 and 1.27 present the normal structure of spleen. Spleen is composed of white pulp, red pulp, cords and sinuses. The white pulp consists of B-cells and

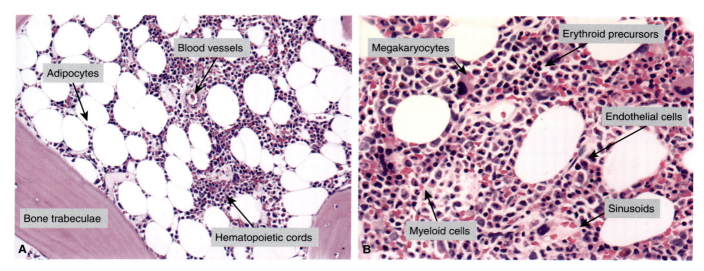

Figure 1.23   Bone marrow – normal histology

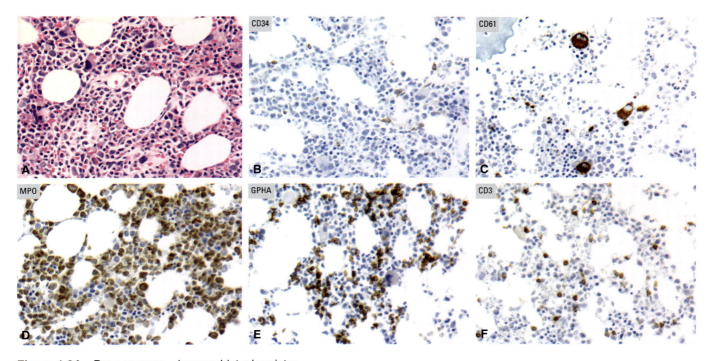

Figure 1.24   Bone marrow – immunohistochemistry

periarteriolar T-cell lymphoid sheaths. The follicles, similarly to the lymph node, can be divided into primary and secondary follicles with similar morphologic characteristics (see above). The red pulp is composed of arterioles, sinusoids and venules. Numerous erythrocytes are responsible for its red color. The sinuses are lined by littoral cells, cells with dual endothelial/macrophage function (they are also present in the medullary sinuses of lymph node). These cells, active in phagocytosis, are positive for CD8 and blood vessel markers (e.g., CD31) as well as histiocyte/macrophage marker CD68.

APPROACH TO THE DIAGNOSIS OF HEMATOPOIETIC TUMORS

Figures 1.28–1.31 present an algorithmic approach to the possible diagnosis of lymphoma, CML, plasma cell myeloma and anemia/MDS, respectively.

WHO CLASSIFICATION OF HEMATOPOIETIC TUMORS

Table 1.12 presents the current WHO classification of the hematolymphoid tumors[72–87].

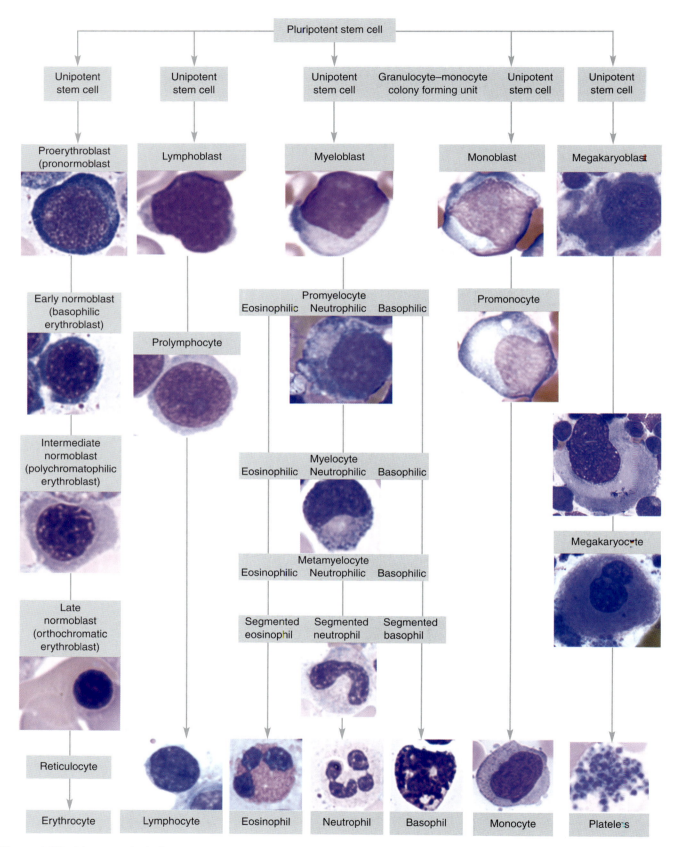

Figure 1.25   Hematopoiesis (see text for details)

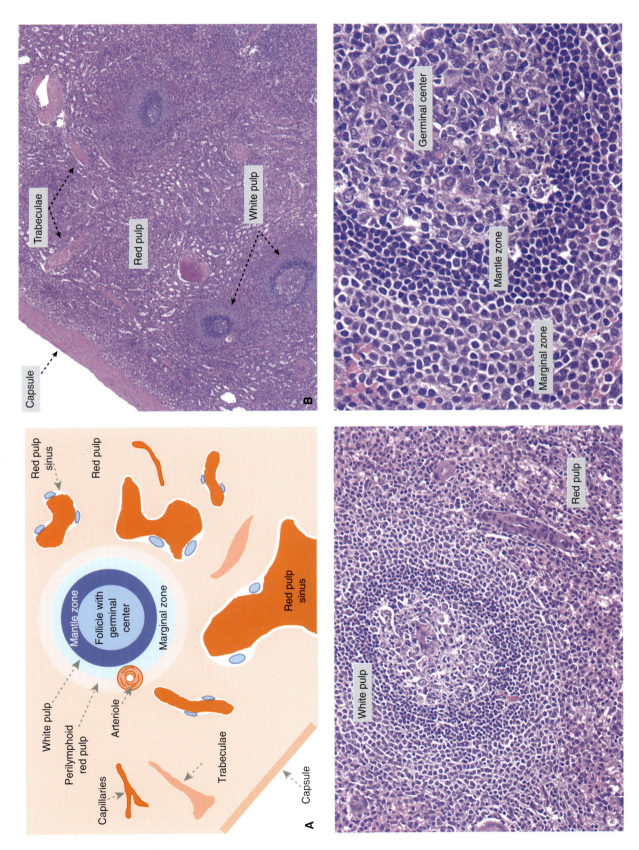

Figure 1.26   Benign spleen – histology

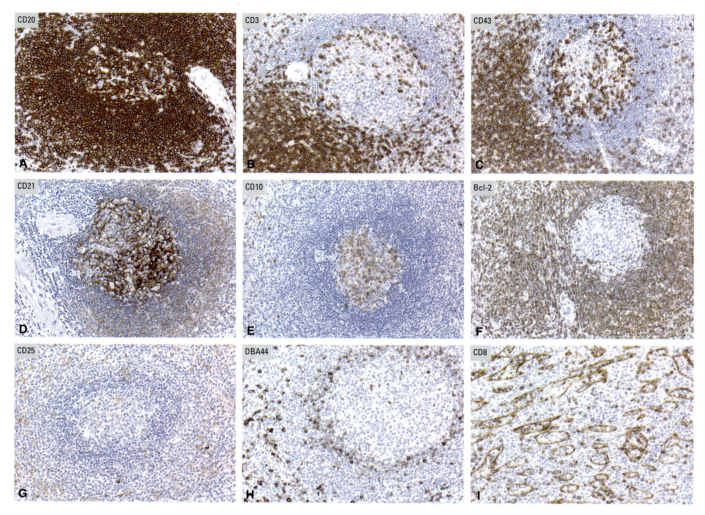

Figure 1.27   Benign spleen – immunohistochemistry

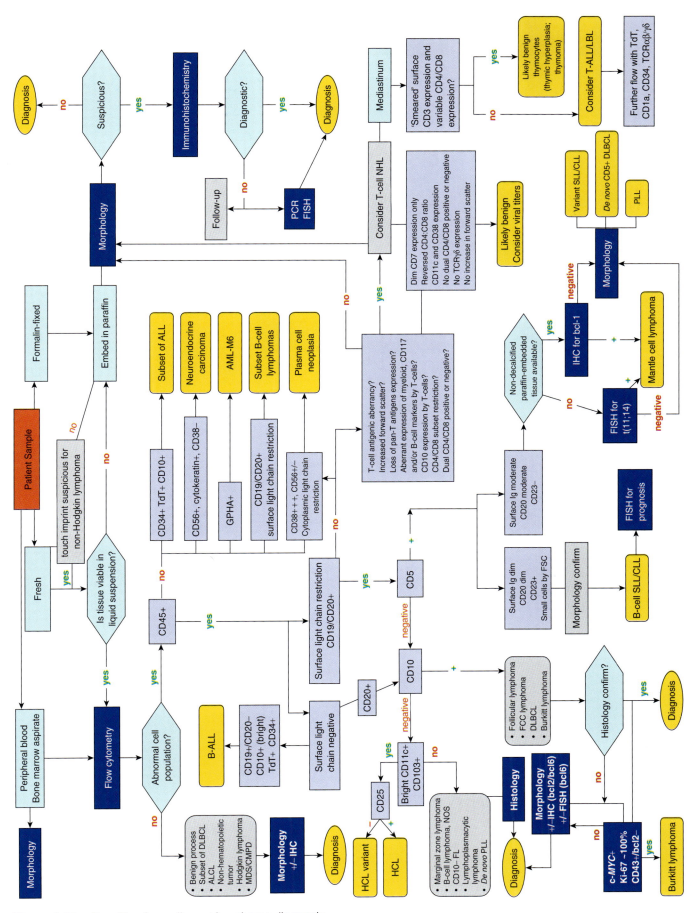

Figure 1.28 Algorithm for malignant lymphoma diagnosis

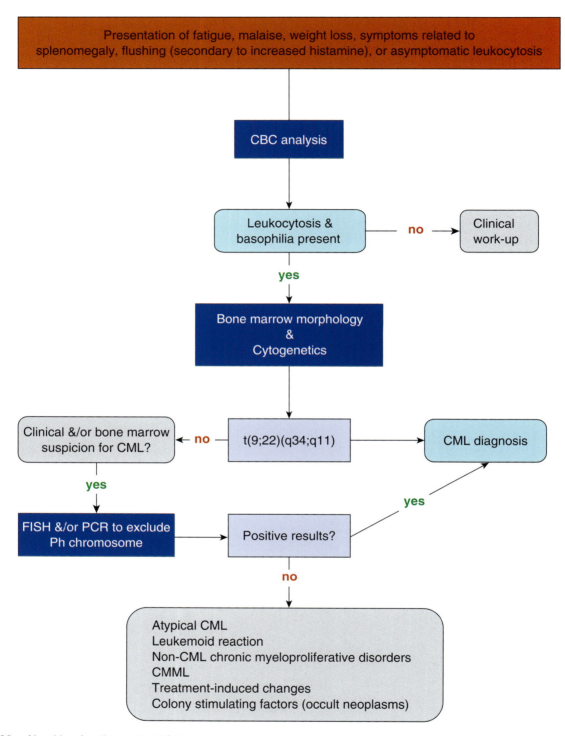

Figure 1.29   Algorithm for diagnosis of CML

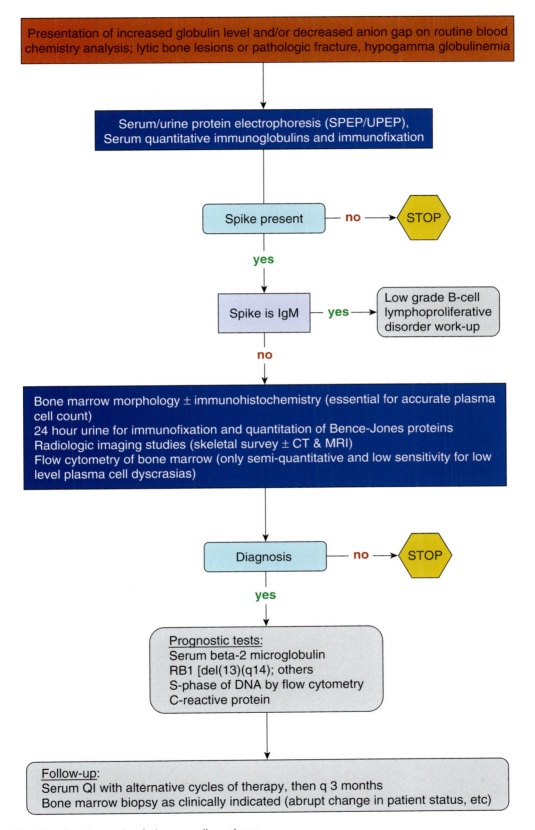

Figure 1.30 Algorithm for diagnosis of plasma cell myeloma

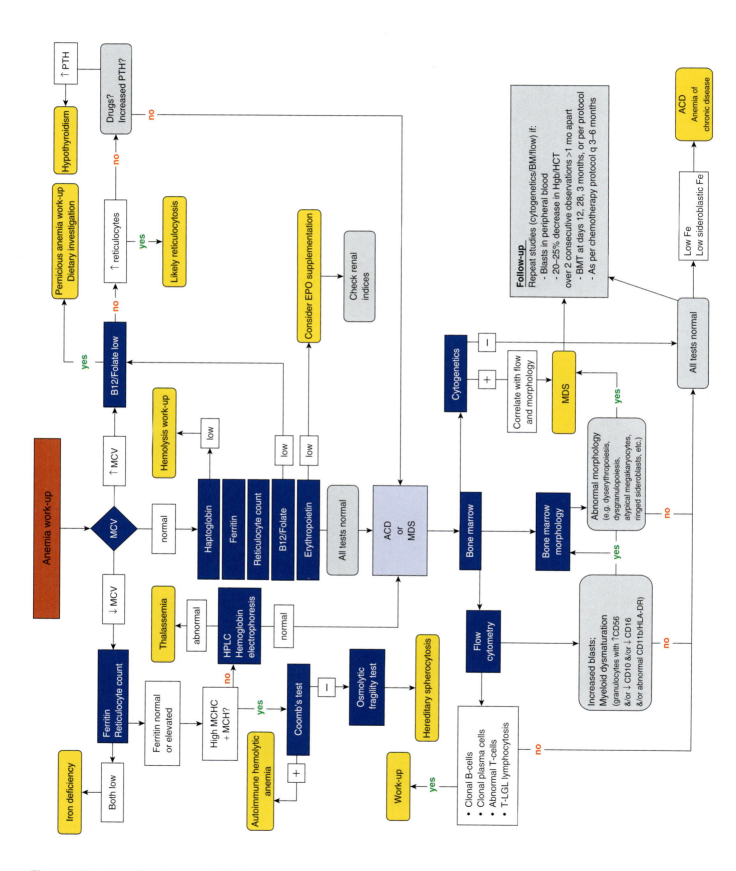

Figure 1.31   Algorithm for anemia/MDS work-up

Table 1.12 WHO classification of tumors of hematopoietic and lymphoid tissues

Mature B-cell neoplasms

Chronic lymphocytic leukemia/small lymphocytic lymphoma (B-CLL/SLL)
B-cell prolymphocytic leukemia (B-PLL)
Lymphoplasmacytic lymphoma
Marginal zone B-cell lymphoma (MZL)
    Splenic marginal zone lymphoma
    Nodal marginal zone lymphoma
    Extranodal marginal zone lymphoma of mucosa-associated lymphoid tissue
Hairy cell leukemia
Plasma cell myeloma/plasmacytoma
Follicular lymphoma (FL)
Mantle cell lymphoma (MCL)
Diffuse large B-cell lymphoma (DLBCL)
Mediastinal (thymic) large B-cell lymphoma
Intravascular large B-cell lymphoma
Primary effusion lymphoma
Burkitt lymphoma/leukemia
B-cell proliferations of uncertain malignant potential
    Lymphomatoid granulomatosis
    Post-transplant lymphoproliferative disorder, polymorphic

Mature T-cell and NK-cell neoplasms

T-cell prolymphocytic leukemia (T-PLL)
T-cell large granular lymphocytic leukemia (T-LGL leukemia)
Aggressive NK-cell leukemia
Adult T-cell leukemia/lymphoma
Extranodal NK/T-cell lymphoma, nasal type
Enteropathy-type T-cell lymphoma
Hepatosplenic T-cell lymphoma
Subcutaneous panniculitis-like T-cell lymphoma
Mycosis fungoides/Sezary syndrome (MF/SS)
Primary cutaneous anaplastic large cell lymphoma
Peripheral T-cell lymphoma, unspecified
Angioimmunoblastic T-cell lymphoma (AILD lymphoma)
Anaplastic large cell lymphoma (ALCL)
T-cell proliferation of uncertain malignant potential
    Lymphomatoid papulosis

Hodgkin lymphoma

Nodular lymphocyte-predominant Hodgkin lymphoma (NLPHL)
Classical Hodgkin lymphoma (HL)
    Nodular sclerosis Hodgkin lymphoma
    Lymphocyte-rich classical Hodgkin lymphoma
    Mixed cellularity Hodgkin lymphoma
    Lymphocyte-depleted Hodgkin lymphoma

Chronic myeloproliferative diseases

Chronic myelogenous leukemia (CML)
Chronic neutrophilic leukemia
Chronic eosinophilic leukemia/hypereosinophilic syndrome
Polycythemia vera (PV)
Chronic idiopathic myelofibrosis (CIMF)
Essential thrombocythemia (ET)
Chronic myeloproliferative disease, unclassifiable

Myelodysplastic/myeloproliferative diseases

Chronic myelomonocytic leukemia (CMML)
Atypical chronic myeloid leukemia
Juvenile myelomonocytic leukemia
Myelodysplastic/myeloproliferative diseases, unclassifiable

Table 1.12 (Continued)

Myelodysplastic syndromes

Refractory anemia (RA)
Refractory anemia with ringed sideroblasts (RARS)
Refractory cytopenia with multilineage dysplasia (RCMD)
Refractory anemia with excess blasts (RAEB)
Myelodysplastic syndrome associated with isolated del(5q)
Myelodysplastic syndrome, unclassifiable

Acute myeloid leukemia (AML)

AML with t(8;21), (AML1/ETO)
AML with inv(16)(p13;q22) or t(16;16)(p13;q22) (acute myelomonocytic leukemia with eosinophilia; AML-M4Eo)
Acute promyelocytic leukemia [AML with t(15;17)(q22;q12)], APL (AML-M3)
Acute myeloid leukemia with multilineage dysplasia
    With prior myelodysplastic syndrome
    Without prior myelodysplastic syndrome
Acute myeloid leukemia and myelodysplastic syndrome, therapy-related
Acute myeloid leukemia, minimally differentiated (AML-M0)
Acute myeloid leukemia without maturation (AML-M1)
Acute myeloid leukemia with maturation (AML-M2)
Acute myelomonocytic leukemia (AML-M4)
Acute monoblastic leukemia (AML-M5)
Acute erythroid leukemia (AML-M6)
Acute megakaryoblastic leukemia (AML-M7)
Acute basophilic leukemia
Acute panmyelosis with myelofibrosis
Myeloid sarcoma

Acute leukemia of ambiguous lineage

Precursor neoplasms

Precursor B-cell neoplasms
    Precursor B lymphoblastic leukemia/lymphoma (B-ALL/LBL)
Precursor T-neoplasms
    Precursor T lymphoblastic leukemia/lymphoma (T-ALL/LBL)
    Blastic NK-cell leukemia/lymphoma (DC2 leukemia)

Histiocytic and dendritic-cell neoplasms

Histiocytic sarcoma
Langerhans cell histiocytosis/Langerhans cell sarcoma
Interdigitating dendritic cell sarcoma
Follicular dendritic cell sarcoma

Mastocytosis

Cutaneous mastocytosis
Indolent systemic mastocytosis
Systemic mastocytosis with associated clonal hematological disease
Aggressive systemic mastocytosis
Mast cell leukemia
Mast cell sarcoma

CHAPTER 2

Mature B-cell neoplasms

Mature B-cell neoplasms, the most common type of malignant lymphoma, are a clonal proliferation of B-cells. They are classified according to the stage of differentiation, histologic architecture, cell size, clinical data and immunophenotype[40,51,72,75–81,84,88–100]. The common types of mature B-cell neoplasms in adults are diffuse large B-cell lymphoma and follicular lymphoma. Table 2.1 presents the current WHO classification of mature B-cell neoplasms. This classification contains defined clinicopathologic entities and, with the exception of hairy cell leukemia, recapitulates stages of normal B-cell differentiation and maturation.

CHRONIC LYMPHOCYTIC LEUKEMIA/SMALL LYMPHOCYTIC LYMPHOMA (B-CLL/SLL)

B-CLL/SLL is a lymphoproliferative disorder composed of small B-lymphocytes positive for CD5 and CD23 involving the bone marrow/peripheral blood (B-CLL) and/or lymph nodes (B-SLL)[99–109].

B-SLL in the lymph node (Figure 2.1) shows effacement of architecture in a diffuse pattern with a characteristic pseudofollicular pattern (Figure 2.1A) caused by admixture of prolymphocytes and paraimmunoblasts in the background of small lymphocytes (Figure 2.1B)[101,110]. Prolymphocytes are medium-sized cells with prominent central nucleoli. They tend to occur in clusters (proliferation centers), which usually stain more strongly with CD20 than the predominant population of small lymphocytes (Figure 2.1D). Apart from CD20, lymphomatous cells are positive for CD5, CD23 and CD43 (Figure 2.1). Bcl-1 is not expressed. Figure 2.2 shows cytologic features of B-SLL. Lymphocytes are small and round with scanty cytoplasm, dense and clumped chromatin and round nuclei without prominent nucleoli or irregular nuclear

Table 2.1 Classification of mature B-cell neoplasms

Chronic lymphocytic leukemia/small lymphocytic lymphoma (B-CLL/SLL)
B-cell prolymphocytic leukemia (B-PLL)
Lymphoplasmacytic lymphoma
Marginal zone B-cell lymphoma (MZL)
    Splenic marginal zone lymphoma
    Nodal marginal zone lymphoma
    Extranodal marginal zone lymphoma of mucosa-associated lymphoid tissue
Hairy cell leukemia
Plasma cell myeloma/plasmacytoma
Follicular lymphoma (FL)
Mantle cell lymphoma (MCL)
Diffuse large B-cell lymphoma (DLBCL)
Mediastinal (thymic) large B-cell lymphoma
Intravascular large B-cell lymphoma
Primary effusion lymphoma
Burkitt lymphoma/leukemia
B-cell proliferations of uncertain malignant potential
    Lymphomatoid granulomatosis
    Post-transplant lymphoproliferative disorder, polymorphic

borders. Occasional cases of B-SLL show an interfollicular pattern or only partial involvement of the lymph node (Figure 2.3). B-SLL with prominent plasmacytic differentiation (Figure 2.4) may have cytomorphologic overlap with lymphoplasmacytic lymphoma. As in lymphoplasmacytic lymphoma, there is a mixed population of clonal B-cells and clonal plasma cells, but B-SLL differs by the phenotype.

B-SLL/CLL has a characteristic phenotype on flow cytometric evaluation: tumor cells have dim expression of CD20 and surface immunoglobulins and coexpress CD5 and CD23 (Figure 2.5). Table 2.2 presents a summary of phenotypic findings in B-SLL/CLL.

On bone marrow and peripheral blood smears (Figure 2.6), B-CLL cells are small with scanty cytoplasm and clumped chromatin. Occasional smudge cells and prolymphocytes are usually also present. Prolymphocytes

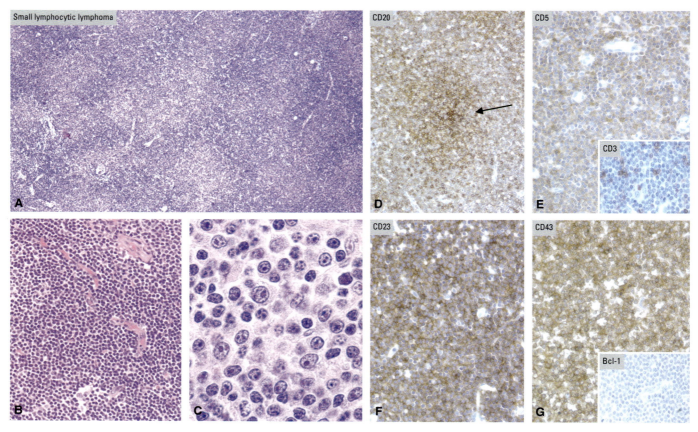

Figure 2.1 B-small lymphocytic lymphoma – histology. (**A**) Low power reveals diffuse lymphoid infiltrate with paler areas (proliferation centers) giving rise to a pseudofollicular pattern. (**B**) Intermediate magnification shows predominance of small lymphocytes. (**C**) Proliferation centers are composed of prolymphocytes with conspicuous nucleoli. The neoplastic cells are typically positive for CD20 (**D**), CD5 (**E**, inset shows negative CD3 staining), CD23 (**F**) and CD43 (**G**, inset shows negative bcl-1 staining). Note that proliferation centers (**D**, arrow) show stronger staining with CD20 than surrounding small lymphocytes

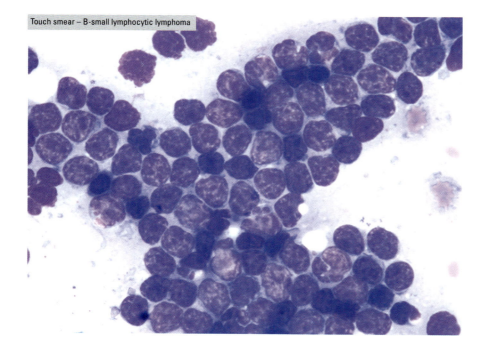

Figure 2.2 B-small lymphocytic lymphoma – cytology (touch smear). The neoplastic lymphocytes are small and round with regular nuclear outlines and compact, darkly stained chromatin

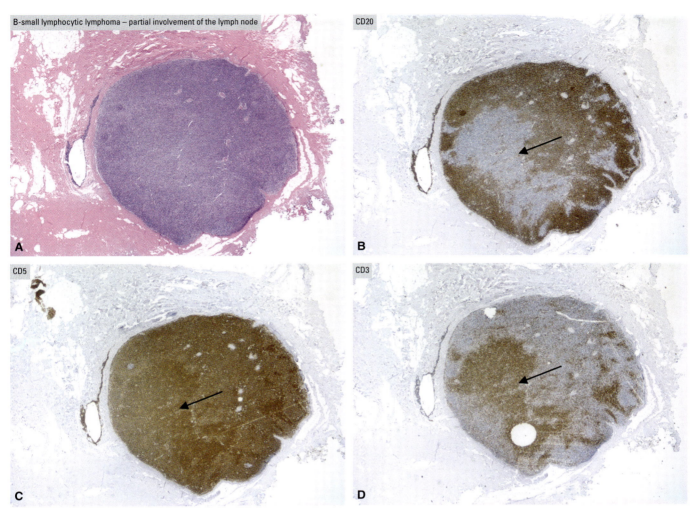

Figure 2.3 B-small lymphocytic lymphoma – partial involvement of the lymph node. The central part of this lymph node (arrow) is not involved by B-SLL: note negative CD20 staining (**B**), positive CD5 (**C**, reactive T-cells are slightly darker than neoplastic B-cells) and CD3 (**D**)

are distinguished from small lymphocytes by their relatively larger size and prominent central nucleoli (Figure 2.7). CLL with > 15% and < 55% prolymphocytes defines B-chronic lymphocytic leukemia/prolymphocytic leukemia (Figure 2.7). B-prolymphocytic leukemia has more than 55% of prolymphocytes. Figure 2.8 presents patterns of bone marrow involvement by B-CLL: nodular (Figure 2.8A and B), interstitial (Figure 2.8C) and diffuse (Figure 2.8D). The pattern of bone marrow involvement correlates with prognosis. Nodular and interstitial patterns are associated with early disease and better prognosis while a diffuse marrow infiltrate is associated with a worse prognosis and advanced disease[109,111,112]. In addition, patients with CD38[+] or ZAP70[+] B-CLL appear to have worse prognosis[35,36,113,114]. The expression of CD38 and ZAP70 in B-CLL is

presented in Figure 1.14 (Chapter 1). Increased numbers of prolymphocytes correlate with a more aggressive disease course and trisomy of chromosome 12[58,111,115,116]. Trisomy 12 (Figure 2.9) is associated with an aggressive clinical course[58,115,117]. Cases with trisomy 12 may present with atypical morphology in the form of prominent nuclear irregularities (Figure 2.10)[58,104,115]. B-CLL with nuclear irregularities, especially indentation of the nuclear membrane (cleaved cells), requires differentiation from mantle cell lymphoma (MCL). Since both disorders may present with aberrant expression of CD23 (e.g., CD23[−] B-CLL or CD23[+] MCL), correlation with bcl-1 or t(11;14) status is required for definite diagnosis.

B-SLL/CLL may undergo transformation into high-grade lymphoma (Richter's syndrome)[47,118–127]. This may take the form of Hodgkin lymphoma (Figure 2.11),

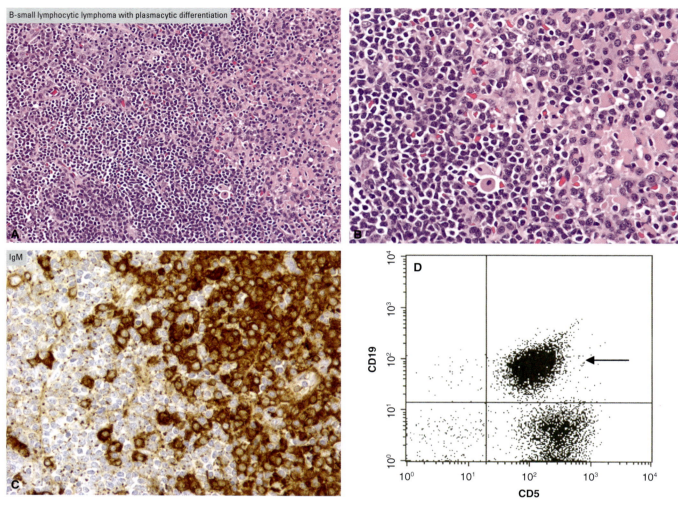

Figure 2.4   B-small lymphocytic lymphoma with plasmacytic differentiation. (**A** and **B**) Low and high power shows a small lymphocytic infiltrate with increased numbers of plasma cells. (**C**) Plasma cells are positive for IgM. (**D**) Flow cytometry of this lymph node reveals coexpression of CD5 by B-cells, which distinguishes this lymphoma from lymphoplasmacytic lymphoma

prolymphocytoid/paraimmunoblastic transformation (Figure 2.12) or diffuse large B-cell lymphoma (Figure 2.13). The cases of CD5+ DLBCL in which patients do not have previous or concomitant evidence of CLL/SLL (or any other low-grade lymphoma) represent *de novo* large B-cell lymphoma, which is distinct from the DLBCL associated with Richter's syndrome[34,121,128].

The differential diagnosis of B-CLL/SLL includes other low-grade B-cell lymphoproliferative disorders (MCL, follicular lymphoma, diffuse follicle center cell lymphoma, marginal zone B-cell lymphoma, and lymphoplasmacytic lymphoma), T-cell lymphomas composed of small cells, lymphocyte-rich and mixed cellularity classic Hodgkin lymphoma, precursor B- and T-lymphoblastic leukemia/lymphoma, and reactive lymphoid infiltrate in extranodal sites. Partial lymph node involvement by B-SLL needs to be distinguished from benign (reactive) processes.

B-CELL PROLYMPHOCYTIC LEUKEMIA

Figure 2.14 presents cytologic and histologic features of B-prolymphocytic leukemia (B-PLL). B-PLL is a *de novo* prolymphocytic neoplasm affecting peripheral blood, bone marrow and spleen in which prolymphocytes exceed 55% of all lymphoid cells in the peripheral blood[78,111]. Patients with a history of B-CLL and more than 55% prolymphocytes in peripheral blood represent disease progression. Only approximately 50% of cases with a history of CLL contain an identical gene rearrangement, meaning that 50% represent a second leukemic clone[120–123,129,130]. Prolymphocytes are medium to large with a moderate amount of cytoplasm, condensed (but more open than in B-CLL) chromatin and prominent central nucleoli. Most *de novo* patients present with marked splenomegaly, but, in contrast to B-SLL/CLL, there is no adenopathy. The differential diagnosis of B-PLL includes splenic marginal zone

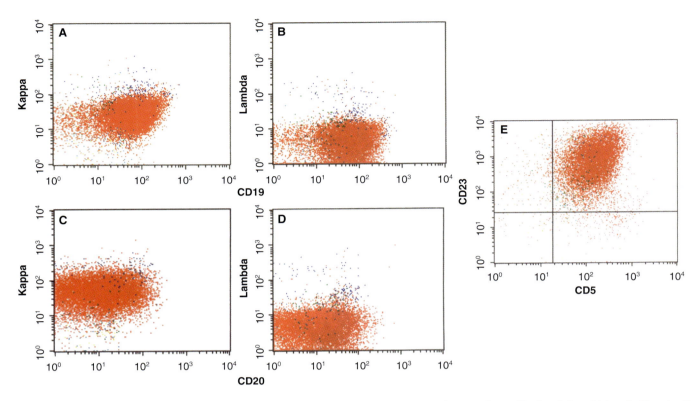

Figure 2.5 B-chronic lymphocytic leukemia – typical flow cytometry immunophenotypic profile (peripheral blood). Neoplastic B-cells show moderate expression of CD19 (**A** and **B**), dim expression of surface immunoglobulins (kappa, **A** and **C**), dim CD20 (**C** and **D**) and coexpression of CD5 with CD23 (**E**)

lymphoma, MCL and B-CLL/PLL. The expression of CD20 and surface immunoglobulins is moderate (not dim, as seen in B-CLL), and a majority of cases are CD23⁻.

LYMPHOPLASMACYTIC LYMPHOMA/ WALDENSTROM MACROGLOBULINEMIA

Lymphoplasmacytic lymphoma is a low-grade lymphoproliferative disorder composed of a spectrum of small lymphocytes, plasmacytoid lymphocytes and plasma cells with a monoclonal serum M-protein (IgM). Waldenstrom macroglobulinemia is a clinical syndrome defined by hyperviscosity and a serum level of IgM above 3 g/dl[82,131–136]. Waldenstrom macroglobulinemia is not synonymous with lymphoplasmacytic lymphoma, since other B-cell lymphomas with plasmacytic differentiation may present with significant serum M-protein (see below)[82,131,132,134–136].

Bone marrow involvement may be diffuse or nodular. Peripheral blood involvement is characterized by a mixture of small lymphocytes, plasmacytoid lymphocytes and plasma cells.

Lymphoplasmacytic lymphoma in lymph nodes (Figure 2.15) shows a diffuse growth pattern of small

Table 2.2 Immunophenotypic profile of B-chronic lymphocytic leukemia

CD5	+
CD10	−
CD11c	+ (dim to moderate)/−
CD19	+ (moderate)
CD20	+ (dim)
CD22	+ (dim)
CD23	+/rare cases −
CD25	+/−
CD30	−
CD38	+/−
CD43	+
CD45	+
CD103	−
CD138	−
Bcl-1	−
Bcl-2	+
Bcl-6	−
BOB-1	+
Light-chain Ig (kappa/lambda)	+ (dim expression)
OCT-2	+
Pax-5	+

lymphocytes, plasmacytoid lymphocytes and plasma cells. The latter often contain prominent intranuclear inclusions (Dutcher bodies), which are PAS⁺ (Figure 2.15C). Lymphoid cells are positive for CD19, CD20, CD22 and Pax-5, whereas plasma cells are usually negative for B-cell

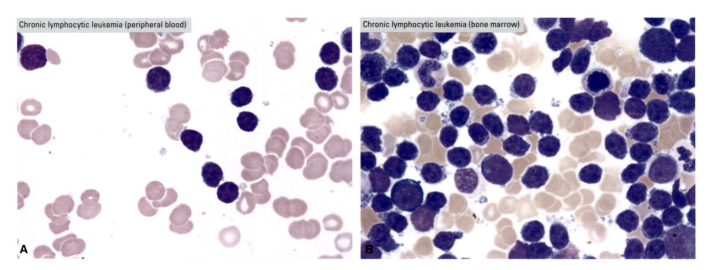

Figure 2.6 B-chronic lymphocytic leukemia – cytology. Peripheral blood (**A**) and bone marrow aspirate (**B**) with marked lymphocytosis of small lymphocytes with scanty cytoplasm and small nuclei with dense, clumped nuclear chromatin

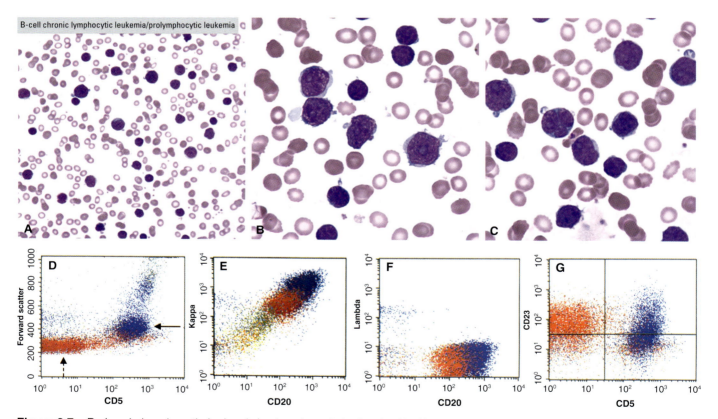

Figure 2.7 B-chronic lymphocytic leukemia/prolymphocytic leukemia. (**A–C**) Peripheral blood smear with lymphocytosis. There is a mixed population of small lymphocytes with dense chromatin and larger cells with prominent nucleoli (prolymphocytes). (**D–G**) Flow cytometry analysis shows two distinct B-cell populations: small cells with low forward scatter (**D**, red dots marked with dotted arrow) and larger cells with higher forward scatter (**D**, blue dots marked with arrow). Larger cells have brighter expression of surface immunoglobulin (**E**), moderate CD20 (**E**, **F**) and only a subset of cells coexpressing CD5 (**D**, **G**). CD23 is positive on both CD5+ and CD5– cells (**G**)

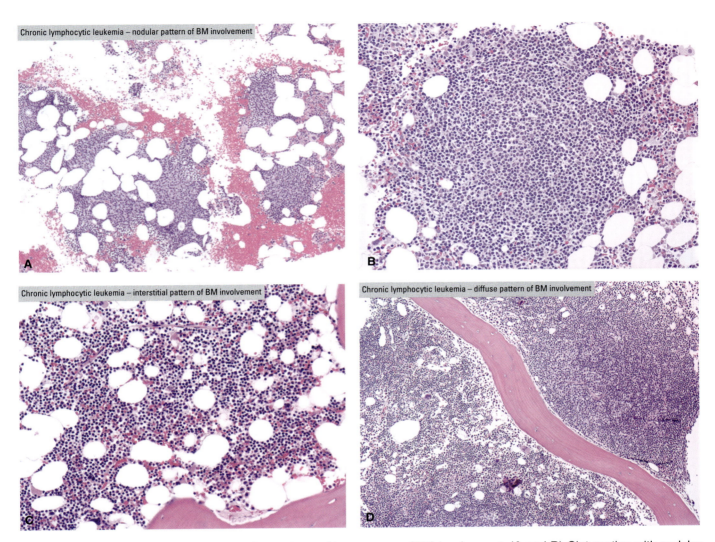

Chronic lymphocytic leukemia – nodular pattern of BM involvement

Chronic lymphocytic leukemia – interstitial pattern of BM involvement

Chronic lymphocytic leukemia – diffuse pattern of BM involvement

Figure 2.8 B-chronic lymphocytic leukemia – pattern of bone marrow (BM) involvement. (**A** and **B**) Clot section with nodular involvement of the bone marrow. Higher magnification (**B**) shows ill-defined lymphoid aggregate composed of mature-appearing lymphocytes. (**C**) Interstitial bone marrow infiltrate. (**D**) Core biopsy with diffuse lymphoid infiltrate

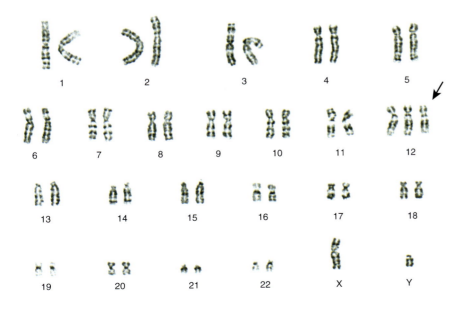

Figure 2.9 Trisomy 12 (arrow) in B-chronic lymphocytic leukemia (cytogenetic studies)

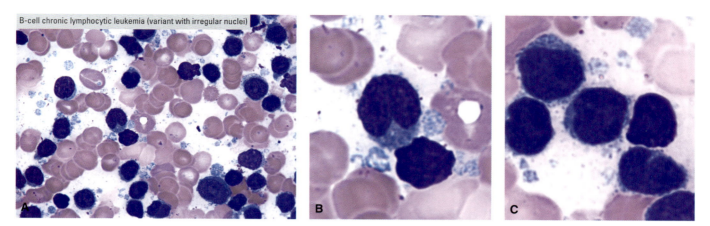

Figure 2.10   B-chronic lymphocytic leukemia with atypical cytologic features (**A**, intermediate magnification; **B–C**, high magnification). Most of the nuclei have irregular (cleaved) nuclear outlines. The phenotype and cytogenetic/molecular studies are similar to classic type of B-CLL (i.e., bcl-1 is negative)

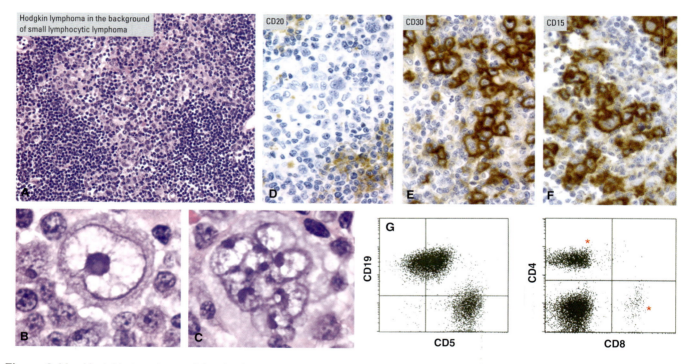

Figure 2.11   Hodgkin lymphoma (classical) in the background of B-small lymphocytic lymphoma. This may be considered a Richter's (large cell transformation) variant. (**A**) Low power shows a diffuse small lymphocytic infiltrate with scattered large atypical cells. (**B** and **C**) High power shows typical Hodgkin cells and multilobated large cells with macronucleoli (Reed–Sternberg cells). Hodgkin component is negative for CD20 (**D**) and positive for CD30 (**E**) and CD15 (**F**). (**G**) Flow cytometry reveals neoplastic B-cells coexpressing CD5 and benign T-cells with predominance of CD4+ cells

markers (except BOB-1 and OCT-2). IgM is positive in plasma cells (strong) and in B-cells (weak). Plasma cells are positive for CD38, CD138 and often bcl-1.

Bone marrow involvement by lymphoplasmacytic lymphoma is usually diffuse (Figure 2.16), but may be nodular as well. Bone marrow aspirate shows lymphocytes, plasmacytoid lymphocytes and plasma cells with Dutcher bodies (Figure 2.17). The lymphocytes range from small cells with scanty cytoplasm to plasmacytoid lymphocytes with abundant cytoplasm and eccentric nuclei.

The most common cytogenetic abnormality is translocation t(9;14). Figure 2.18 shows complex karyotypic changes including t(9;14). Abnormal/complex cytogenetic findings in lymphoplasmacytic lymphoma are associated

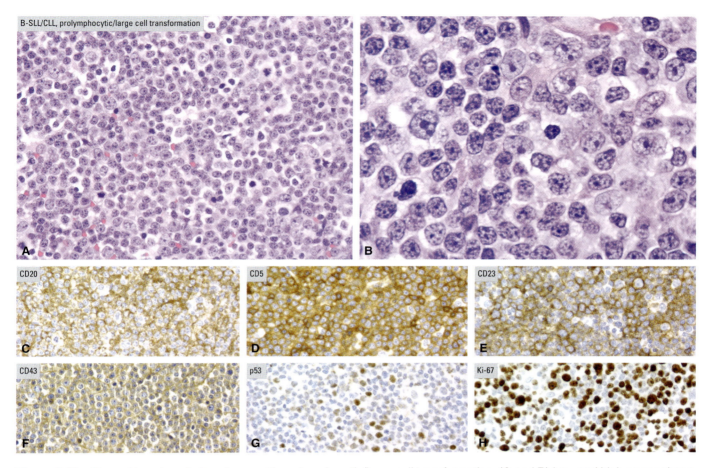

Figure 2.12 B-small lymphocytic lymphoma with prolymphocytic/large cell transformation. (**A** and **B**) Low and high power shows a diffuse lymphoid infiltrate composed of medium to large cells with occasionally prominent nucleoli. The neoplastic cells are positive for CD20 (**C**), CD5 (**D**), CD23 (**E**), and CD43 (**G**), as in typical B-SLL. A subset of cells is positive for p53 (**G**). (**H**) In contrast to B-SLL, the fraction of proliferating cells (as determined by Ki-67/MIB-1 staining) is very high

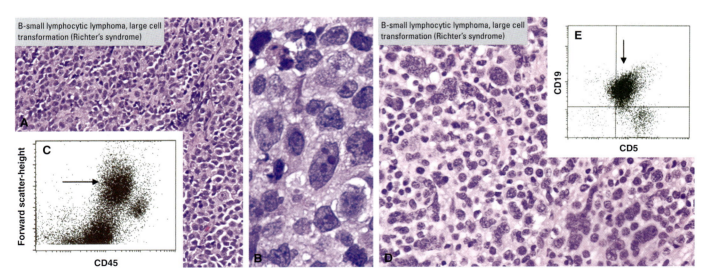

Figure 2.13 Richter syndrome. Two cases of large cell transformation (Richter's syndrome) of B-SLL/CLL. (**A**) Histologic section shows diffuse large cell infiltrate. (**B**) High magnification shows large lymphocytes with several nucleoli. (**C**) Flow cytometry revealed predominance of lymphoid cells with increased forward scatter (FS, arrow) indicating large size. Normal (small) lymphocytes with bright CD45 have lower FS. (**D**) Lymph node with highly pleomorphic lymphoid infiltrate which still displays coexpression of CD19 and CD5 by flow cytometric analysis (**E**)

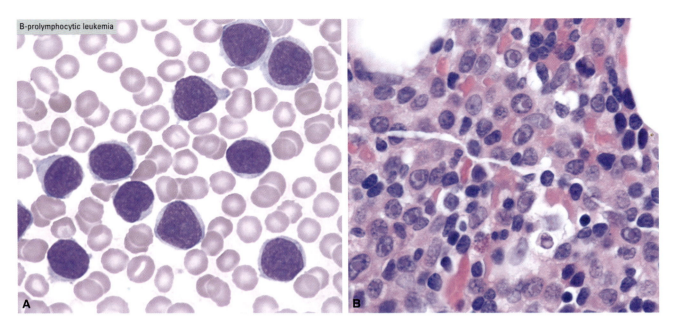

Figure 2.14   B-prolymphocytic leukemia. (**A**) Peripheral blood smear shows typical cytologic features of B-PLL with prominent nucleoli. (**B**) Bone marrow involvement. Lymphoid cells with prominent nucleoli

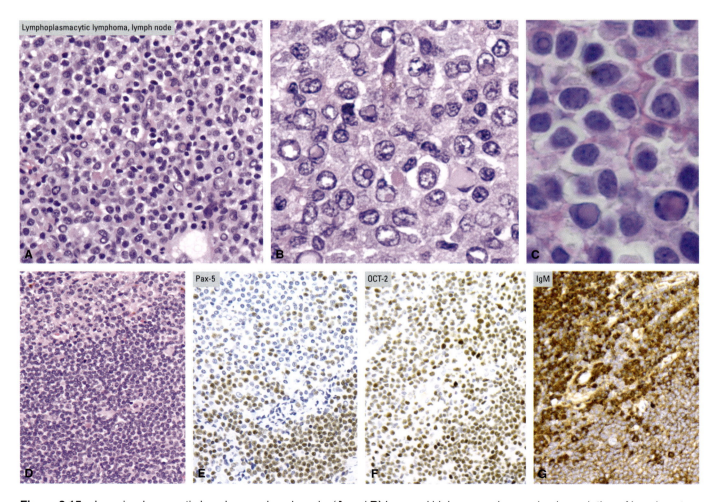

Figure 2.15   Lymphoplasmacytic lymphoma – lymph node. (**A** and **B**) Low and high power shows mixed population of lymphocytes, plasmacytoid lymphocytes and plasma cells with numerous Dutcher bodies. Dutcher bodies are PAS$^+$ (**C**). Plasma cell component (**D**, upper part) is negative for Pax-5 (**E**), is positive for OCT-2 (**F**) and displays strong staining with IgM (**G**). Lymphoid component (**C**, lower portion) is Pax-5 positive (**E**)

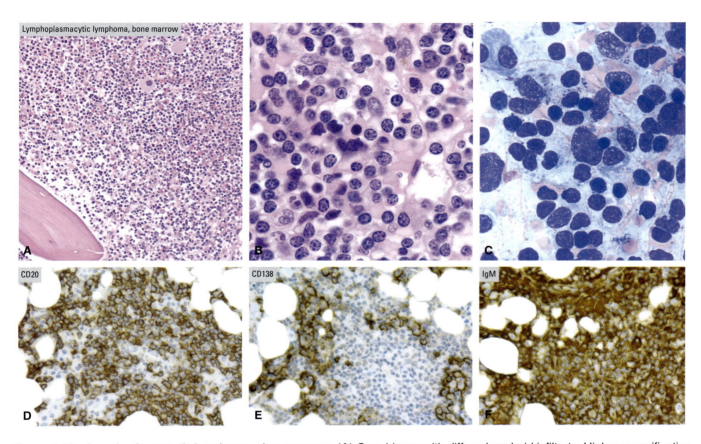

Figure 2.16   Lymphoplasmacytic lymphoma – bone marrow. (**A**) Core biopsy with diffuse lymphoid infiltrate. Higher magnification (**B**) and bone marrow aspirate (**C**) show mixed population of lymphocytes and plasma cells. Lymphocytes are positive for CD20 (**D**) and are negative for CD138 (**E**). Plasma cells display reverse immunoreactivity. Both lymphocytes and plasma cells are positive for IgM (**F**)

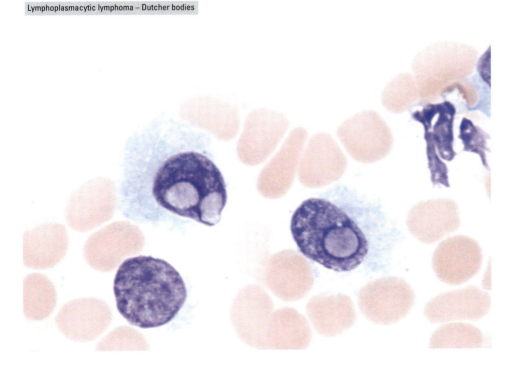

Figure 2.17   Lymphoplasmacytic lymphoma. Prominent intranuclear inclusions (Dutcher bodies)

Lymphoplasmacytic lymphoma with complex chromosomal abnormalities: +3, del(7)(q22q34), del(14)(q32), t(9;14)

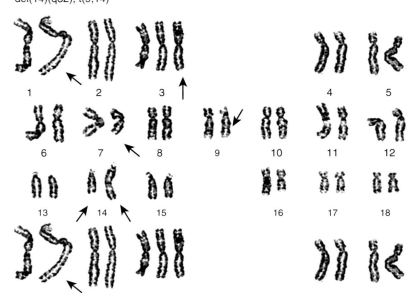

Figure 2.18 Lymphoplasmacytic lymphoma – cytogenetics. Complex chromosomal abnormalities, including +3, del(7), del(14), and t(9;14), are present (arrows)

with poor prognosis. An example of a flow cytometry immunophenotype (Figure 2.19) shows two distinct clonal populations. B-cells have moderate to bright expression of surface immunoglobulin (Figure 2.19C and D) and dim to moderate expression of cytoplasmic IgM (Figure 2.19F). They do not express CD5, CD10, CD23 and CD38. The plasma cell population is usually smaller and is negative for surface immunoglobulins, brightly positive for cytoplasmic immunoglobulins (of the same isotype as B-cells; Figure 2.19C–H) and positive for CD38/CD138.

Rare cases of lymphoplasmacytic lymphoma (and plasma cell myeloma) may be associated with crystal-storing histiocytosis (Figure 2.20). The intracellular crystal formation is almost always accompanied by the expression of kappa light chains[137–139]. Patients usually present with marked paraproteinemia and symptoms of hyperviscosity. Lymphoplasmacytic lymphoma is a low-grade B-cell malignancy[133], but the overall prognosis may be worse than for other types of small B-cell lymphomas[131,140].

The differential diagnosis of lymphoplasmacytic lymphoma includes other B-cell lymphomas with plasmacytic differentiation, mainly, marginal zone B-cell lymphoma and B-chronic lymphocytic leukemia/small lymphocytic lymphoma[1,78,91,134,141–143]. Other B-cell lymphomas, such as follicular lymphoma and diffuse large B-cell lymphoma, only rarely display plasmacytic differentiation. Patients with splenic marginal zone lymphoma may have a serum monoclonal IgM spike, but in much smaller titers than in lymphoplasmacytic lymphoma. The immunophenotype helps to distinguish this entity from B-CLL/SLL. Crystal-storing histiocytosis has to be distinguished from plasma cell neoplasms, granular cell tumor and other lesions, (pseudo-) Gaucher cells, and rhabdomyoblasts.

MARGINAL ZONE B-CELL LYMPHOMA (MZL)

The rubric of MZL encompasses splenic marginal zone lymphoma, nodal marginal zone lymphoma, and MALT lymphoma, each of which is discussed below.

Splenic marginal zone B-cell lymphoma

Splenic marginal zone lymphoma (SMZL) is a low-grade B-cell neoplasm involving the spleen, and may have involvement of the splenic hilar lymph node(s), bone marrow and peripheral blood[141,142,144–158]. Involvement of hilar splenic lymph nodes may be observed, but peripheral adenopathy is uncommon[148]. A subset of patients may have a small monoclonal serum M-protein, but marked hyperviscosity and hypergammaglobulinemia are uncommon[141,153,154]. Progression to large B-cell lymphoma is rare[144].

SMZL involves the white pulp of the spleen (Figure 2.21A–C) and usually has spillover into the red pulp. Prominent nodules of white pulp are composed of residual germinal centers colonized by small lymphomatous cells and an expanded pale marginal zone with characteristic abundant pale cytoplasm. There is no clear demarcation between the mantle and marginal zones as seen in benign splenic follicle (Figure 2.21D). Circulating cells in peripheral blood often present as villous lymphocytes (Figure 2.22). In the bone marrow, the most common

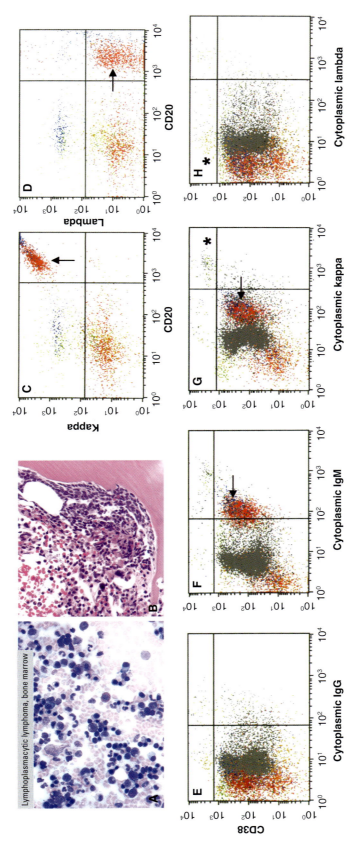

Figure 2.19 Lymphoplasmacytic lymphoma – flow cytometry. Lymphoplasmacytic lymphoma (**A**, aspirate; **B**, core biopsy) when analyzed by flow cytometry (**C–H**) shows clonal B-cells and plasma cells. B-cells (arrow) display strong expression of surface immunoglobulins (kappa, **C** and **D**) and dim to moderate expression of cytoplasmic IgM (**F**). Plasma cells (*) are relatively rare. They have bright expression of cytoplasmic IgM (**F**, compare with cytoplasmic IgG on **E**) and bright cytoplasmic kappa (**G**, compare with cytoplasmic lambda on **H**)

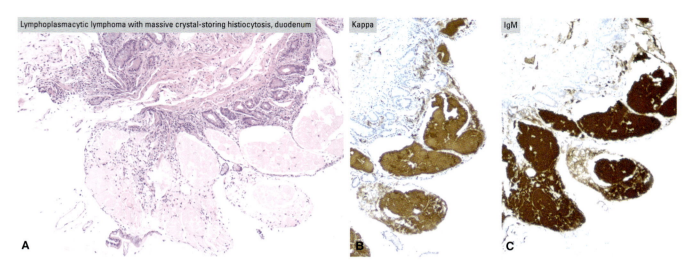

Figure 2.20 Crystal-storing histiocytosis associated with lymphoplasmacytic lymphoma – duodenum. (**A**) Histologic section shows amorphous material within cystic-like spaces. Plasma cells express kappa immunoglobulins (**B**). The amorphous material is strongly positive for IgM (**C**)

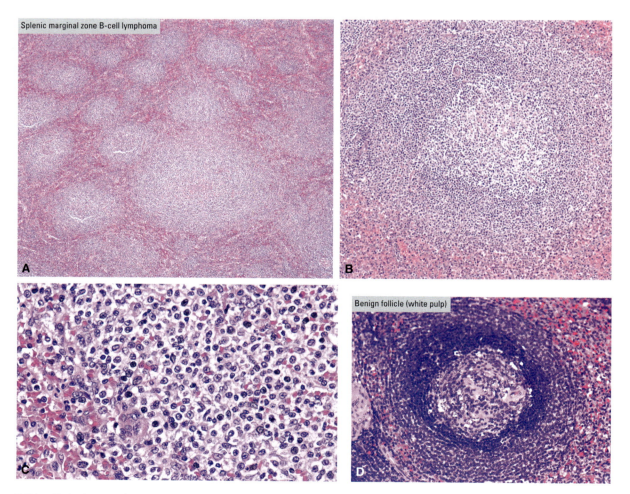

Figure 2.21 Splenic marginal zone B-cell lymphoma. (**A**) Low magnification shows expansion of the white pulp. (**B**) Higher magnification of the nodule shows a residual germinal center surrounded by small lymphocytes merging at the periphery with slightly larger cells with pale cytoplasm. (**C**) High magnification shows monocytoid features. (**D**) Benign follicle in the spleen. Note germinal center with mild sclerosis surrounded by well-demarcated mantle and marginal zones

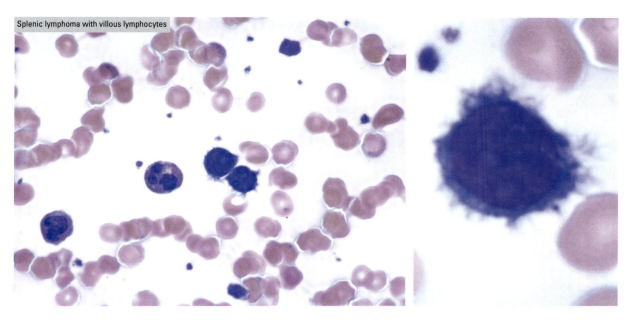

Splenic lymphoma with villous lymphocytes

Figure 2.22   Splenic lymphoma with villous lymphocytes – peripheral blood. Small to medium-sized lymphocytes with bipolar irregular cytoplasmic borders

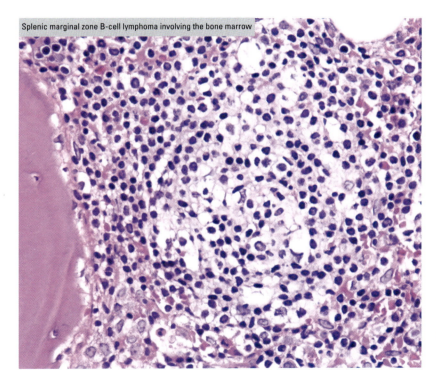

Splenic marginal zone B-cell lymphoma involving the bone marrow

Figure 2.23   Splenic marginal zone B-cell lymphoma – bone marrow. Interstitial lymphoid aggregate in the bone marrow is composed of small to medium-sized lymphocytes with pale cytoplasm

pattern of involvement is that of a nodular interstitial lymphoid infiltrate composed of small to medium-sized lymphocytes with pale cytoplasm (Figure 2.23).

The differential diagnosis includes other low-grade B-cell lymphoproliferative disorders composed of small cells, such as B-CLL/SLL, MCL, and follicular lymphoma[1,141,156,159–162]. Hairy cell leukemia (HCL) does not display a nodular pattern of splenic involvement and therefore can be easily excluded on a morphologic basis. T-cell lymphoproliferative disorders, such as T-cell prolymphocytic leukemia (T-PLL), may have dense red pulp infiltration.

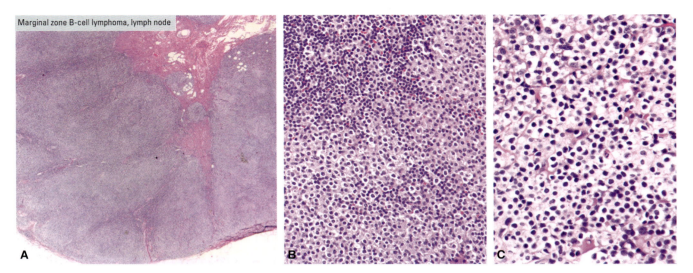

Figure 2.24   Nodal marginal zone B-cell lymphoma. (**A**) Low power of the lymph node shows vague nodularity. (**B** and **C**) Intermediate and high magnification shows atypical lymphocytes with pale, clear cytoplasm, and irregular nuclei

Nodal marginal zone B-cell lymphoma

Nodal marginal zone B-cell lymphoma is a primary B-cell lymphoma of the lymph node[141,163–168]. By definition, there is no evidence of involvement of the spleen or other extranodal sites, such as gastrointestinal tract, skin, lung, salivary gland or ocular adnexae. Nodal involvement by MZL has either a diffuse or vaguely nodular pattern (Figure 2.24). Residual germinal centers are usually preserved, but are disrupted. The lymphoid cells are small to medium in size with scattered large B-cells with prominent nucleoli (immunoblast-like). In many cases, B-cells have a monocytoid appearance (Figure 2.24C) with abundant pale or eosinophilic cytoplasm.

Phenotypically, MZL has a non-specific phenotype without expression of CD5, CD10 and CD103. Often, there is dim to moderate expression of CD11c (Figure 2.25). CD25 may be positive. Some cases display aberrant coexpression of CD43, a useful criterion in identifying neoplastic processes. Immunohistochemical evaluation of the lymph node shows disruption of the follicular dendritic cell meshwork (CD21 and CD23 staining, Figure 2.26B and C) caused by follicle colonization as well as lack of CD5 and CD10 expression. Plasma cells are often monotypic (Figure 2.26F). Occasional cases of MZL show an extensive plasmacytic differentiation (Figure 2.27). Figure 2.28 compares the follicular dendritic cell (FDC) meshwork in a normal lymph node, MCL, marginal zone lymphoma and follicular lymphoma. Note the prominent, asymmetrical disruption of the FDC in MZL.

The differential diagnosis of nodal MZL lymphoma includes a reactive lymph node with monocytoid B-cell hyperplasia (Figure 2.29A), mantle zone hyperplasia (Figure 2.29B), follicular lymphoma, especially with a reversed pattern (Figure 2.29C), low-grade B-cell lymphomas, such as lymphoplasmacytic lymphoma, and other lymphoproliferations with increased number of monocytoid B-cells (e.g., unusual case of classical Hodgkin lymphoma with clusters of monocytoid B-cells; Figure 2.29D).

Extranodal marginal zone B-cell lymphoma of mucosa-associated lymphoid tissue (MALT lymphoma)

The gastrointestinal tract is most often involved by MZL of MALT-type, followed by lung, salivary gland, thyroid, ocular adnexae, skin, breast and other locations[92,127,141,162, 169–181]. In the stomach, the most common site of MALT in the USA, lymphomagenesis is associated with antigenic drive due to *Helicobacter pylori* infection[177,182–190]. Gastric MALT lymphoma may be associated with t(11;18). MALT lymphomas without t(11;18), which may have numerous allelic imbalances, similar to those of diffuse large B-cell lymphoma, are more likely to transform into high-grade DLBCL than tumors with t(11;18)[191–193]. Gastric MALT shows an expansion of the mucosa and submucosa by a diffuse infiltrate of B-lymphocytes (Figure 2.30A and B). Small to medium-sized cells predominate (Figure 2.30C), but there is a variable proportion of large lymphocytes. Many cases have a typical monocytoid appearance with abundant clear cytoplasm. There is often plasmacytic differentiation subjacent to the surface epithelium, which may or may

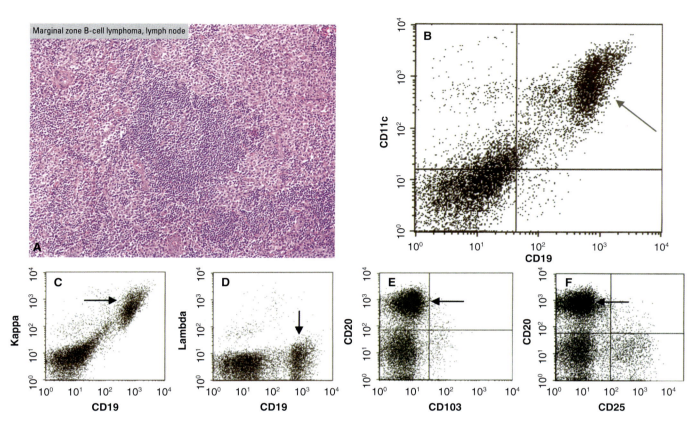

Figure 2.25 Nodal marginal zone B-cell lymphoma – flow cytometry. (**A**) Histology of the lymph node shows a residual germinal center surrounded by small lymphocytic infiltrate with plasma cells. Neoplastic B-cells are positive for CD11c (**B**) and kappa immunoglobulins (**C**, **D**), and are negative for CD103 (**E**) and CD25 (**F**)

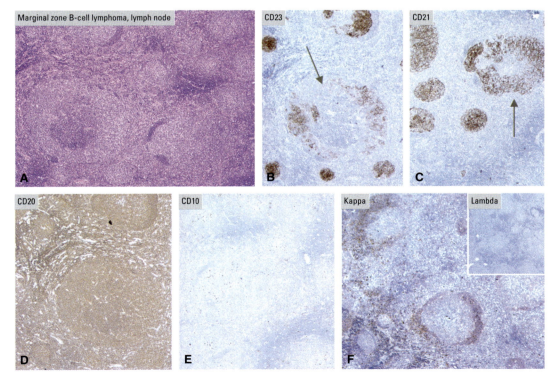

Figure 2.26 Nodal marginal zone B-cell lymphoma – immunohistochemistry. (**A**) Typical histologic pattern of marginal zone lymphoma. (**B** and **C**) Expanded and disrupted follicular dendritic cell meshwork visualized by staining with CD23 (**B**) and CD21 (**C**). Neoplastic and non-neoplastic B-cells are positive for CD20 (**D**), negative for CD10 (**E**) and show plasmacytic differentiation with kappa restriction (**F**)

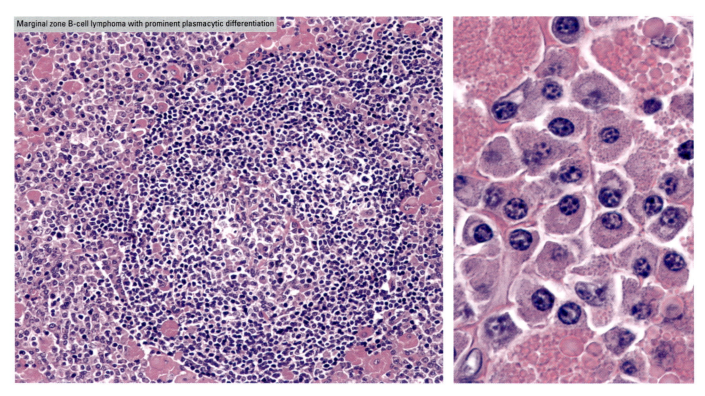

Figure 2.27   Marginal zone B-cell lymphoma with prominent plasmacytic differentiation (low and high magnification)

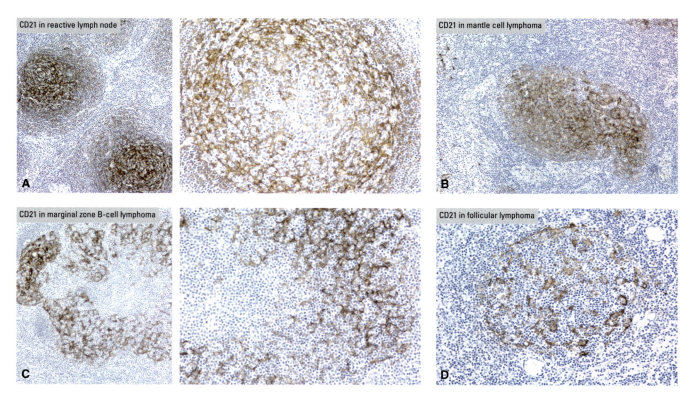

Figure 2.28   The pattern of CD21 immunohistochemical staining in a reactive lymph node (**A**), mantle cell lymphoma (**B**), marginal zone lymphoma (**C**) and follicular lymphoma (**D**). Colonization of follicles by neoplastic B-cells in marginal zone lymphoma causes disruption of follicular dendritic cells (**C**)

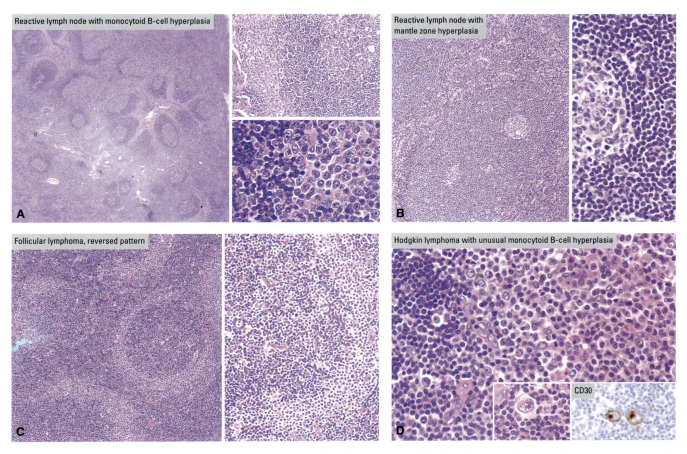

Figure 2.29 Differential diagnosis of nodal marginal zone B-cell lymphoma. (**A**) Reactive lymph node with prominent germinal centers and foci of monocytoid B-cells. (**B**) Reactive lymph node with mantle zone hyperplasia. (**C**) Follicular lymphoma with reversed pattern. (**D**) Classical Hodgkin lymphoma with unusual large foci of monocytoid B-cells mimicking marginal zone lymphoma (inset, higher magnification shows large cells which are positive for CD30)

not be monotypic. A subset of cases shows coexpression of CD43 by CD20+ B-cells (Figure 2.30D–F; compare with CD5 staining). Reactive and/or residual follicles are often present and may show a colonization by lymphomatous cells with disruption of follicular dendritic cell meshwork (Figure 2.30G–I). Infiltration and destruction of the glandular structures by neoplastic lymphocytes with formation of lymphoepithelial lesions (Figure 2.31) is characteristically identified, and this may be better visualized with an anticytokeratin immunohistochemical stain (Figure 2.31D). The presence of lymphoepithelial lesions is a diagnostic criterion chiefly in the stomach and the salivary gland; in other extranodal locations, it is not significant. Differential diagnosis of gastric MALT lymphoma includes reactive processes such as chemical gastropathy, chronic active gastritis associated with *H. pylori* infection (Figure 2.32), low-grade B-cell lymphomas and T-cell lymphomas[194–196]. Differential diagnosis of MALT lymphoma in small and large intestine include reactive

processes, such as inflammatory bowel disease and low-grade lymphoproliferative disorders[197]. Reactive processes differ by showing more prominent germinal centers with well-preserved mantle/marginal zones, well-defined separation of follicles, lack of lymphoepithelial lesions, lack of B-cells spillover from the follicles, lack of aberrant expression of CD43 by B-cells, lack of monotypic plasma cells, and lack of monocytoid appearance and cytologic atypia.

Figures 2.33 and 2.34 show MZL of MALT-type in large intestine and salivary gland, respectively. There is prominent monocytoid appearance of neoplastic B-cells, which infiltrate epithelial elements.

MALT lymphomas are indolent and often regress with treatment, which includes among others, antibiotics (gastric MALT) and local treatment with radiation. Rare cases may undergo transformation to large cell lymphoma. The presence of t(11;18) in gastric MALT predicts autonomous behavior and lack of the response

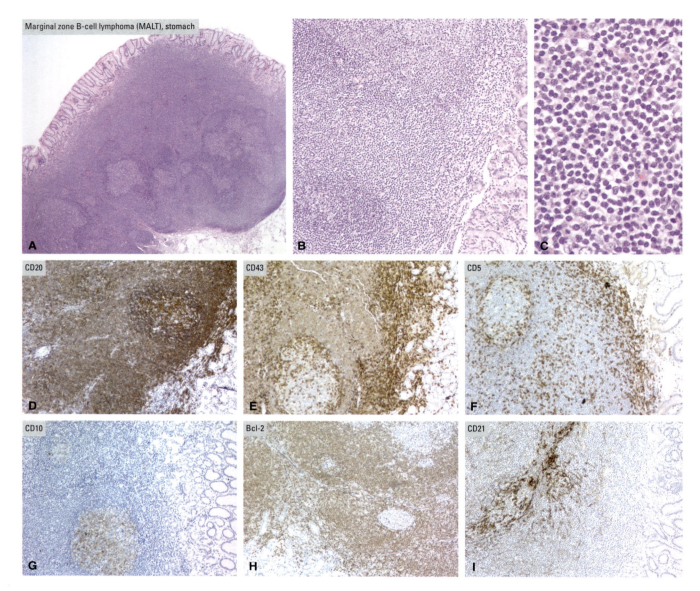

Figure 2.30 Gastric marginal zone B-cell lymphoma (MALT lymphoma). (**A**) Low magnification shows prominent lymphoid infiltrate with tumor cells surrounding reactive follicles. (**B** and **C**) Higher magnifications show monotonous lymphoid cells with pale cytoplasm. Neoplastic B-cells are positive for CD20 (**D**) and show aberrant expression of CD43 (**E**). The expression of CD43 is dimmer than in residual small T-cells (compare with CD5 staining, **F**). Residual (benign) germinal centers are positive for CD10 (**G**) and negative for bcl-2 (**H**). Follicular dendritic cell meshwork is distorted (CD21 staining, **I**)

to *H. Pylori* eradication therapy. Figure 2.35 shows a marginal zone lymphoma in the lung, which 1 year later transformed into diffuse large B-cell lymphoma (PCR tests revealed a clonal peak at the same location, which confirmed clonal evolution rather than secondary malignancy).

HAIRY CELL LEUKEMIA (HCL)

HCL is a B-cell lymphoproliferative disorder composed of small lymphocytes with characteristic hairy-like

cytoplasmic protrusions (Figure 2.36), bright expression of CD11c and CD20, and positive expression of CD103[198–203]. Neoplastic B-cells are medium-sized with pale cytoplasm, oval and often reniform or bean-shaped nuclei, and clumped or evenly dispersed chromatin. In the bone marrow (Figure 2.37), the leukemic infiltrate is always diffuse without aggregates and may be inconspicuous due to small, widely spaced lymphoid cells with pale cytoplasm. Immunohistochemical staining with CD20 helps to identify the extent of the disease. The infiltrate may be patchy with typical 'streaming' on low magnification

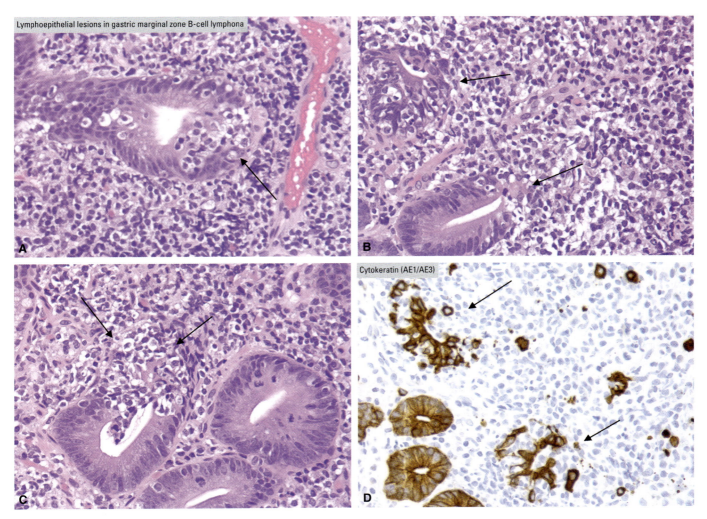

Figure 2.31 Gastric marginal zone B-cell lymphoma (MALT lymphoma) with prominent lymphoepithelial lesions (**A–C**). The lymphoepithelial lesions can be easily identified by immunohistochemical staining for cytokeratin (arrows) (**D**)

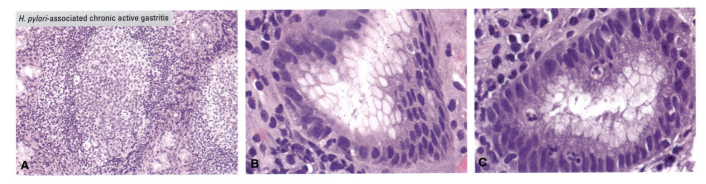

Figure 2.32 Chronic active ('follicular') gastritis. (**A**) Prominent reactive follicles with well-preserved mantle and marginal zones. (**B**) Numerous *H. pylori*-like structures are present. (**C**) In contrast to MALT lymphoma, no lymphoepithelial lesions are present

(Figure 2.37). Higher power shows lymphoid cells with irregular nuclei (Figure 2.37C) and abundant cytoplasm. There is variable reticulin fibrosis.

Flow cytometry (Figure 2.38) shows increased side scatter, placing leukemic cells in the 'monocytic' region (Figure 2.38A), bright expression of CD20 and surface immunoglobulins (Figure 2.38C and D), bright expression of CD11c (Figure 2.38E) and coexpression of CD25 with CD103 (Figure 2.38G and H). Table 2.3 presents phenotypic findings in HCL.

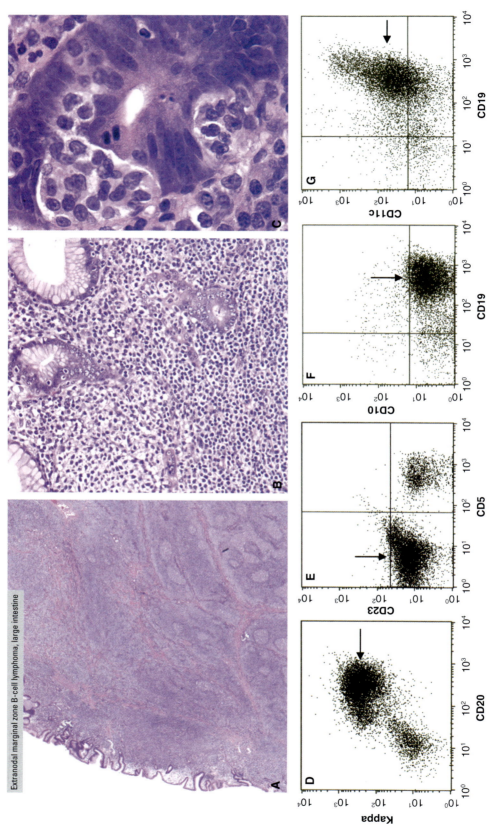

Figure 2.33 Extranodal marginal zone B-cell lymphoma (MALT lymphoma) – large intestine. (**A**) Prominent lymphoid infiltrate with follicles. (**B**) Atypical lymphoid cells with clear cytoplasm predominate. (**C**) Lymphoepithelial lesions are easily identified. (**D–G**) Flow cytometry analysis revealed clonal kappa⁺ B-cells (**D**, **E**) which lack CD10 (**F**) and coexpress CD11c (**G**)

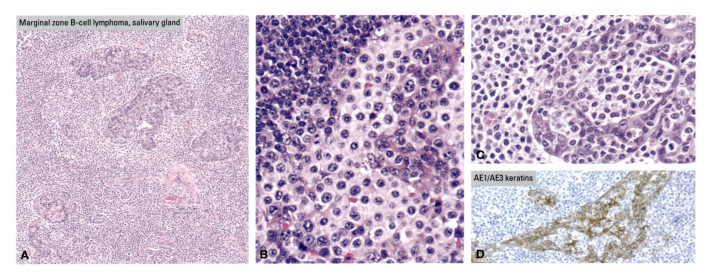

Figure 2.34 Extranodal marginal zone B-cell lymphoma – salivary gland. (**A**) Low magnification shows a prominent lymphoid infiltrate and lymphoepithelial islands. (**B**) Higher magnification shows neoplastic B-cells with abundant eosinophilic cytoplasm. (**C**) Prominent lymphoepithelial lesions are present, highlighted by anti-cytokeratin stain (**D**)

Figure 2.39 shows an electron photomicrograph of HCL with typical ribosome–lamellar complexes.

HCL involves predominantly the bone marrow and spleen, and presents with leukopenia and mono-cytopenia[199]. Lymph node infiltration may occur[204] (Figure 2.40) and is predominantly paracortical with sparing of follicles. Other locations may include skin and liver[198–203]. Immunohistochemistry (Figure 2.40D–H) shows the expression of B-cell markers, CD25 and DBA44. Bcl-1 (cyclin D1) is often positive. In the spleen (Figure 2.41), the leukemic cells involve the red pulp with inconspicuous (atrophic) white pulp. Collections of pooled red cells in the form of blood lakes are typical for HCL splenic involvement.

Variants of HCL[198,201,203,205,206] include the CD25-negative form, HCL with blastoid appearance (Figure 2.42A and B) and HCL with irregular nuclear contours (Figure 2.42C) or spindle cells. Since the phenotype, clinical presentation, prognosis and response to treatment in patients with CD25⁻ HCL differs from classical HCL, the former may represent a variant of marginal zone lymphoma[203].

The differential diagnosis of HCL includes other lymphoproliferative disorders composed of small to medium-sized lymphocytes especially when associated with splenomegaly, such as splenic lymphoma with villous lymphocytes, B-CLL/SLL, B-cell prolymphocytic leukemia, T-cell prolymphocytic leukemia, and other T-cell disorders with involvement of spleen.

PLASMA CELL NEOPLASMS

Plasma cell myeloma is a multifocal clonal plasma cell proliferation infiltrating the bone marrow[207–212], characterized by lytic bone lesions (Figures 2.43–2.45) and serum monoclonal protein (M-protein; Figure 2.46). Neoplastic transformation in plasma cell myeloma most likely originates in immunoglobulin heavy chain (IgH) switch recombinations, resulting in the translocation of oncogenes (e.g., *BCL-1/PRAD-1*/cyclin D1) to the IgH locus on 14q32[213–219]. The clinical features vary from indolent (smoldering) to aggressive disseminated disease with leukemic blood involvement[2,207–212,219–221]. The extent of the bone marrow involvement correlates with clinical presentation. Apart from local symptoms related to direct bone destruction by tumor cells, patients may present with anemia, hypercalcemia, infections and renal insufficiency. Monoclonal gammopathy of undetermined significance (MGUS) is defined by the presence of a monoclonal (M-) protein without fulfilling diagnostic criteria for plasma cell myeloma, Waldenstrom macroglobulinemia or primary amyloidosis. Approximately 25% of patients with MGUS develop plasma cell myeloma or other lymphoproliferative disorders after follow-up for more than 20 years[2,57,78,222]. Plasmacytoma is a clonal plasma cell proliferation with localized osseous or extraskeletal presentation (solitary plasmacytoma of bone and extraosseous plasmacytoma)[223]. Cytologic and immunophenotypic features are similar to plasma cell myeloma.

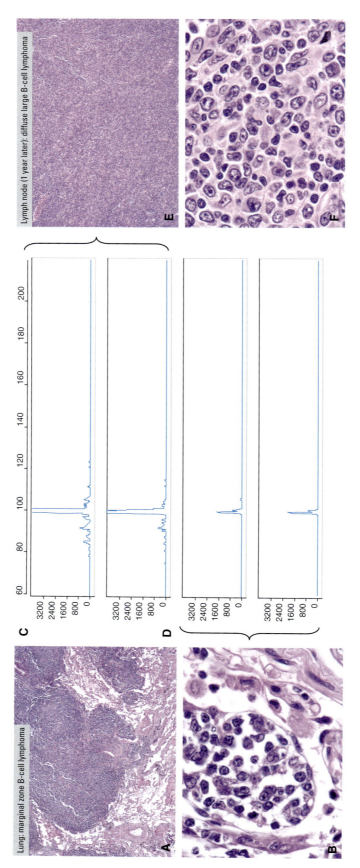

Figure 2.35   Extranodal marginal zone B-cell lymphoma involving lung (**A**, **B**) with transformation into large B-cell lymphoma 1 year later (**E**, **F**). Molecular analysis confirmed a clonal IgH gene rearrangement, which is identical in both the primary pulmonary low-grade lymphoma and transformed nodal large cell lymphoma (**C**, **D**)

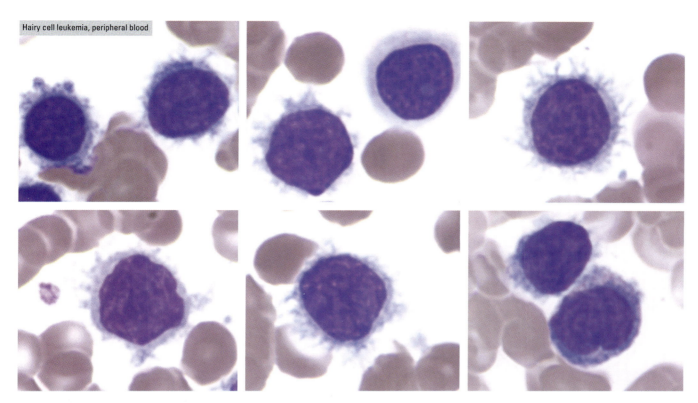

Hairy cell leukemia, peripheral blood

Figure 2.36 Hairy cell leukemia – cytology

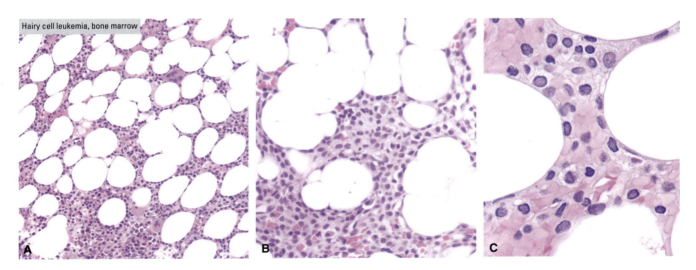

Hairy cell leukemia, bone marrow

Figure 2.37 Hairy cell leukemia – histology (bone marrow). Subtle interstitial lymphoid infiltrate of hairy cells

The diagnosis and subclassification of the various plasma cell dyscrasias depends on correlation of radiologic imaging data (bone lesions) and laboratory data (M-protein type and amount) with morphologic, cytogenetic and phenotypic findings[2,57,135,207,209–211,213,214,219,221,224]. Cytologic features of plasma cell myeloma vary from mature forms resembling benign plasma cells to highly anaplastic cells. Mature plasma cells (Figure 2.47) are round or oval with abundant basophilic cytoplasm, perinuclear cytoplasmic clearing and an eccentric nucleus. Binucleation is common. On histologic examination, plasma cells may occur in clusters, sheets or as a diffuse interstitial infiltrate replacing normal marrow elements (Figure 2.48). Some cases show prominent cytoplasmic

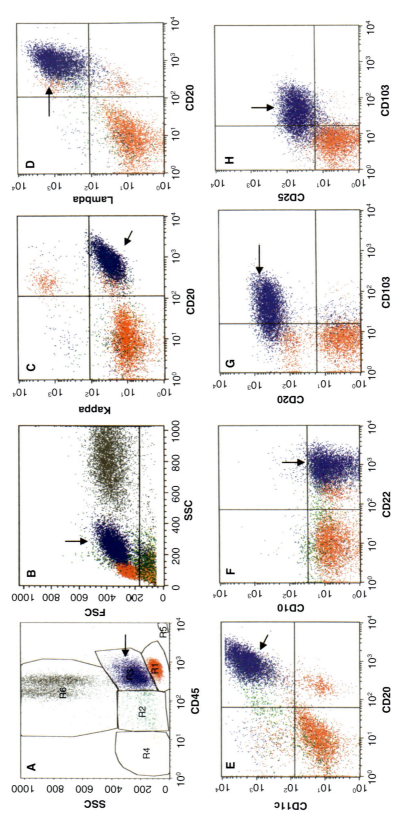

Figure 2.38   Hairy cell leukemia – flow cytometry. (**A**) Leukemic cells show increased orthogonal side scatter (SSC, arrow), which places the cells in the 'monocytic region', above normal lymphocytes (red). (**B**) Dot plots display increased side scatter (SSC) and forward scatter (FSC) in HCL (blue; arrow) as compared to benign lymphocytes (red). Neoplastic cells show moderate to bright expression of CD20 (**C–E**), surface immunoglobulin (lambda, **D**), bright expression of CD11c (**E**), bright expression of CD22 (**F**) and coexpression of CD25 and CD103 (**G** and **H**)

Table 2.3   Immunophenotypic profile of hairy cell leukemia

CD5	–/(very rare +)
CD10	–/(rare +)
CD11c	+ (bright)
CD20	+ (bright)
CD25	+/subset – (HCL variant)
CD45	+
CD79a	+
CD103	+
Bcl-1	–/+
Bcl-2	+
Bcl-6	–
Light-chain Ig (kappa/lambda)	+ (bright)
Pax-5	+/–

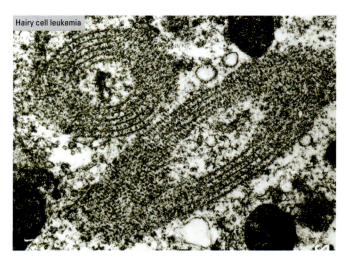

Figure 2.39   Hairy cell leukemia – electron microscopy, showing characteristic ribosome–lamellar complex

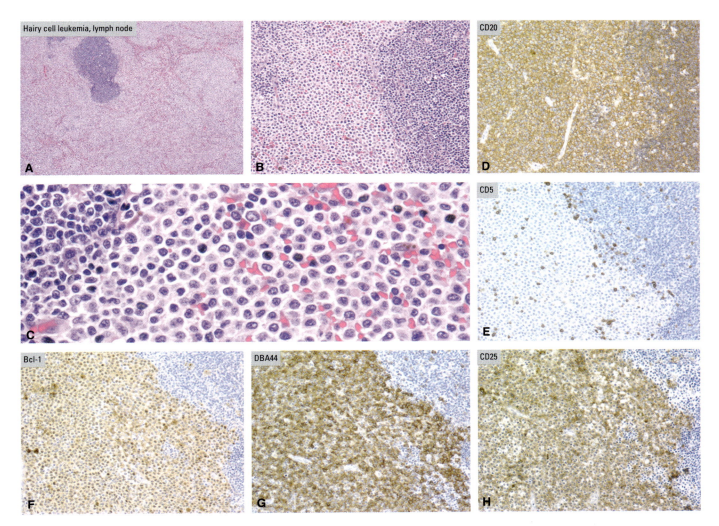

Figure 2.40   Hairy cell leukemia – lymph node. (**A**) Low magnification shows prominent perifollicular/paracortical infiltrate. (**B** and **C**) Higher magnification shows atypical lymphoid cells with moderate amount of pale cytoplasm and irregular nuclei. Hairy cell leukemia cells are positive for CD20 (**D**), negative for CD5 (**E**) and positive for bcl-1 (**F**), DBA44 (**G**) and CD25 (**H**)

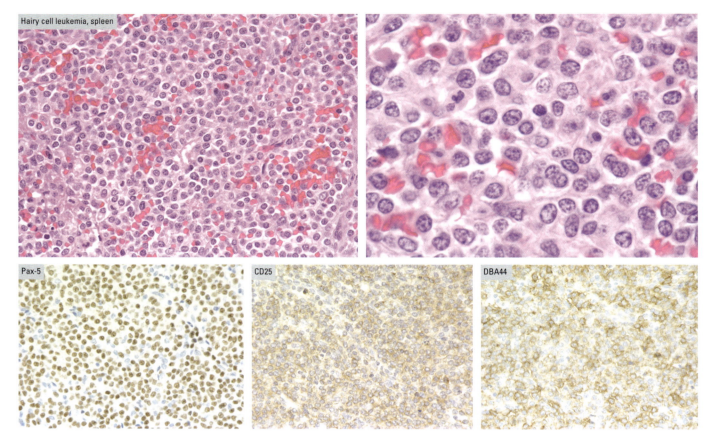

Figure 2.41   Hairy cell leukemia – spleen. Effacement of splenic architecture by monotonous lymphoid infiltrate with occasional red cell lakes. Leukemic cells are positive for Pax-5, CD25 and DBA44

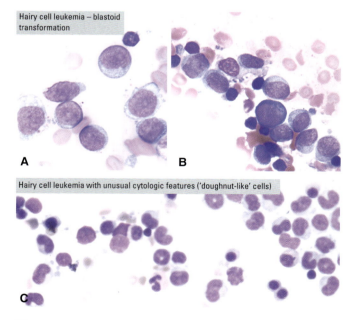

Figure 2.42   Hairy cell leukemia – unusual cytologic features. (**A** and **B**) Blastoid transformation of hairy cell leukemia. (**C**) Leukemic cells with irregular nuclei ('doughnut-like' cells)

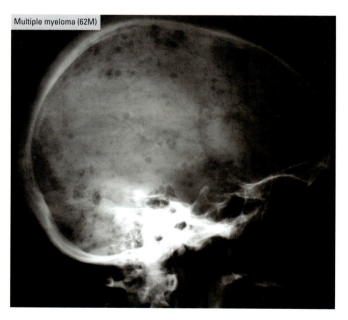

Figure 2.43   Plasma cell myeloma – radiograph of the skull demonstrating lytic bone lesions

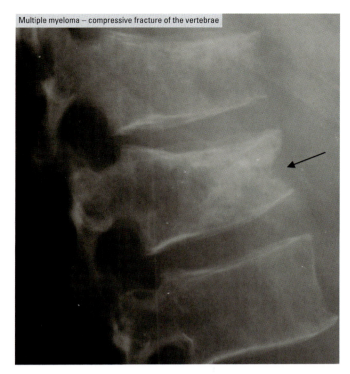

Figure 2.44 Plasma cell myeloma – radiograph of the vertebrae demonstrating compression fracture (arrow)

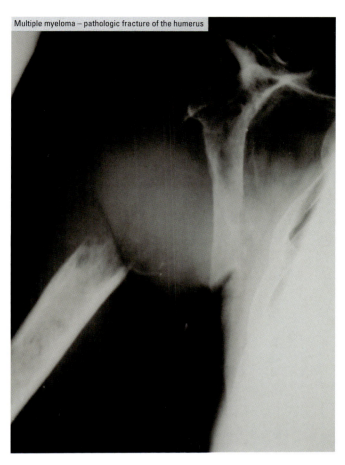

Figure 2.45 Plasma cell myeloma – radiograph of the humerus with pathologic fracture

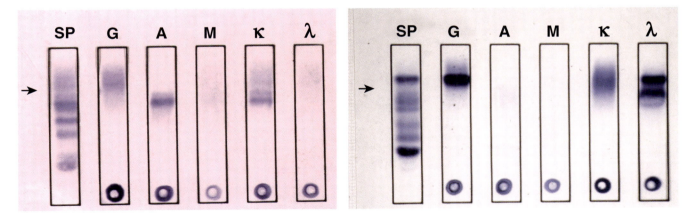

Figure 2.46 Plasma cell myeloma – serum immunofixation electrophoretogram showing IgA-kappa band (left) and IgG-lambda with free light chains (right)

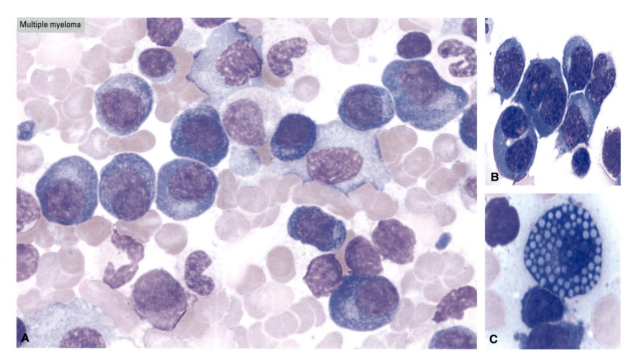

Figure 2.47   Plasma cell myeloma – cytology. (**A**) Mature plasma cells have abundant cytoplasm and eccentric nuclei with clumped chromatin. (**B**) Binucleated cells. (**C**) Mott cell with numerous cytoplasmic vacuoles

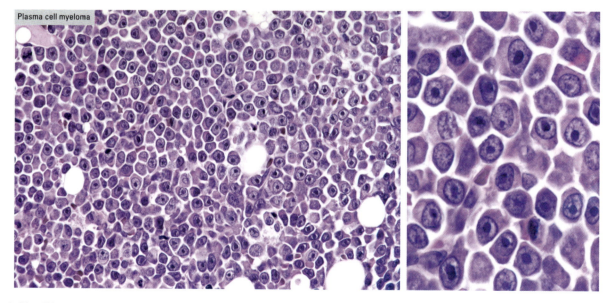

Figure 2.48   Plasma cell myeloma – histology

inclusions (Russell bodies; Figure 2.49A) or intranuclear inclusions (Dutcher bodies; Figure 2.49B). Immature plasma cell myelomas (Figure 2.50) exhibit marked pleomorphism with multinucleation and prominent nucleoli ('anaplastic plasma cell myeloma')[224].

In early or post-treatment lesions, plasma cells may be difficult to note and distinguish from reactive plasmacytosis. Immunohistochemistry helps in identifying plasma cells and confirming their clonality (Figure 2.51).

Plasma cells are usually positive for CD138, light- and heavy-chain immunoglobulins, OCT-2 and BOB-1 (Figure 2.51). Table 2.4 presents the immunophenotypic profile of plasma cell myeloma. Immunophenotyping by flow cytometry (Figure 2.52) reveals typical monotypic expression of cytoplasmic immunoglobulins. Surface immunoglobulins are usually negative, but occasional cases display dim expression of light chains. IgG is most commonly heavy chain, followed by IgA, no heavy chain,

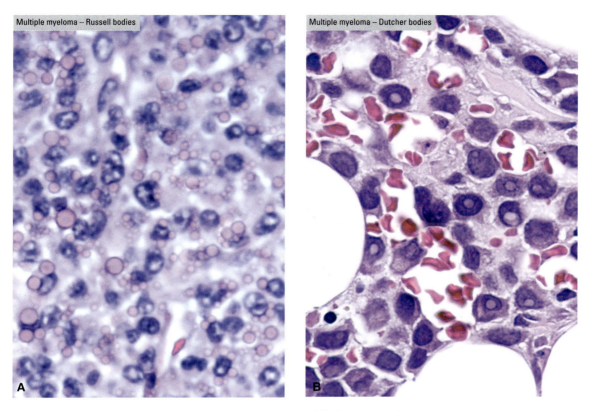

Figure 2.49 Plasma cell myeloma – histology. (**A**) Russell bodies. (**B**) Dutcher bodies

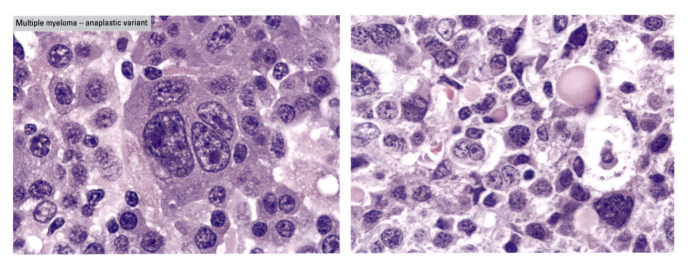

Figure 2.50 Anaplastic (immature) variants of plasma cell myeloma (two cases). Note prominent nuclear pleomorphism, hyperchromasia, macronucleoli and multinucleation

IgM, and IgD. Table 2.4 summarizes the phenotype of plasma cell neoplasms. More than 50% of tumors express CD43, CD117 and/or CD56 and approximately one-third of cases are positive for bcl-1, Pax-5, CD20 and/or EMA. Pax-5 expression correlates with CD20 and bcl-1 expression: the majority of Pax-5+ plasma cell neoplasms express also CD20 and/or bcl-1. Multiple myeloma with t(11;14)(q13;q32) displays upregulation of bcl-1 (cyclin D1), often has 'lymphoplasmacytic morphology' and is much less likely to be hyperdiploid[213–217]. Plasma cell neoplasms may be associated with deposition of amyloid (primary amyloidosis). Amyloid stains pink in HE sections (Figure 2.53B) and pink-orange in Congo red preparations (Figure 2.53C). Factors associated with worse prognosis in patients with plasma cell myeloma include anaplastic/immature morphology (plasmablastic

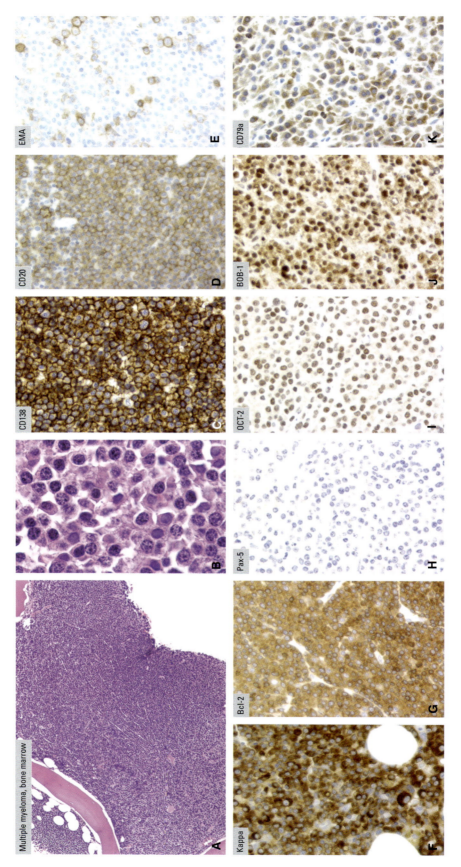

Figure 2.51   Plasma cell myeloma – immunohistochemistry. (**A** and **B**) Diffuse, extensive bone marrow involvement by plasma cell myeloma. Neoplastic plasma cells are positive for CD138 (**C**), CD20 (**D**), focally EMA (**E**), light chain (kappa, **F**), bcl-2 (**G**), OCT-2 (**I**), BOB-1 (**J**) and CD79a (**K**). Pax-5 is not expressed (**H**)

features), extensive bone marrow involvement (> 50%), high proliferation fraction (S-phase or Ki-67 index), deletions of 13q14 and 17p13 and leukemic peripheral blood involvement. Figure 2.54 presents 'plasma cell leukemia'.

The differential diagnosis of plasma cell myeloma (Figure 2.55) includes both reactive and neoplastic lesions which either morphologically or phenotypically resemble plasma cell neoplasms. Plasmablastic lymphoma (Figure 2.55A) usually differs from plasma cell myeloma by clinical presentation and positive expression of EBV/EBER and negative expression of light- and heavy-chain

Table 2.4 Immunophenotypic profile of plasma cell neoplasms

Marker (antigen)	% positive	Marker (antigen)	% positive
CD19	6.5	Heavy chains	
CD20	30.9	IgG	56.4
CD38	98.4	IgA	20.0
CD138	96.2	IgM	5.5
CD43	51.5	IgD	1.8
CD45	21.4	No heavy chains	11.0
CD56	53.8	Light chains	
CD79a	26.7	Kappa	57.3
CD117	63.2	Lambda	41.2
Bcl-1	34.1	No light chains	1.5
Bcl-2	53.3	PAX-5	29.6
EMA	34.0		

immunoglobulins. However, the distinction between plasmablastic lymphoma and plasma cell neoplasm may be occasionally difficult, since both the cytomorphologic and phenotypic features often overlap. Metastatic carcinoma, especially from breast and prostate, may mimic plasma cell tumors (Figure 2.55B and D). Bone marrow with reactive plasmacytosis exhibits polytypic immunoglobulin expression (Figure 2.55C). In trephine core biopsy, reactive plasma cells tend to occur individually or in small groups around blood vessels. Malignant plasma cells form larger clusters and are not perivascular. Osteoblasts may resemble atypical plasma cells (Figure 2.55E). Malignant lymphomas with extensive plasmacytic differentiation may be indistinguishable morphologically from plasma cell neoplasms, especially when plasma cells predominate (e.g., after treatment which eliminated the B-cell component or in limited biopsy specimens which reflect plasma cell-rich areas). Lymphoplasmacytic lymphoma and other types of B-cell lymphomas, especially marginal zone B-cell lymphoma, can be differentiated from plasma cell neoplasms by demonstration of a clonal B-cell component with monotypic expression of the same light-chain immunoglobulin. Marginal zone B-cell lymphoma (Figure 2.55F) differs by clinical presentation and lack of a significant serum M-protein. Occasional cases of marginal zone lymphomas may be difficult to distinguish from extraosseous

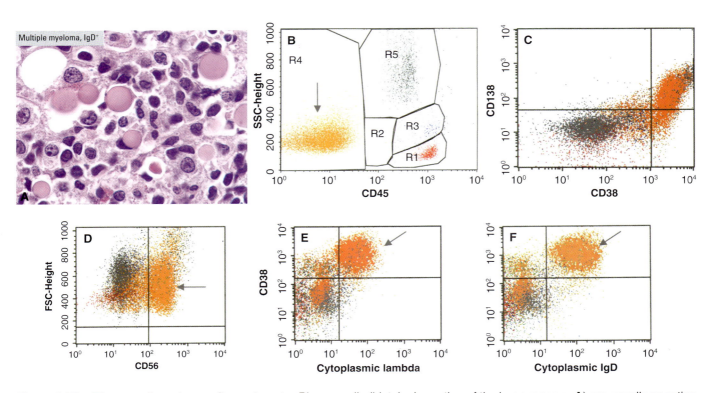

Figure 2.52 Plasma cell myeloma – flow cytometry. Plasma cells (histologic section of the bone marrow, **A**) are usually negative for CD45 (**B**), are positive for CD38/CD138 (**C**), CD56 (**D**) and show clonal expression of light and heavy chains (**E**, **F**); see Table 2.4 for details

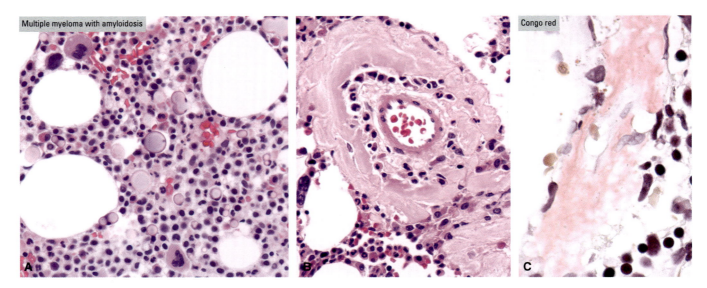

Figure 2.53   Primary amyloidosis. (**A**) Bone marrow with neoplastic plasma cells. (**B**) Characteristic amorphous eosinophilic deposits around the blood vessels. (**C**) Deposits are congophilic in a Congo red stain

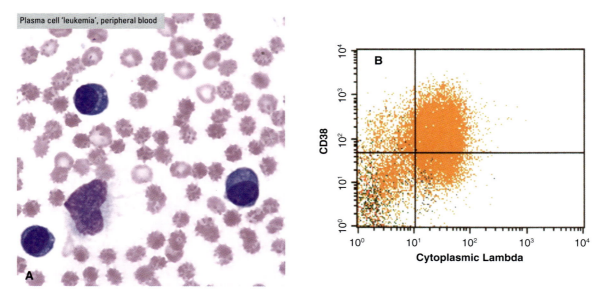

Figure 2.54   Plasma cell leukemia – peripheral blood. Atypical plasma cells in peripheral blood film (**A**) are positive for CD38 and cytoplasmic lambda immunoglobulins (**B**)

plasmacytoma. Lymphoplasmacytic lymphoma shows intranuclear inclusions and gradual transition from small lymphocytes to plasma cells. The latter may have a 'flame cell' appearance (Figure 2.55I) often associated with the IgA isotype. Poorly differentiated carcinoma with neuroendocrine features shares positive CD56 expression and lack of CD45 (Figure 2.55G). Plasmacytoma (Figure 2.55H) is distinguished from plasma cell myeloma by radiologic and clinical data. Occasional cases of Castleman's disease, plasma cell type (Figure 2.55J), may display monotypic (IgA/lambda) plasma cells and requires differentiation

from plasma cell tumors. Acute myeloid leukemias (Figure 2.55K) or acute erythroleukemia may histologically mimic plasma cell myeloma. They may also share phenotypic antigens, including CD38, CD43, CD56 and CD117. Rare variants of large B-cell lymphomas, including ALK+ large B-cell lymphoma and primary effusion lymphoma (PEL), may have cytologic or phenotypic features resembling plasma cell myeloma. ALK+ large B-cell lymphoma (Figure 2.55L) differs from plasma cell tumor by cytoplasmic staining with ALK-1. PEL (Figure 2.55M) may be indistinguishable cytologically from high-grade

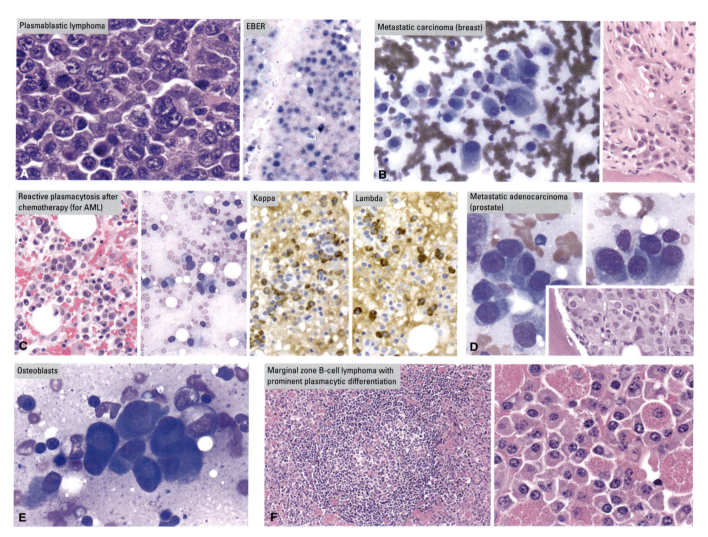

Figure 2.55   Plasma cell myeloma – differential diagnosis. (**A**) Plasmablastic lymphoma. (**B**) Metastatic breast carcinoma. (**C**) Reactive plasmacytosis. (**D**) Metastatic adenocarcinoma (prostate). (**E**) Osteoblasts. (**F**) Marginal zone lymphoma with extensive plasmacytic differentiation. (**G**) Metastatic small cell carcinoma. (**H**) Solitary plasmacytoma. (**I**) Lymphoplasmacytic lymphoma. (**J**) Castleman's disease (plasma cell type). (**K**) Acute myeloid leukemia. (**L**) Diffuse large B-cell lymphoma with ALK expression. (**M**) Primary effusion lymphoma

plasma cell tumors involving body cavities. It may lack B-cell markers but usually is positive for CD45. It differs from plasma cell tumors by expression of HHV-8.

FOLLICULAR LYMPHOMA (FL)

FL is one of the most common types of malignant lymphoma in adults and is defined as a B-cell neoplasm of follicle center cell origin which usually displays a nodular pattern of growth[78,225,226]. FL is composed of a variable proportion of small and large centrocytes (cleaved cells) and centroblasts (large non-cleaved cells).

The follicular nodules (Figure 2.56) are usually closely packed with a back-to-back arrangement and have comparable size and shape, differing from florid follicular hyperplasia. The neoplastic follicles most often lack a well-defined mantle zone, polarization or tingible-body macrophages (Figure 2.56A). Occasional cases show a vague nodularity (Figure 2.56B), with nodules of variable size (Figure 2.56C) or shape (Figure 2.56D). High-grade FL may have a starry-sky pattern, which, together with lack of bcl-2 expression, imitates a reactive pattern. Typical cases of FL show positive expression of CD10, bcl-6 and bcl-2 (Figure 2.57). The expression of bcl-2 is usually dimmer than in residual benign small T-cells. Some cases, however, show very strong bcl-2 positivity (Figure 2.58). This is especially common in cases with partial involvement by FL (FL '*in situ*'). FL, even those with distinct

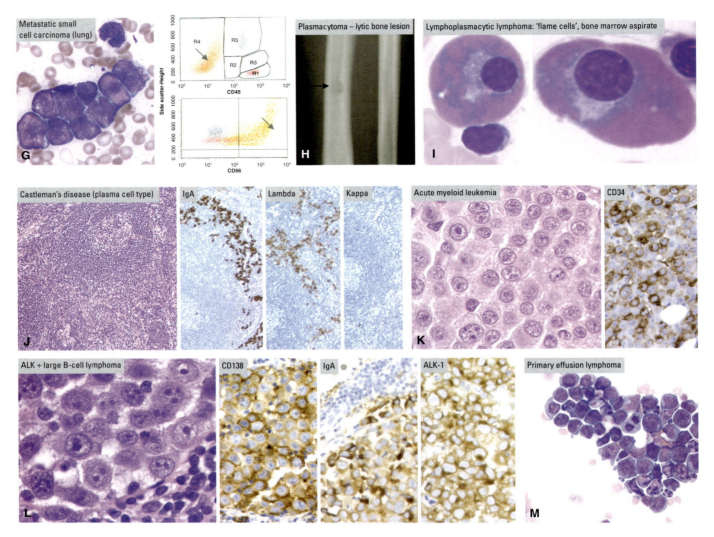

Figure 2.55   *(Continued)*

nodular architecture, may show a significant proportion of CD10/bcl-6+ B-cells in the interfollicular areas.

FL is graded by the proportion of large non-cleaved cells with nucleoli (centroblasts). WHO recommends a three-grade system (grades 1, 2 and 3) based on the number of centroblasts per × 40 high-power field (hpf). Grade 1 is defined by 5 or fewer centroblasts/hpf (Figure 2.59A), grade 2 has 6–15 centroblasts/hpf (Figure 2.59B) and grade 3 has more than 15 centroblasts/hpf (Figure 2.59C-D)[68,78]. FL grade 3 is a heterogeneous group, which may be further subdivided into 3a (with centrocytes) and 3b (without centrocytes)[68,78]. Since the cytomorphologic features often vary among follicles, the whole lymph node must be sampled and carefully evaluated. Centroblasts need to be differentiated from other large cells such as histiocytes, endothelial cells, follicular dendritic cells and large centrocytes. It is also necessary to exclude any areas with diffuse large cell infiltrate.

Immunophenotypically, FL is most often positive for CD45 (LCA), B-cell markers (CD19, CD20, CD22, CD79a, Pax-5), CD10, bcl-2 and bcl-6. Most cases are negative for CD43. A subset of FL is negative for either CD10 and/or bcl-2 (Figure 2.60). Rare cases may be positive for CD5 or CD43[37,227]. Bcl-2 negative tumors are usually of higher grade. Lack of both bcl-2 and CD10 expression is often observed in FL without t(14;18) and with bcl-6 rearrangement[228,229]. FL may show only partial involvement of the lymph node (Figure 2.61). The areas of FL differ by showing larger, closely packed nodules, which, in contrast to reactive follicles, show positive expression of bcl-2. Virtually all cases of FL have chromosomal abnormalities[51,228–230], the most common being t(14;18)(q32;q21), which involves the rearrangement of the *BCL-2* gene (Figure 2.62 and 2.63). Other changes include *BCL-6* rearrangement and 17p abnormalities.

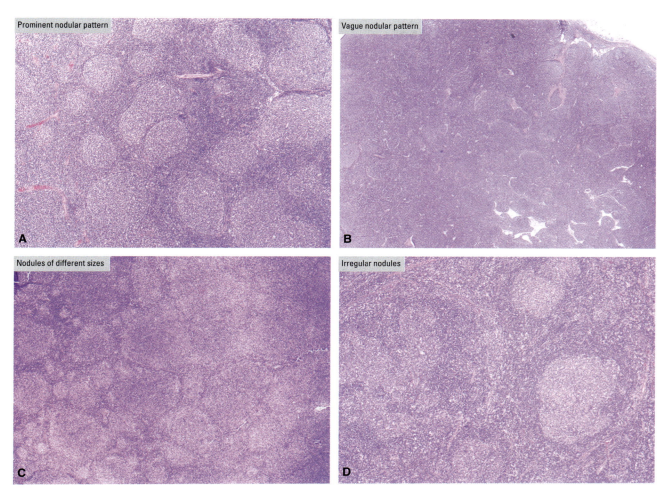

Figure 2.56 Follicular lymphoma (FL) – lymph node. (**A**) FL with prominent nodular pattern. (**B**) FL with vague nodularity. (**C**) FL with nodules of different sizes. (**D**) FL with irregular nodules

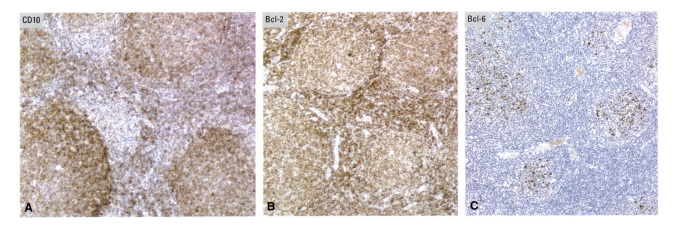

Figure 2.57 Follicular lymphoma (FL) – immunohistochemistry. Typical FL is positive for CD10 (**A**), bcl-2 (**B**) and bcl-6 (**C**)

Flow cytometry (FC) (Figure 2.64) shows monotypic expression of surface immunoglobulins, moderate to bright expression of CD20, dim expression of CD19 and positive expression of CD10. Often, FC reveals two B-cell populations: a neoplastic population with monotypic expression of surface immunoglobulins and a subpopulation of residual benign (polytypic) B-cells. Dim expression of CD19 and coexpression of CD10 and bcl-2

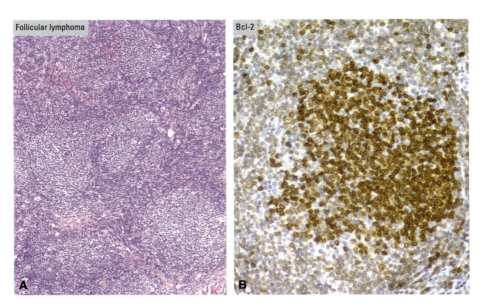

Figure 2.58 Follicular lymphoma (**A**, histology) with overexpression of bcl-2 (**B**). Compare the bcl-2 expression in neoplastic cells (center) with that of benign small lymphocytes (periphery)

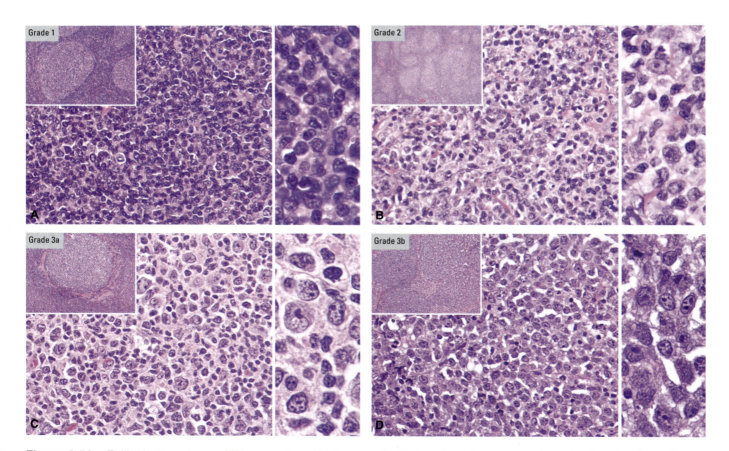

Figure 2.59 Follicular lymphoma (FL) – grading. (**A**) Low-grade FL (grade 1) is composed predominantly of small cells with irregular nuclei. (**B**) Intermediate grade FL (grade 2) has mixture of small (centrocytes) and (5–15) larger (centroblasts) lymphocytes. (**C** and **D**) High-grade FL (grade 3) has predominantly large lymphocytes. Depending on the presence of few scattered small lymphocytes, grade 3 FL can be subdivided into 3a (small cells present) and 3b (small cells absent)

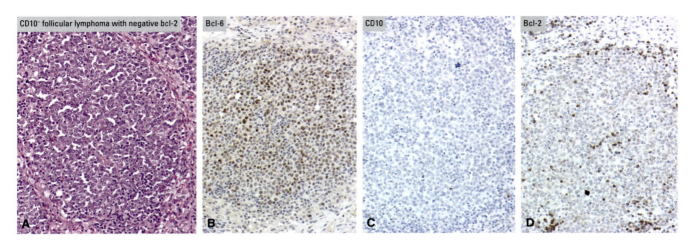

Figure 2.60   CD10 negative and bcl-2 negative follicular lymphoma. Follicular lymphoma (grade 3, **A**) positive for bcl-6 (**B**) with lack of CD10 (**C**) and bcl-2 (**D**)

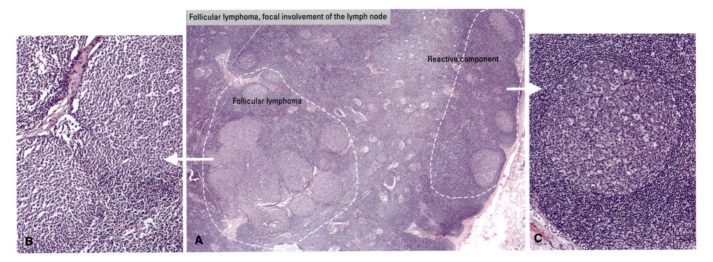

Figure 2.61   Follicular lymphoma – partial lymph node involvement. (**A**) Low magnification shows cluster of atypical follicles. (**B**) Higher magnification of that area shows follicles composed of monotonous lymphoid cells without tingible-body macrophages. (**C**) Higher magnification of reactive component with tingible-body macrophages

usually confirm a malignant process in these cases. A subset of FL may lack surface light-chain immunoglobulins. Table 2.5 summarizes the phenotype of FL.

Most patients with FL have stage IV disease with bone marrow and even peripheral blood ('leukemic') involvement. In the bone marrow, FL typically shows a paratrabecular pattern (Figure 2.65A), but nodular interstitial infiltrates may be also seen (Figure 2.65B). Discrepancy between the grade of nodal and bone marrow compartments is not uncommon. Peripheral blood involved by FL shows small to medium-sized lymphocytes with prominent nuclear cleavage (Figure 2.66).

Morphologic and phenotypic variants of FL include the floral variant (Figure 2.67A), monocytoid variant (Figure 2.67B), FL with reversed pattern (neoplastic cells ringing benign nodules; Figure 2.67C), FL with prominent sclerosis (Figure 2.67D), signet-ring cell variant (Figure 2.67E), surface immunoglobulin negative FL (Figure 2.68) and diffuse follicle center cell lymphoma (Figure 2.69). The latter has all the cytomorphologic and phenotypic features of FL except for a diffuse pattern of growth. Diffuse follicle center cell lymphoma is composed of centrocytes (grade 1) or centrocytes and centroblasts (grade 2). If centroblasts predominate, it is classified as diffuse large B-cell

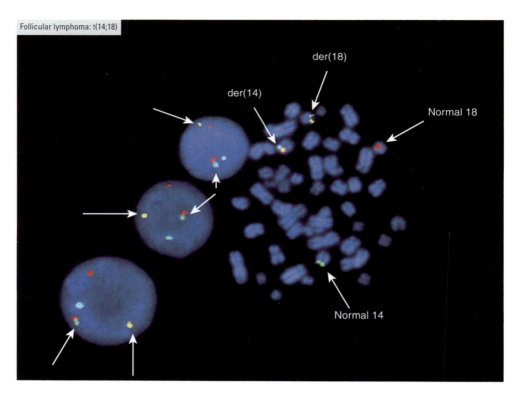

Figure 2.62   Follicular lymphoma with t(14;18) – FISH

Follicular lymphoma: t(14;18)

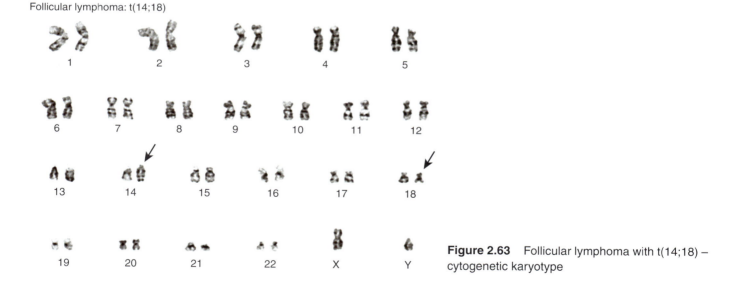

Figure 2.63   Follicular lymphoma with t(14;18) – cytogenetic karyotype

lymphoma. Positive expression of CD10, bcl-6 and negative expression of CD5 and bcl-1 distinguish diffuse follicle center cell lymphoma from other types of low-grade lymphomas with a diffuse pattern.

FL may undergo large cell transformation (Figure 2.70). The proportion of diffuse and follicular areas in the lymph node should be included in a pathologic report; e.g., FL, predominantly follicular (> 75% follicular) or FL, follicular and diffuse (50% follicular), or focally follicular

(< 25% follicular)[78,231]. Progression of FL to a higher-grade malignancy frequently heralds a poor prognosis. Occasional cases of transformed FL may have blastoid morphology[232]. Rare cases of FL may undergo transformation into precursor B-lymphoblastic leukemia/lymphoma with t(14;18).

FL occurs predominantly in lymph nodes, but may be seen also in the spleen, bone marrow, and peripheral blood and in non-hematopoietic locations (gastrointestinal tract,

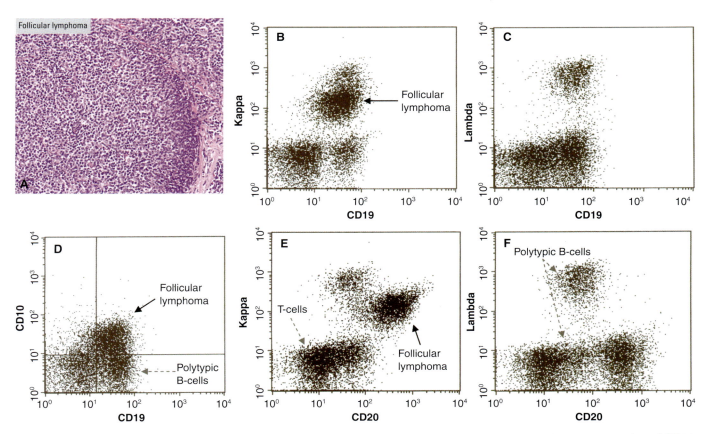

Figure 2.64 Follicular lymphoma – flow cytometry. Follicular lymphomas (**A**, histology) may display dimmer expression of CD19 (**B**, arrow) and slightly brighter expression of CD20 (**E**, arrow) when compared to benign B-cells (**F**, arrow). CD10 is positive in most cases (**D**). In contrast to other B-cell lymphomas, polytypic B-cells are often present (**B, C, E, F**). Note dimmer expression of kappa by neoplastic cells when compared to benign B-cells (**B, C, E, F**)

Table 2.5 Immunophenotypic profile of follicular lymphoma

CD5	–
CD10	+/–
CD11c	–/+
CD19	+ (dim)
CD20	+ (moderate)
CD22	+ (moderate)
CD23	+/–
CD25	–
CD30	–
CD38	+/rare –
CD43	–/very rare cases +
CD45	+
CD103	–
CD138	–
Bcl-1	–
Bcl-2	+/subset – (usually higher grade)
Bcl-6	+
BOB-1	+
Ki-67	+ (scattered cells, no polarization)
Light-chain Ig (kappa/lambda)	+/–*
OCT-2	+
Pax-5	+

*Follicular lymphomas comprise the largest group of surface immunoglobulin-negative B-cell lymphomas

skin, soft tissue, orbit/ocular adnexae)[233–238]. Primary FL of the skin represents one of the most common types of cutaneous lymphoma[239]. Figure 2.71 shows extranodal FL. In the gastrointestinal tract, the small intestine is most frequently involved. FL involving skin may show monocytoid features and bcl-2 negativity.

The differential diagnosis of FL includes reactive follicular hyperplasia and other low-grade B-cell lymphomas with a nodular pattern of growth (Figures 2.72–2.74). The morphologic and immunophenotypic differences between follicular hyperplasia and FL are illustrated in Figure 2.72. Hyperplastic follicles (Figure 2.72A) show polarization, well-preserved mantle and marginal zones, and the presence of tingible-body macrophages. Follicles often have irregular size and shape and are located predominantly in the cortex. Benign follicles, similarly to FL are CD10+ (Figure 2.72B and B′) and bcl-6+, but do not stain with bcl-2 (Figure 2.72C and C′). Polarization can be best visualized by staining with Ki-67 (Figure 2.72D)

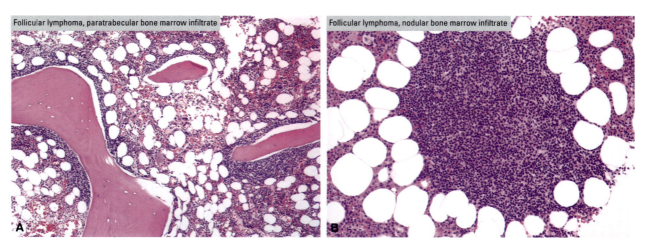

Figure 2.65   Follicular lymphoma – patterns of bone marrow involvement. **(A)** Characteristic paratrabecular pattern of involvement. **(B)** Nodular interstitial lymphoid infiltrate

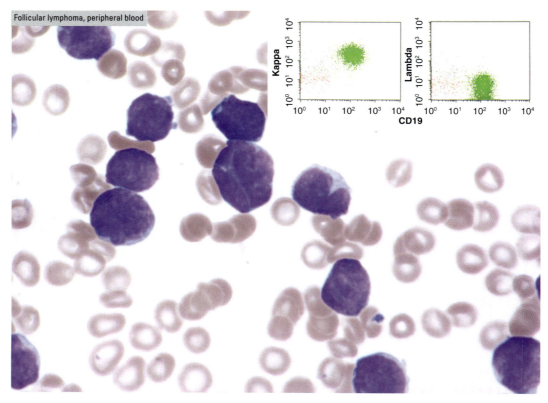

Figure 2.66   Leukemic peripheral blood involvement by follicular lymphoma (inset: flow cytometry with clonal expression of kappa Ig)

and CD23 (Figure 2.72F). Staining with CD21 for follicular dendritic cells (Figure 2.72E and E′) shows well-preserved meshworks. Neoplastic follicles, even in high-grade FL, contain lower number of Ki-67+ cells, which are haphazardly distributed (Figure 2.73). Thus, Ki-67 staining may be useful in confirming high-grade FL with negative bcl-2 and starry-sky pattern.

Toxoplasmic lymphadenitis (Figure 2.74A) shows reactive follicular hyperplasia with clusters of monocytoid B-cells around the follicles and epithelioid histiocytes aggregates. Progressive transformation of germinal centers (PTGC) (Figure 2.74B) is a benign process, which is associated with nodular lymphocyte-predominant Hodgkin lymphoma. PTGC are larger than nodules in follicular

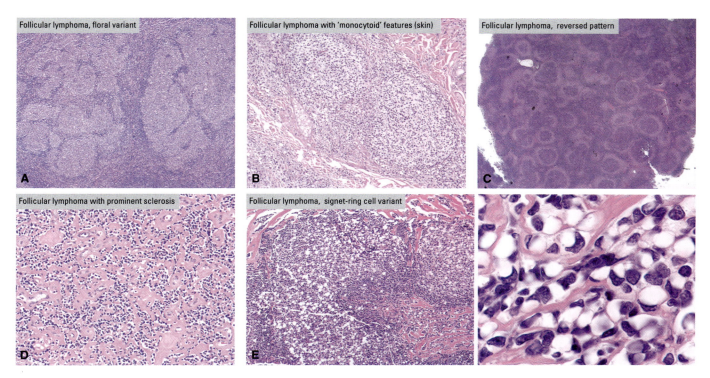

Figure 2.67 Morphologic variants of follicular lymphoma (FL). (**A**) Floral variant. (**B**) FL with pale (clear) cytoplasm (monocytoid B-cell appearance). (**C**) Reversed pattern. (**D**) FL with prominent sclerosis, obliterating nodular architecture. (**E**) Signet-ring cell variant (low and high magnification)

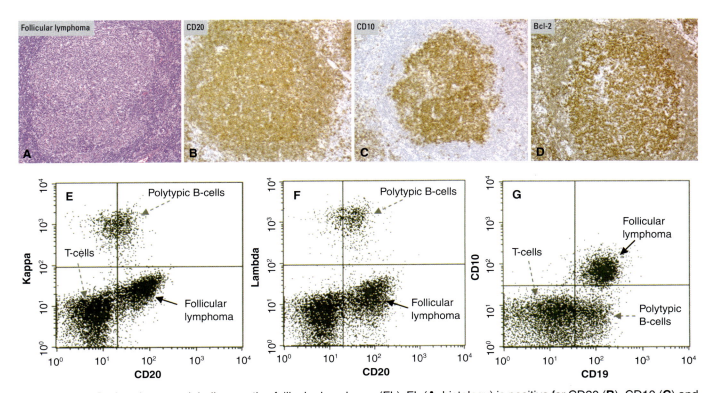

Figure 2.68 Surface immunoglobulin negative follicular lymphoma (FL). FL (**A**, histology) is positive for CD20 (**B**), CD10 (**C**) and bcl-2 (**D**) by immunohistochemical staining. Flow cytometry (**E–G**) shows lack of surface immunoglobulins (**E**, **F**; solid arrow) and positive expression of CD10 (**G**, solid arrow; polytypic B-cells are CD10 negative). Note mixture of polytypic B-cells (**E**, **F**; broken arrow)

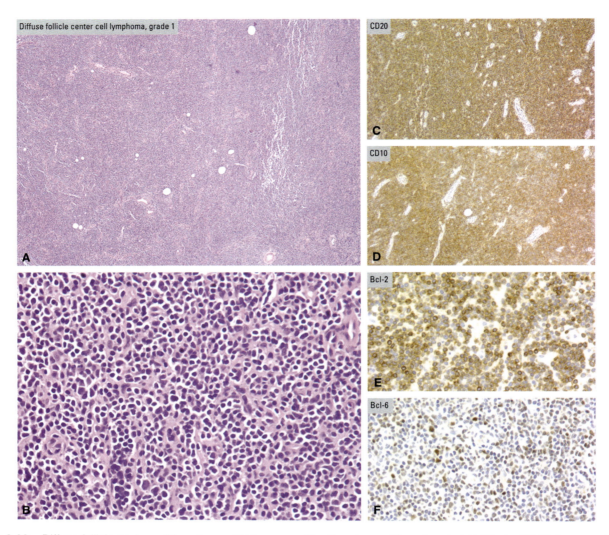

Figure 2.69   Diffuse follicle center cell lymphoma. (**A**) Low magnification shows diffuse lymphoid infiltrate. (**B**) Higher magnification shows predominance of small lymphocytes with irregular nuclei. Immunohistochemistry depicts the typical phenotype: CD20⁺ (**C**), CD10⁺ (**D**), bcl-2⁺ (**E**) and bcl-6⁺ (**F**)

lymphoma and are composed of small B-lymphocytes. Castleman's disease, plasma cell type (Figure 2.74C), shows reactive follicles and prominent interfollicular sheets of plasma cells. HHV-8 staining may be positive. Castleman's disease, hyaline-vascular type (Figure 2.74D), is characterized by reactive follicles with a broad mantle zone in typical concentric arrangement ('onionskin' pattern). Occasional follicles contain more than one small germinal center, with hyalinized vessels. Mantle zone hyperplasia (Figure 2.74E) shows a prominent mantle zone of monotonous small B-cells, which are CD5/bcl-1 negative. Kimura disease (Figure 2.74F) is characterized by reactive follicles accompanied by pools of eosinophils. Occasional large multinucleated cells are present within expanded germinal centers.

Low-grade B-cell lymphomas may have a distinct nodular pattern, which mimics FL. Marginal zone lymphoma (Figure 2.74G) differs from FL by lack of CD10

expression. The pseudofollicular pattern of B-small lymphocytic lymphoma (Figure 2.74H) is a result of clusters of prolymphocytes (proliferation centers). Mast cell infiltrates (Figure 2.74I) may be nodular and are positive for CD117 and mast cell tryptase. MCL (Figure 2.74J) often has a nodular pattern.

Nodular lymphocyte-predominant Hodgkin lymphoma (Figure 2.74K) is recognized by large atypical cells with multilobated nuclei with prominent nucleoli (L&H cells or popcorn cells) scattered among small B-cells. Rosettes of CD57⁺ small T-cells are often identified.

MANTLE CELL LYMPHOMA (MCL)

MCL is a B-cell lymphoma of small to medium-sized lymphocytes with irregular nuclei characterized by expression of bcl-1[51,99,240–251]. MCL occurs in lymph nodes,

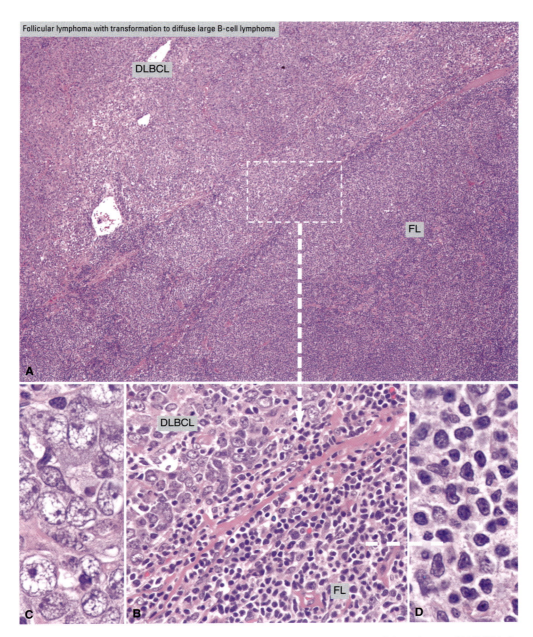

Figure 2.70   Follicular lymphoma (FL) with transformation into diffuse large B-cell lymphoma (DLBCL). Low magnification (**A**) shows two well-demarcated areas: one composed of small lymphocytes with nodular architecture (lower right corner, FL) and the other composed of large cells (DLBCL, left side). (**B**) Higher magnification of the transition zone. (**C** and **D**) High magnification shows clear difference in the size of the lymphocytes of two components (DLBCL, **C**; FL, **D**)

bone marrow, the gastrointestinal tract (lymphomatous polyposis), and spleen, and rarely involves peripheral blood[252–254].

Histology reveals a monomorphic lymphoid infiltrate with scattered histiocytes (Figure 2.75). The lymphomatous infiltrate may be diffuse (Figure 2.75), with a mantle zone distribution (Figure 2.76), or nodular (Figure 2.77). The nuclei are characteristically irregular or cleaved (Figure 2.78), and may resemble centrocytes. Phenotypically, typical MCL is CD5+ and CD23− with nuclear expression of bcl-1 (Figures 2.75–2.77). Virtually all cases demonstrate

the t(11;14) translocation between IgH and cyclin D1 (*BCL-1*) genes by using fluorescent *in situ* hybridization (Figure 2.80). Flow cytometry (Figure 2.79) shows moderate expression of CD20 and surface immunoglobulins. Occasional cases may display an unusual phenotype such as lack of CD5[255] (Figure 2.81), aberrant expression of CD10 (Figure 2.82) or coexpression of bcl-6 (Figure 1.16; Chapter 1). Table 2.6 presents a summary of the immunophenotypic characteristics of MCL.

Mantle cell lymphoma may display blastoid morphology[256–260] (Figure 2.83). Blastoid variants may be either

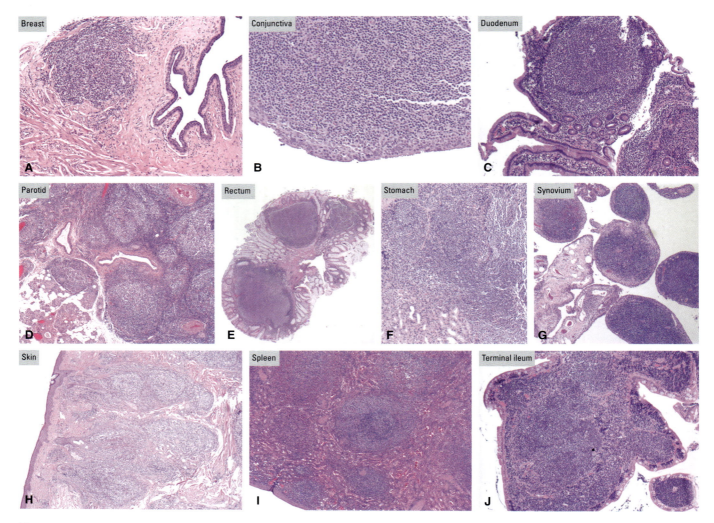

Figure 2.71   Follicular lymphoma – extranodal. (**A**) Breast. (**B**) Conjunctiva. (**C**) Duodenum. (**D**) Parotid. (**E**) Rectum. (**F**) Stomach. (**G**) Synovium. (**H**) Skin. (**I**) Spleen. (**J**) Terminal ileum

pleomorphic with irregular nuclei (Figure 2.83A) or monomorphic (classic) with lymphoblast-like cells, a high mitotic rate and prominent nucleoli (Figure 2.83B). Figure 2.84 shows an unusual variant of MCL with 'prolymphocytoid-like' transformation. Two cell types are present: small lymphocytes with irregular nuclei and inconspicuous nucleoli surrounded by larger cells with nucleoli and a geographic-like distribution. Both populations are positive for CD20, CD5 and bcl-1, but larger cells display dimmer CD20 staining (Figure 2.84D) and brighter CD5 staining (Figure 2.84E), and are positive for Ki-67 (Figure 2.84H) and p53 (Figure 2.84I).

Bone marrow involvement varies histologically (Figure 2.85) and may be diffuse and/or nodular, with or without a paratrabecular component. Occasional cases display intrasinusoidal involvement[13]. Bcl-1 immunohistochemical analysis on decalcified trephine core biopsy material may result in a falsely negative staining.

The differential diagnosis of MCL includes B- and T-cell lymphoproliferative disorders and other hematopoietic tumors. Based on the cytology, MCL must be differentiated from follicle center cell lymphoma (FL and diffuse follicle center cell lymphoma), which show irregular nuclear contours. The blastoid variant of MCL has to be distinguished from DLBCL, peripheral T-cell lymphoma, granulocytic sarcoma and precursor B- or T-lymphoblastic leukemia/lymphoma.

By the expression of CD5, MCL has to be distinguished from B-CLL/SLL (especially atypical variants of B-CLL/SLL, which may lack CD23 expression and may show moderate expression of CD20 and surface immunoglobulins), *de novo* CD5+ DLBCL, and other B-cell lymphoproliferations which may occasionally show aberrant expression of CD5.

Bcl-1 expression is not specific for MCL (Figure 14.2; Chapter 14). Plasma cell neoplasms, subset of HCL and epithelial tumors may be bcl-1 positive.

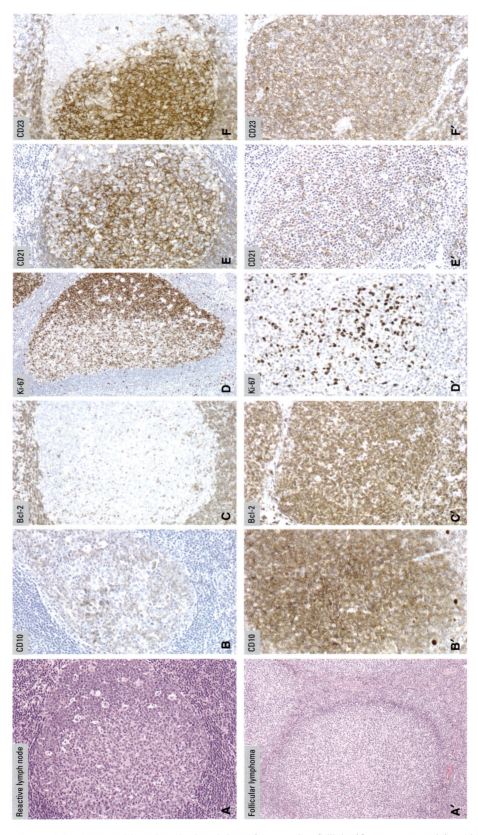

Figure 2.72   Comparison of the immunohistochemical staining of a reactive follicle (**A**, upper panels) and follicular lymphoma (**A′**, lower panels). Both benign and neoplastic follicles are positive for CD10 (**B**, **B′**). In contrast to benign processes, follicular lymphomas are most often bcl-2 positive (**C**, **C′**). Occasional cases of FL may be bcl-2 negative. Ki-67 is useful in differentiating reactive from neoplastic follicles. Reactive follicles (**D**) have a higher number of proliferating cells and display distinct polarization with dense accumulation of Ki-67+ cells at one pole of the follicle. A majority of FL have a low number of proliferating cells (**D′**). Follicular dendritic cell meshwork (visualized by CD21 staining) is delicate in FL (**E′**). Staining with CD23 shows polarization in reactive follicles (**F**), a feature usually absent in FL (**F′**)

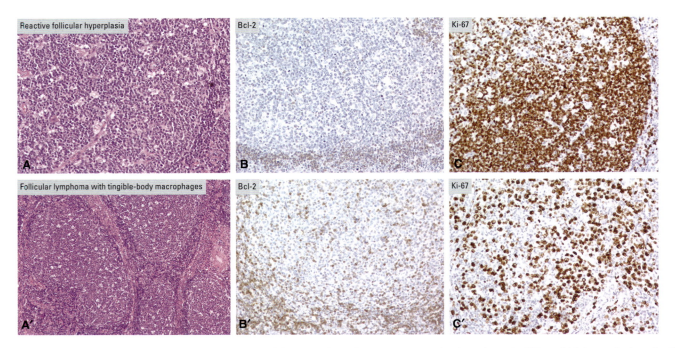

Figure 2.73 Comparison of histology and immunohistochemistry between a reactive lymph node (**A**) and high-grade (grade 3) follicular lymphoma (FL; **A′**) with tingible-body macrophages and lack of bcl-2 expression (**B′**). In some cases, the distinction between reactive and neoplastic process may be difficult, especially in cases which lack bcl-2 expression. Low-power features (back-to-back arrangement of follicles), atypia of lymphoid cells and a different pattern of immunoreactivity with Ki-67 (**C**, **C′**) help to differentiate the two proliferations. FL lack a polarized distribution of Ki-67+ cells (compare **C** and **C′**) and have fewer proliferating cells which are haphazardly distributed (**C′**)

DIFFUSE LARGE B-CELL LYMPHOMA (DLBCL)

Diffuse large B-cell lymphoma (DLBCL), the single largest category of lymphoma, is a heterogeneous group of malignant lymphomas with several morphologic variants, which include centroblastic, immunoblastic, T-cell/histiocyte-rich, anaplastic and plasmablastic, and those with cytoplasmic ALK expression[92–96,98,229,261–268].

DLBCL usually express CD45 and pan-B-cell antigens, such as CD19, CD20, CD22, CD79a and Pax-5. Pax-5 is detected as nuclear staining in very early B-cell progenitors and in subsequent stages of B-cell differentiation until the plasma cell stage, where it is downregulated (approximately 30% of plasma cell tumors are Pax-5+). Terminally differentiated DLBCL, such as immunoblastic or plasmablastic lymphomas and DLBCL treated with anti-CD20 antibodies (rituximab), may lack the expression of CD20. A small subset of DLBCL expresses CD5 (*de novo* CD5+ DLBCL) or CD43. Patients with *de novo* CD5+ DLBCL have a survival curve significantly inferior to that for patients with CD5− DLBCL[34,128]. Expression of bcl-2, a protein involved in control of apoptosis, is observed in 30–50% of DLBCL[229,269]. Bcl-6 and CD10, stage-specific markers of germinal center cell differentiation, are expressed by 50–70% DLBCL[90–92,262]. The prognostic implications of bcl-6 and/or CD10 expression in DLBCL are not certain. The coexpression of bcl-6 and CD10 is often associated with t(14;18) translocation. Expression of MUM1 protein in DLBCL may indicate post-germinal center differentiation (up to plasma cell)[92,262].

DLBCL with centroblastic morphology (centroblastic lymphoma) is the most common variant (Figure 2.86). It is composed of large lymphoid cells with vesicular nuclei and several nucleoli located at the periphery close to the nuclear membrane, often antiparallel to the long axis of the cell. The nuclei may be irregular. Neoplastic cells are positive for CD45, B-cell markers and often bcl-6 and CD10.

DLBCL with immunoblastic morphology (immunoblastic lymphoma) is characterized by large nuclei with fine chromatin and a single, centrally located prominent macronucleolus (Figure 2.87) with variable amounts of eosinophilic to amphophilic cytoplasm. Those with abundant cytoplasm and an eccentric nucleus are termed 'immunoblastic/plasmacytoid'. Neoplastic cells are strongly positive for CD45 and B-cell markers, and are negative for TdT, CD34, CD138, CD56, EMA and bcl-1. Table 2.7 presents a summary of phenotypic characteristics of DLBCL.

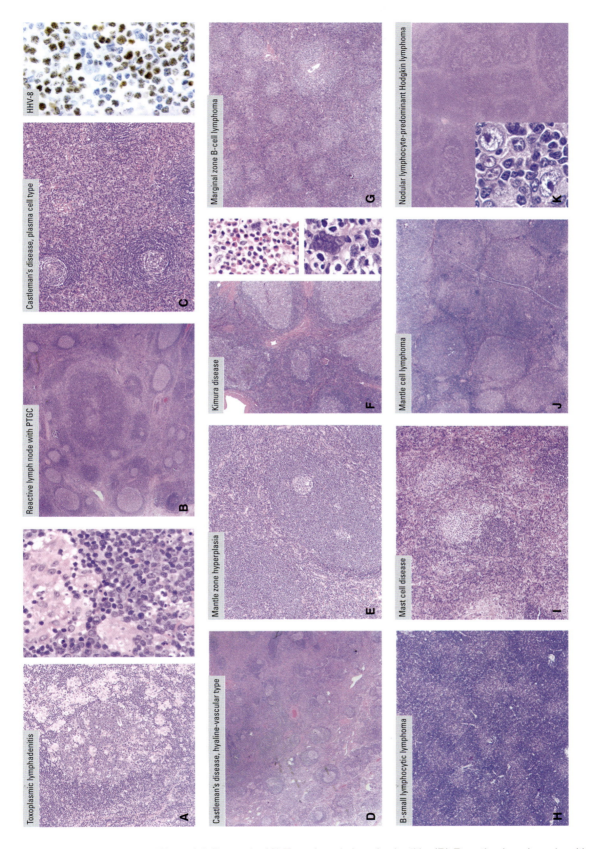

Figure 2.74   Follicular lymphoma – differential diagnosis. (**A**) Toxoplasmic lymphadentitis. (**B**) Reactive lymph node with progressive transformation of germinal centers (PTGC). (**C**) Castleman's disease, plasma cell type. (**D**) Castleman's disease, vascular type. (**E**) Mantle zone hyperplasia. (**F**) Kimura disease. (**G**) Marginal zone B-cell lymphoma. (**H**) B-cell small lymphocytic lymphoma. (**I**) Mast cell disease (**J**) Mantle cell lymphoma. (**K**) Nodular lymphocyte-predominant Hodgkin lymphoma

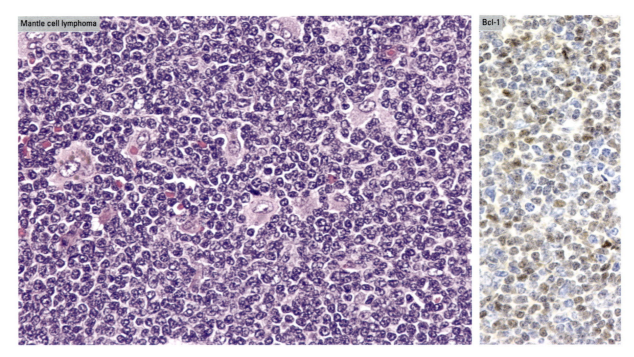

Figure 2.75   Mantle cell lymphoma (MCL) – histology. Diffuse lymphoid infiltrate composed of lymphocytes with irregular nuclear contours. Note the presence of histiocytes, often present in MCL

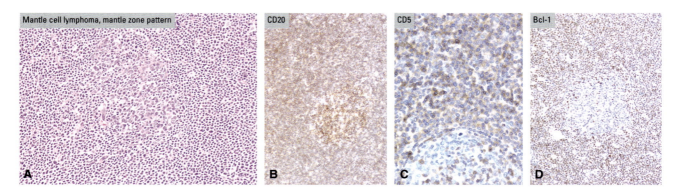

Figure 2.76   Mantle cell lymphoma (MCL) with classic mantle zone pattern. Neoplastic B-cells surround residual germinal center (**A**). MCL is characterized by coexpression of CD20 (**B**) with CD5 (**C**) and bcl-1 (**D**)

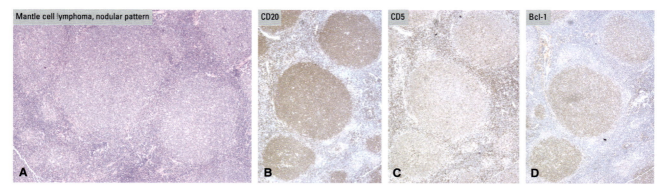

Figure 2.77   Mantle cell lymphoma with nodular pattern (**A**), mimicking follicular lymphoma. Neoplastic lymphocytes are positive for CD20 (**B**), CD5 (**C**) and bcl-1 (**D**)

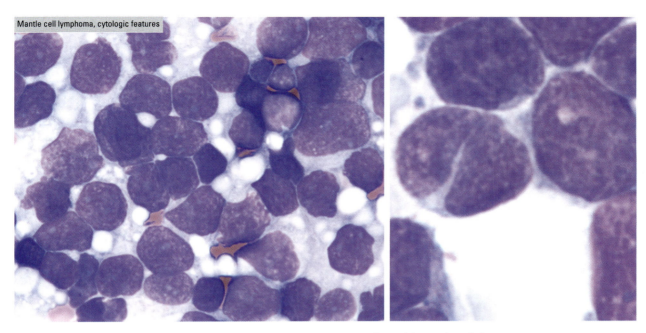

Figure 2.78   Mantle cell lymphoma – cytology. Note irregular nuclear outlines (cleaved nuclei)

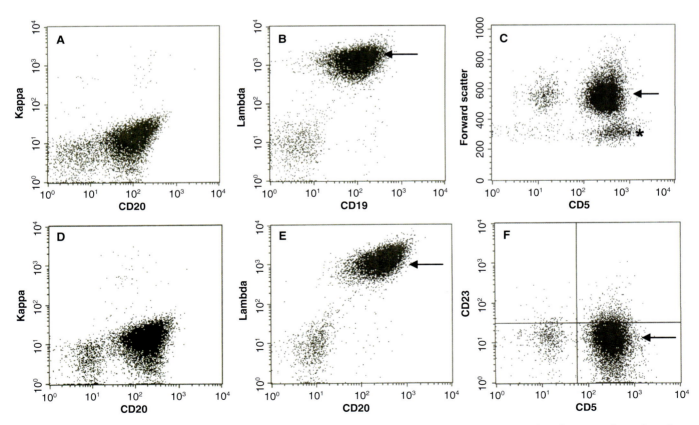

Figure 2.79   Mantle cell lymphoma – flow cytometry. (**A** and **B**) Lymphoma cells display clonal expression of surface immunoglobulin. The expression of light-chain immunoglobulin is moderate to bright (**B**), which helps to differentiate MCL from B-small lymphocytic lymphoma/chronic lymphocytic leukemia. (**C**) Forward scatter is increased (arrow) when compared to benign lymphocytes (*). (**D** and **E**) The expression of CD20 is moderate. (**F**) Typical MCL is positive for CD5 (arrow) and lacks CD23

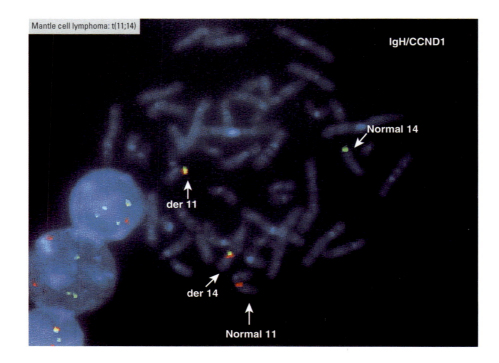

Figure 2.80   Mantle cell lymphoma – FISH shows 2 fusion signals of t(11;14)

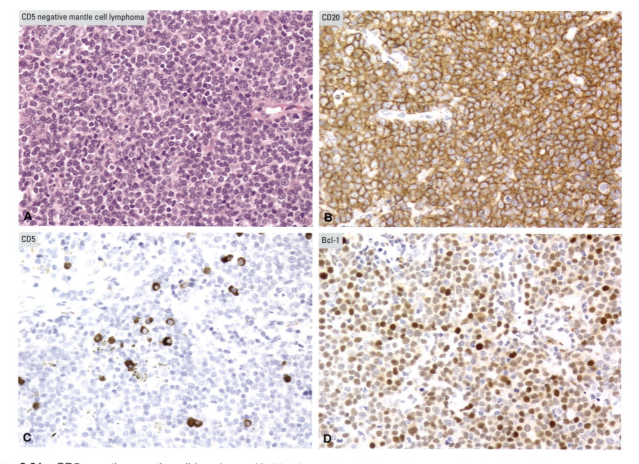

Figure 2.81   CD5 negative mantle cell lymphoma (**A**, histology). Neoplastic cells are positive for CD20 (**B**) and bcl-1 (**D**). They lack CD5 (**C**). CD5 negative MCL comprise approximately 11% of all cases (see Table 2.6 for details)

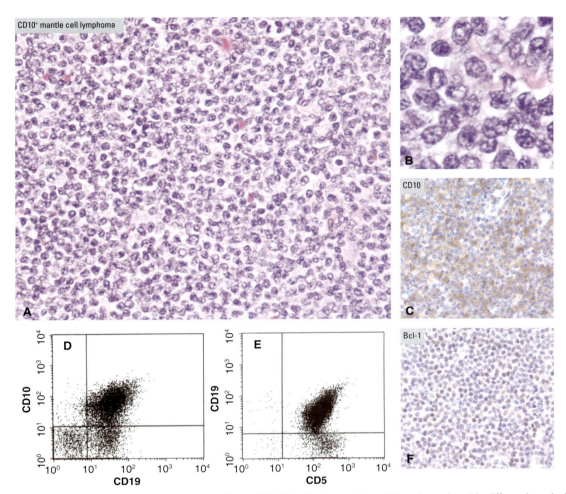

Figure 2.82 CD10 positive mantle cell lymphoma. (**A** and **B**) Histologic section of lymph node with diffuse lymphoid infiltrate composed of atypical cells with irregular nuclear contours. Immunohistochemistry and flow cytometry show expression of CD10 (**C** and **D**, respectively). Positive expression of CD5 (**E**, flow cytometry) and bcl-1 (**F**, immunohistochemistry) confirms the diagnosis of MCL

Table 2.6 Immunophenotypic profile of mantle cell lymphoma

CD5	+/rarely – (11%)*
CD10	–/rarely + (6%)*
CD20	+ (moderate expression)
CD23	–/rarely + (6%)*
CD25	–
CD30	–
CD45	+
CD103	–
CD138	–
Bcl-1	+
Bcl-2	+
Bcl-6	–
BOB-1	+
EBV/EBER	–
EMA	–
HHV-8	–
Heavy-chain Ig (IgG/IgA/IgM)	+
Light-chain Ig (kappa/lambda)	+ (moderate expression)
OCT-2	+
Pax-5	+

*Classic phenotype (CD5+/CD10–/CD23–) is seen in 80% of cases. CD5– MCL comprise 11% and CD10+ MCL 6% (majority of them are CD5+). CD23+ MCL are seen in 6% (majority of them are CD5+).

T-cell/histiocyte-rich variant of DLBCL (Figure 2.88) is composed of rare large B-cells and a predominance of reactive elements, such as small T-cells and histiocytes[270–274]. The neoplastic B-cells are atypical and may resemble Reed–Sternberg cells or popcorn cells (L&H cells) of NLPHL. They are surrounded by small T-cells and histiocytes with scanty (if any) small B-cells. There is no apparent nodularity or expanded and disrupted follicular dendritic cell meshwork. Tumor cells are positive for CD45 and B-cell markers, and negative for CD15, EMA and EBV/EBER.

DLBCL with anaplastic features (Figure 2.89) shows marked pleomorphism of tumor cells, which may resemble Reed–Sternberg cells or carcinoma cells[264,275]. Large B-cells tend to form cohesive clusters with an intrasinusoidal distribution[276]. Neoplastic cells are positive for at least some B-cell markers and are negative for cytokeratin, EMA, ALK-1, S100, pan-T antigens, CD15 and EBV/EBER. CD45 may be negative, and many cases are CD30 positive. The term 'anaplastic large cell lymphoma'

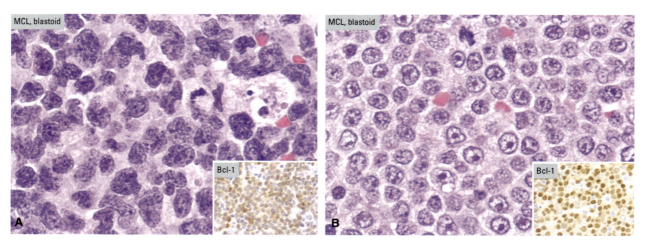

Figure 2.83   Blastoid variants of mantle cell lymphoma. (**A**) Blastoid mantle cell lymphoma with pleomorphic nuclei and few inconspicuous nucleoli. (**B**) This blastoid variant shows prominent nucleoli

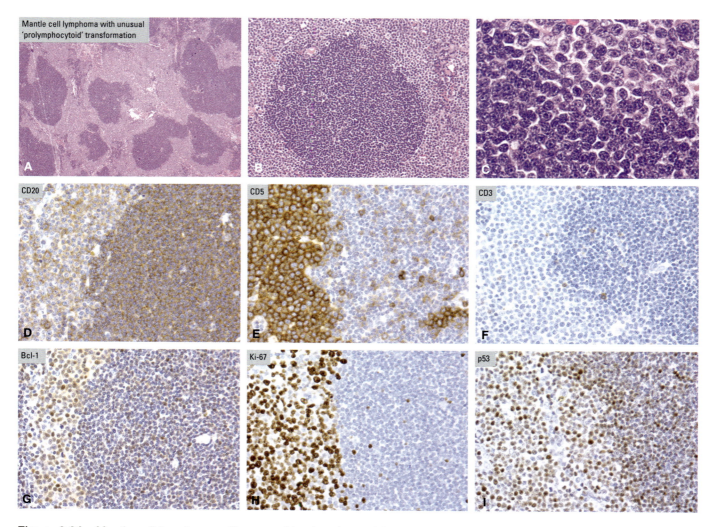

Figure 2.84   Mantle cell lymphoma with unusual 'prolymphocytoid' transformation. (**A**) Low magnification shows two distinct populations of cells: darkly stained small lymphocytes surrounded by larger cells with more abundant eosinophilic cytoplasm. (**B**) Intermediate magnification shows sharp demarcation of two types of lymphoid cells. (**C**) Larger cells have nucleoli and resemble prolymphocytes. Both small and larger cells are positive for CD20 (**D**) and CD5 (**E**). Small lymphocytes are weakly positive for CD5 (compare with negative expression of CD3, **F**). Bcl-1 is positive on both cell populations (**G**), whereas Ki-67 is strongly positive only on large, transformed cells (**H**). p53 is strongly positive (**I**), a feature rarely observed in typical mantle cell lymphoma

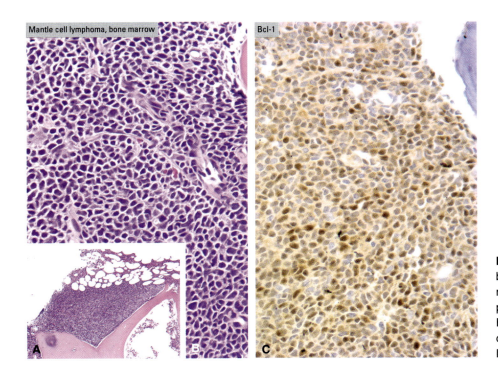

Figure 2.85 Mantle cell lymphoma – bone marrow. (**A**) Histology of bone marrow core biopsy shows a dense paratrabecular lymphoid infiltrate. (**B**) Higher magnification displays nuclear contour irregularities. (**C**) Neoplastic lymphocytes are positive for bcl-1

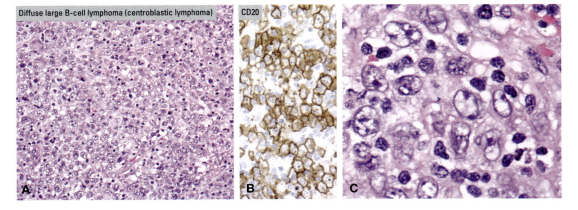

Figure 2.86 Diffuse large B-cell lymphoma (DLBCL) – centroblastic variant. (**A**) Lymph node with diffuse large cell lymphoid infiltrate. (**B**) Neoplastic cells are positive for CD20. (**C**) High magnification shows large atypical cells with up to three nucleoli

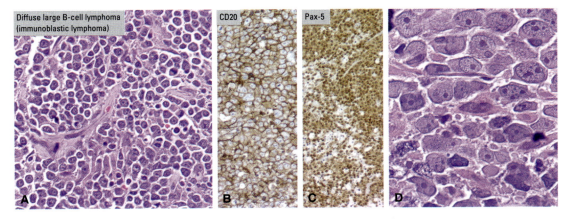

Figure 2.87 Diffuse large B-cell lymphoma (DLBCL) – immunoblastic variant. (**A**) Lymph node with diffuse large cell lymphoid infiltrate. Neoplastic cells are positive for CD20 (**B**) and Pax-5 (**C**). **D** High magnification shows large monomorphic cells with prominent central nucleoli

Table 2.7   Immunophenotypic profile of diffuse large B-cell lymphoma

CD5	–/rare + (*de novo* CD5⁺ DLBCL)
CD10	+/–
CD19	+
CD20	+/very rare may be –
CD22	+
CD23	–/+ (rare)
CD25	–/rare +
CD30	–/+
CD43	–/+
CD45	+/very rare may be –
CD56	–/rare cases +*
CD79a	+
CD103	–/very rare may be + (usually on subset)
Bcl-1	–
Bcl-2	+/–
Bcl-6	–/+
Ki-67	+ (less than 90%)
Light-chain Ig (kappa/lambda)	+/rare –
Pax-5	+
TdT	–

*CD56⁺ DLBCL are usually CD10⁺. EMA and ALK are negative in those cases.

is restricted to large T-cell lymphoma, which is unrelated to the anaplastic variant of DLBCL.

Occasional cases of DLBCL form cohesive sheets of large cells with an amorphous myxoid background (Figure 2.90) resembling metastatic carcinoma. A subset of DLBCL may coexpress CD5 (Figure 2.91). These lymphomas, without any antecedent history of low-grade CD5⁺ B-cell lymphoma, are termed *de novo* CD5⁺ DLBCL and may have a more aggressive clinical behavior[34,121,128]. Another group of DLBCL may be positive for CD56 (Figure 2.92), an NK-cell-associated antigen.

Plasmablastic lymphoma (Figure 2.93) is a rare variant of DLBCL, which usually presents in HIV⁺ patients[277–281]. It was originally described in the oral cavity, and less often presents in lymph nodes, skin, soft tissues and extranodal sites. Disseminated presentation is not uncommon. The presence of large macronucleoli and moderate cytoplasm mimics immunoblastic lymphoma or plasma cell myeloma

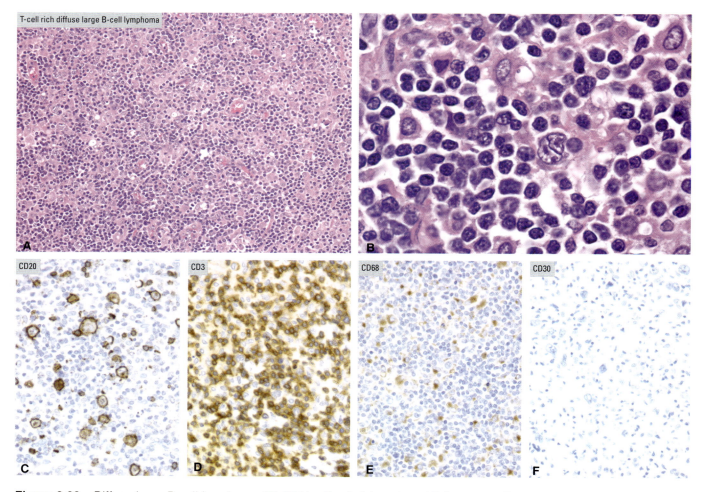

Figure 2.88   Diffuse large B-cell lymphoma (DLBCL) – T-cell-rich variant. (**A**) Low magnification shows effaced lymph node architecture with predominance of small lymphocytes. (**B**) High magnification shows scattered large atypical lymphocytes with nucleoli. Large tumor cells are positive for CD20 (**C**) and are associated with numerous small CD3⁺ T-cells (**D**) and rare histiocytes (**E**, CD68 staining). CD30 is not expressed (**F**)

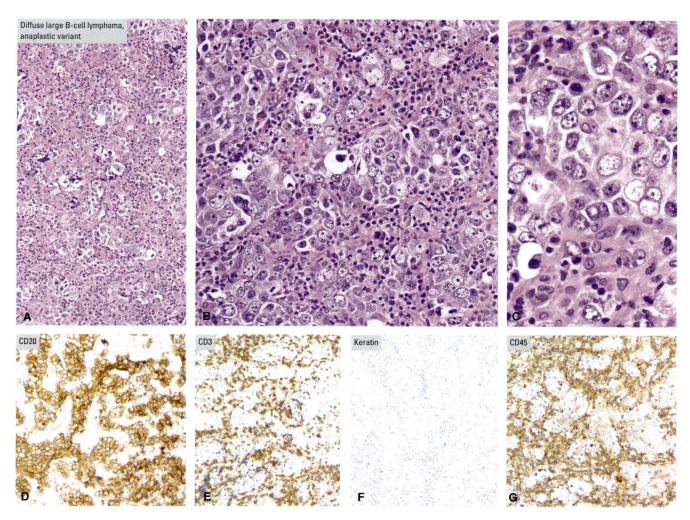

Figure 2.89 Diffuse large B-cell lymphoma (DLBCL) – anaplastic variant. (**A** and **B**) Histologic section shows intrasinusoidal clusters of large lymphoma cells. (**C**) Neoplastic cells have pleomorphic nuclei with irregularly distributed chromatin and nucleoli. (**D**) Large tumor cells show strong membranous staining with CD20. (**E**) Scattered small T-cells are positive for CD3. Tumor cells are negative for cytokeratin (**F**) and CD45 (**G**)

with anaplastic features. Plasmablastic lymphomas are negative for light- and heavy-chain immunoglobulins, CD20, CD79a and bcl-6, and are usually negative for CD43. They are strongly positive for CD138 and are usually positive for CD10 and EBV/EBER (Table 2.8). Positive expression of EBV/EBER and lack of CD20 and bcl-6 distinguish it from DLBCL. EBV/EBER positivity distinguishes it from plasma cell tumors (both plasmablastic lymphoma and plasma cell neoplasms may be positive for CD138, CD56, bcl-1, EMA, CD10 and Pax-5). A variant of plasmablastic lymphoma may occur in the setting of multicentric Castleman's disease (Figure 2.94). The neoplastic cells form vague nodules which are surrounded by polytypic plasma cells. Lymphomatous cells are positive for CD20 (dim), CD45, HHV8 and lambda immunoglobulins.

Diffuse large B-cell lymphoma with expression of ALK (Figure 2.95) is a rare form of DLBCL composed of large, immunoblastic-like cells with prominent nucleoli. This variant of DLBCL is defined by cytoplasmic expression of ALK-1 (Figure 2.95D). There is no evidence of t(2;5) translocation[261,263,282]. Tumor cells have a characteristic phenotype: CD20[-], CD30[-], CD45[+], CD56[+] CD138[+], IgA[+], lambda immunoglobulin[+], kappa immunoglobulin[-] and EMA[+]. Expression of ALK differentiates this lymphoma from plasma cell tumors, plasmablastic lymphoma and immunoblastic lymphoma. Negative CD30 and pan-T antigens exclude anaplastic large cell lymphoma.

The differential diagnosis of DLBCL in the lymph node (Figure 2.96) includes a wide range of primary and secondary lymph node tumors. Anaplastic large cell lymphoma (Figure 2.96A) and peripheral T-cell lymphoma,

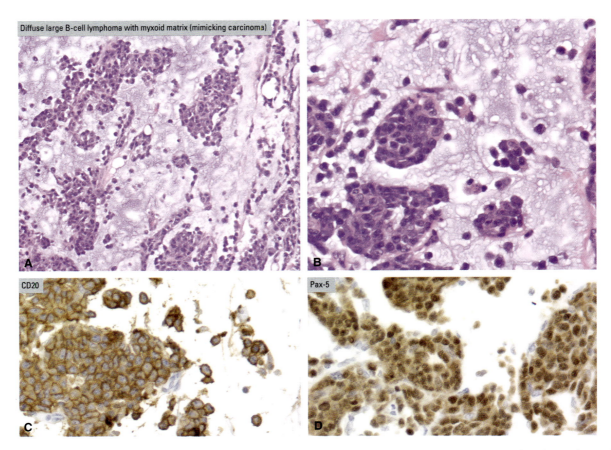

Figure 2.90   Diffuse large B-cell lymphoma with myxoid stroma. (**A** and **B**) Low and high magnifications show clusters of lymphoma cells surrounded by amorphous, basophilic stroma. Large lymphoma cells are positive for CD20 (**C**) and Pax-5 (**D**)

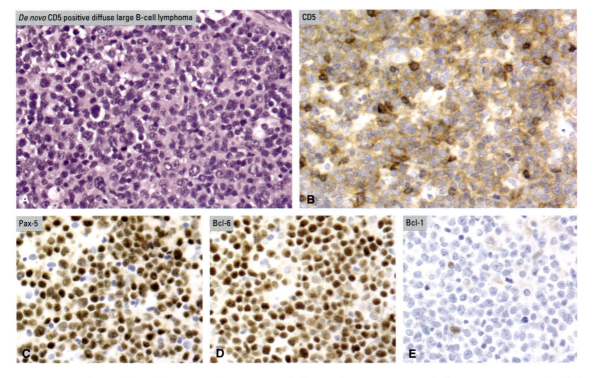

Figure 2.91   *De novo* CD5⁺ diffuse large B-cell lymphoma. Diffuse infiltrate composed of large lymphoid cells (**A**). They are positive for CD5 (**B**), Pax-5 (**C**), and bcl-6 (**D**). Bcl-1 is not expressed (**E**), excluding blastoid variant of mantle cell lymphoma

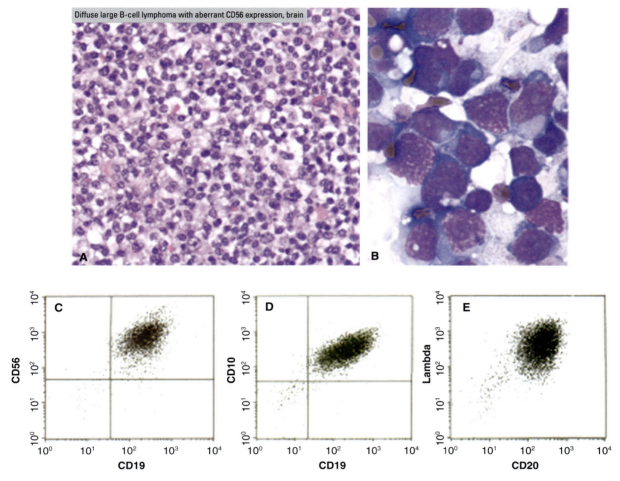

Figure 2.92 Diffuse large B-cell lymphoma with aberrant expression of CD56 – brain. (**A**) Diffuse lymphoid infiltrate composed of large pleomorphic cells. (**B**) Touch smear shows highly atypical cells with high nuclear/cytoplasmic ratio and coarse chromatin. (**C–E**) Flow cytometry shows coexpression of CD19 with CD56 (**C**), CD10 (**D**) and lambda surface immunoglobulin (**E**). A majority of DLBCL with aberrant expression of CD56 are CD10 positive

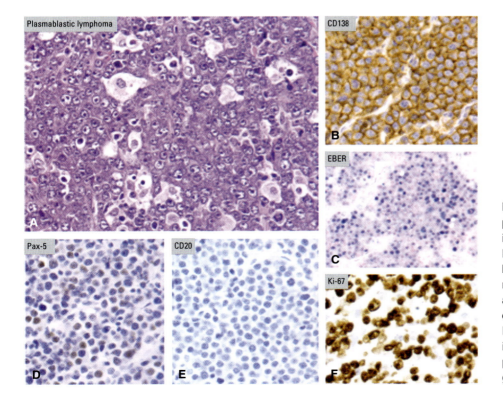

Figure 2.93 Plasmablastic lymphoma. (**A**) Diffuse large cell lymphoid infiltrate with scattered histiocytes. Lymphomatous cells have dense basophilic cytoplasm, vesicular chromatin with thick nuclear membranes and prominent nucleoli. Neoplastic cells are positive for CD138 (**B**), EBER (**C**), and dimly Pax-5 (**D**). CD20 is not expressed (**E**). Ki-67 is strongly positive, which confirms the high-grade nature of this lymphoma (**F**)

Table 2.8 Immunophenotypic profile of plasmablastic lymphoma

CD10	+/(rarely –)
CD20	–
CD30	+ (may be focal)/–
CD43	–
CD45	+/–
CD56	+/–
CD79a	–
CD138	+ (strong)
ALK-1	–
Bcl-1	–/+
Bcl-2	–
Bcl-6	–
BOB-1	+
EBV/EBER	+
EMA	+ (may be focal and dim)
HHV-8	–/*
Heavy-chain Ig (IgG/IgA/IgM)	–
Light-chain Ig (kappa/lambda)	–
OCT-2	+
Pax-5	+/–

*Plasmablastic lymphoma in the background of Castleman's disease shows HHV-8⁺ cells.

unspecified (Figure 2.96B) are distinguished by positive expression of pan-T antigens and lack of B-cell antigens. Blastoid variant of MCL (Figure 2.96C) is distinguished by positive nuclear staining for bcl-1 (cyclin D1). Precursor T-cell lymphoma (Figure 2.96D) is negative for B-cell markers and positive for pan-T antigens, especially CD7 and blastic markers such as TdT. Blastic NK-cell lymphoma (Figure 2.96E) is positive for CD4 and CD56, as well as CD7 in most cases. Metastatic tumors, such as PNET/Ewing sarcoma (Figure 2.96F), poorly differentiated carcinoma (Figure 2.96F and G), or melanoma, are distinguished by lack of CD45, B-cell markers and positive expression of CD99 (PNET), cytokeratin (carcinoma) and S100/HMB-45 (melanoma). Hodgkin lymphoma, especially lymphocyte depleted and the syncytial variant of nodular sclerosis types (Figure 2.96H and M), may be difficult to distinguish from DLBCL, since both tumors may share CD20, CD30 and Pax-5 expression[69,271,283–291]. Expression of CD15, EBV/EBER and negative staining

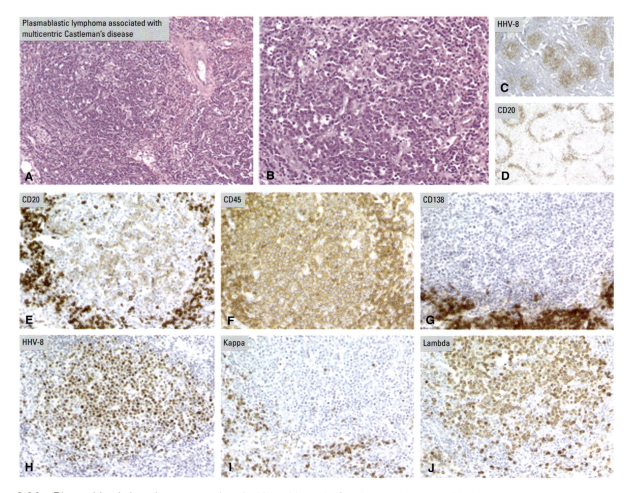

Figure 2.94 Plasmablastic lymphoma associated with multicentric Castleman's disease. (**A**) Low magnification shows a nodular lymphoid infiltrate. (**B**) Higher magnification shows large atypical lymphocytes in the center of the nodules, surrounded by plasma cells. The nodular pattern is best appreciated by immunostaining with HHV-8 (**C**) and CD20 (**D**). Neoplastic B-cells are positive for CD20 (**E**, focal and dim expression), CD45 (**F**), HHV-8 (**H**) and lambda (**J**). Plasma cells are positive for CD138 (**G**). They are polytypic (**I** and **J**)

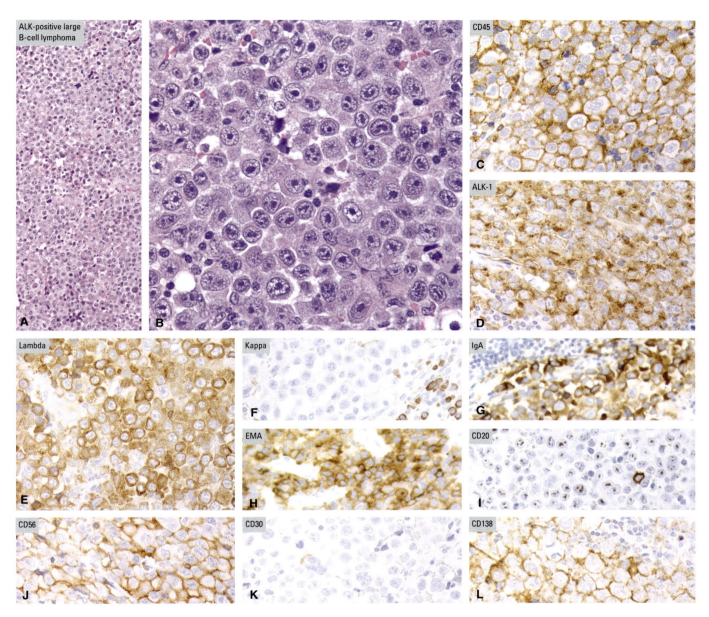

Figure 2.95   ALK positive diffuse large B-cell lymphoma. This is a rare variant of DLBCL with morphologic features resembling plasmablastic lymphoma and immunoblastic lymphoma. Its hallmark is expression of full length ALK-protein. (**A** and **B**) Histologic section shows a diffuse large cell lymphoid infiltrate with prominent central nucleoli. Neoplastic cells are positive for CD45 (**C**), ALK-1 (**D**, cytoplasmic staining), lambda (**E**), IgA (**G**), EMA (**H**), CD56 (**J**) and CD138 (**L**). CD20 (**I**) and CD30 (**K**) are not expressed

for CD45 (LCA) and CD79a, in conjunction with cytomorphologic features (typical Reed–Sternberg cells) and the presence of scattered eosinophils, favors Hodgkin lymphoma. Extramedullary myeloid tumor (granulocytic sarcoma) (Figure 2.96I) is differentiated by expression of pan-myeloid antigens (CD13, CD33, MPO), CD117, CD34, muramidase and/or CD68, and lack of B-cell markers. Nodular lymphocyte-predominant Hodgkin lymphoma (NLPHL) (Figure 2.96J) may be difficult to differentiate from DLBCL, especially the T-cell/histiocyte-rich variant[271,283,284,293–294]. The presence (at least focally)

of a nodular pattern with nodules composed of small B-lymphocytes, with rare large popcorn cells (L&H cells) and preserved (and expanded) follicular dendritic cell meshwork, favors the diagnosis of NLPHL. T-cell/histiocyte-rich DLBCL contains few small B-cells (T-lymphocytes and histiocytes predominate) and does not display a nodular pattern. Immunohistochemical studies may be helpful by documenting positive expression of EMA by popcorn (L&H) cells and the presence of T/NK-cell rosettes around large neoplastic cells, and by confirming the B-cell phenotype of small lymphocytes in

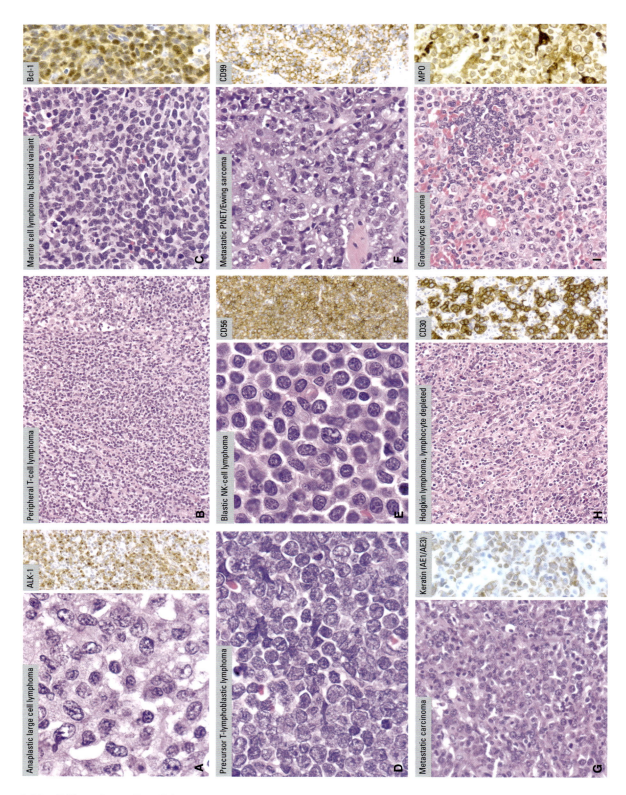

Figure 2.96   Diffuse large B-cell lymphoma – differential diagnosis (lymph node). (**A**) Anaplastic large cell lymphoma. (**B**) Peripheral T-cell lymphoma, unspecified. (**C**) Blastoid variant of mantle cell lymphoma. (**D**) Precursor T-lymphoblastic lymphoma. (**E**) Blastic NK-cell lymphoma. (**F**) Metastatic PNET/Ewing's sarcoma. (**G**) Metastatic poorly differentiated carcinoma. (**H**) Lymphocyte-depleted classical Hodgkin lymphoma. (**I**) Extramedullary myeloid tumor (granulocytic sarcoma). (**J–L**) Nodular lymphocyte-predominant Hodgkin lymphoma (**J**, low magnification; **K**, high magnification; **L**, CD20 staining). (**M**) Syncytial variant of nodular sclerosis Hodgkin lymphoma. (**N**) Histiocytic sarcoma. (**O**) Dendritic cell sarcoma

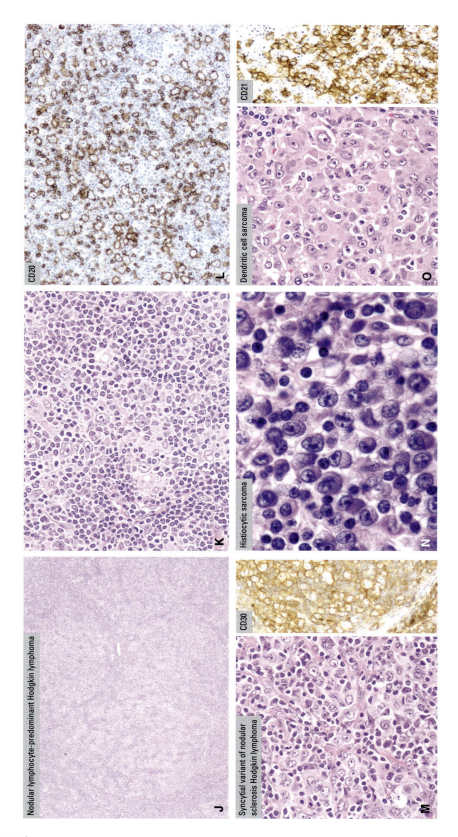

Figure 2.96   (*Continued*)

the background of large neoplastic cells in NLPHL. Both histiocytic sarcoma (Figure 2.96N) and follicular dendritic cell sarcoma are very rare tumors, which are distinguished from DLBCL by lack of B-cell markers, including Pax-5.

The differential diagnosis of DLBCL in the bone marrow includes (among others) plasma cell myeloma (Figure 2.97A), peripheral T-cell lymphoma (Figure 2.97B), precursor B- or T-cell lymphoma/leukemia (Figure 2.97C), anaplastic large cell lymphoma (Figure 2.97D), Langerhans cell histiocytosis (Figure 2.97E), small cell carcinoma (Figure 2.97F), acute myeloid leukemia (Figure 2.97G), alveolar rhabdomyosarcoma (Figure 2.97H) and malignant melanoma (Figure 2.97I). Involvement of the bone marrow by DLBCL may be associated with hemophagocytic syndrome[295].

MEDIASTINAL LARGE B-CELL LYMPHOMA

Mediastinal large B-cell lymphoma is a subtype of diffuse large B-cell lymphoma arising in the mediastinum (thymus) with localized disease and characteristic histomorphologic features[69,78,90,296–307]. Patients present with anterior mediastinal mass (Figure 2.98A) and may have superior vena cava syndrome. Response to treatment is good (Figure 2.98B) but prognosis depends on the initial stage of the disease. On histologic examination (Figure 2.99) there is a diffuse large cell infiltrate with prominent fibrosis, which often separates individual cells. The lymphomatous cells may vary in size and shape, but most cases display abundant clear cytoplasm (Figure 2.99B). Phenotypically, tumor cells are positive for CD45, B-cell markers and often CD30[308] and bcl-6.

INTRAVASCULAR LARGE B-CELL LYMPHOMA

Intravascular large B-cell lymphoma (formerly known as malignant hemangioendotheliomatosis) is a variant of DLBCL characterized by intravascular distribution of tumor cells[66,309]. The disease is most often disseminated and involves skin, brain and other extranodal sites. Bone marrow and lymph nodes may be involved. Neoplastic cells are large with irregular nuclei and prominent nucleoli. They are distributed in the lumina of small to medium-sized vessels (Figure 2.100). Occasional cases (Figure 2.101) have anaplastic features and may resemble metastatic carcinoma on HE examination. Tumor cells are positive for CD45, B-cell markers and occasionally CD5 (Figure 2.100H) and CD30.

PRIMARY EFFUSION LYMPHOMA (PEL)

PEL is a human herpes virus 8 (HHV-8)-associated, body cavity-based, large B-cell lymphoma involving the pleura, peritoneum, pericardium and scrotum, usually in immunocompromised patients[129,310–318]. Patients usually have a serous effusion without adenopathy.

Tumor cells are large with either immunoblastic or plasmablastic features (Figure 2.102). Cytoplasm is densely basophilic and moderate to abundant. Nuclei are large and often irregular with prominent nucleoli. Histology (either cell block preparations or pleural biopsy) reveals large closely packed neoplastic cells with abundant cytoplasm, large nuclei with coarse unevenly distributed chromatin and prominent nucleoli (Figure 2.103). Phenotypically, PEL is positive for HHV-8 and EBER (Figure 2.103B and C). Most cases express CD45, CD30, CD38/CD138 and EMA. B-cell markers, including CD19, CD20, CD22 and CD79a, are negative, but occasional cases are positive for Pax-5, BOB-1 and OCT-2 and may show aberrant cytoplasmic expression of T-cell antigen CD3 (Figure 2.103E).

The differential diagnosis of PEL includes large B-cell lymphomas, plasma cell neoplasms, anaplastic large cell lymphoma and other T-cell lymphomas, mesothelioma and poorly differentiated carcinoma[319,320]. Plasma cell tumors differ in positive staining with cytoplasmic immunoglobulins and lack of HHV-8 and EBER. Anaplastic large cell lymphoma can be excluded by lack of ALK-1, pan-T antigens (except CD3) and positive HHV-8 and EBER. Metastatic carcinoma and mesothelioma are distinguished by the expression of epithelial markers.

BURKITT LYMPHOMA

Burkitt lymphoma is a high-grade B-cell neoplasm composed of medium-sized lymphocytes forming a monotonous and diffuse infiltrate with a characteristic starry-sky pattern[51,96,321–324]. The hallmark of Burkitt lymphoma is a translocation involving c-myc. Burkitt lymphoma occurs endemically or sporadically in children and young adults, with an increased incidence in HIV+ patients.

Burkitt lymphoma occurs more often in extranodal locations: jaw tumors are common in the endemic variant and an abdominal location prevails in sporadic cases.

Regardless of the site of involvement, Burkitt lymphoma exhibits monotonous infiltrate of medium-sized lymphocytes with minimal variation in cell size and shape (Figures 2.104 and 2.105). The infiltrate contains numerous mitotic figures and apoptotic cells.

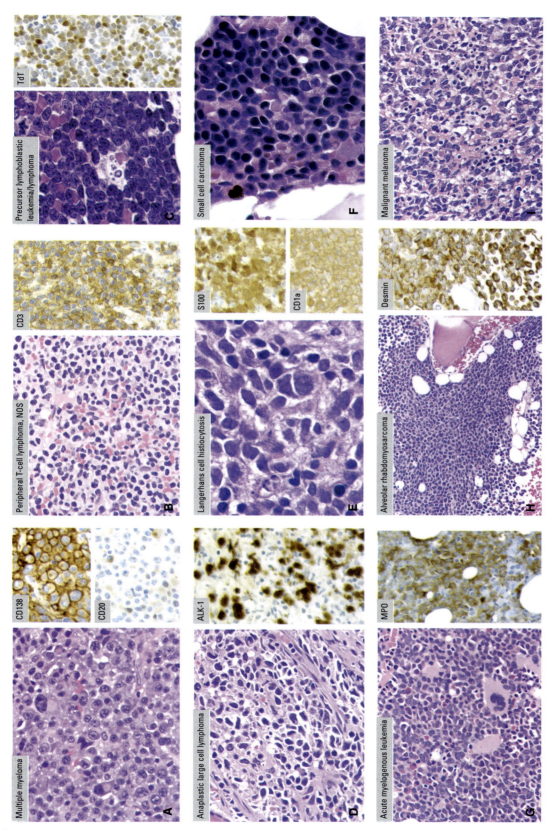

Figure 2.97   Diffuse large B-cell lymphoma – differential diagnosis (bone marrow). **(A)** Plasma cell myeloma. **(B)** Peripheral T-cell lymphoma, unspecified. **(C)** Precursor lymphoblastic leukemia. **(D)** Anaplastic large cell lymphoma. **(E)** Langerhans cell histiocytosis. **(F)** Metastatic small cell carcinoma. **(G)** Acute myeloid leukemia. **(H)** Metastatic alveolar rhabdomyosarcoma. **(I)** Metastatic malignant melanoma

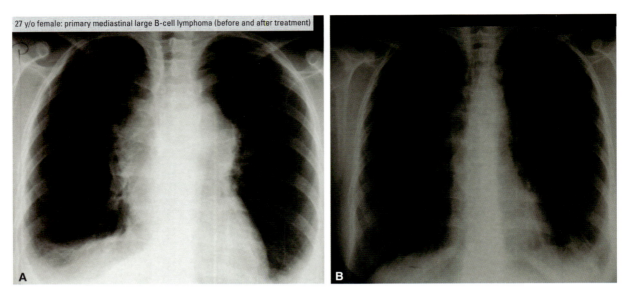

Figure 2.98 Radiographs of mediastinum demonstrating primary mediastinal large B-cell lymphoma (**A**, at diagnosis; **B**, after treatment)

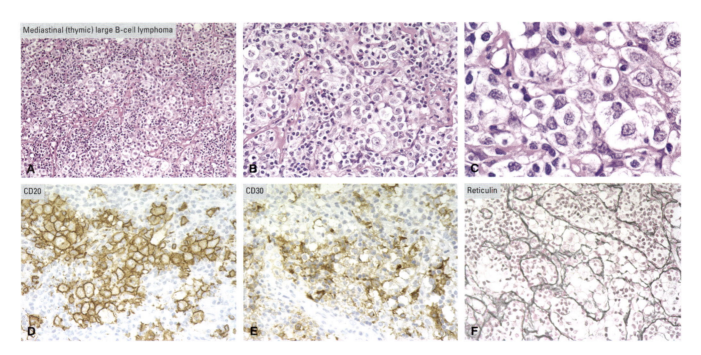

Figure 2.99 Primary mediastinal large B-cell lymphoma. (**A–C**) Histologic sections show diffuse large cell infiltrate. Neoplastic cells have abundant pale (clear) cytoplasm and irregular nuclei with nucleoli, which resemble centroblasts. (**D** and **E**) Immunohistochemical staining demonstrates positive expression of CD20 (**D**) and CD30 (**E**). (**F**) Reticulin staining shows delicate fibrosis around tumor cell clusters

The presence of tingible-body macrophages creates a starry-sky pattern (Figure 2.104A). Medium-sized nuclei (comparable to nuclei of histiocytes) and lack of pleomorphism to help distinguish Burkitt lymphoma from DLBCL.

Phenotypic characteristics of Burkitt lymphoma are summarized in Table 2.9. Tumor cells are positive for CD45, B-cell markers, CD10, CD43 and bcl-6 (Figures 2.104 and 2.105). They lack bcl-2 expression. CD21 expression is variable and is more often associated with the endemic form. Blastic markers (TdT and CD34) are negative. The proliferation index determined by Ki-67 staining (MIB1) approaches 100%. Burkitt lymphoma in immunocompromised patient is often EBER positive. The diagnosis of Burkitt lymphoma requires confirmation of c-*myc* expression (Figure 2.105G).

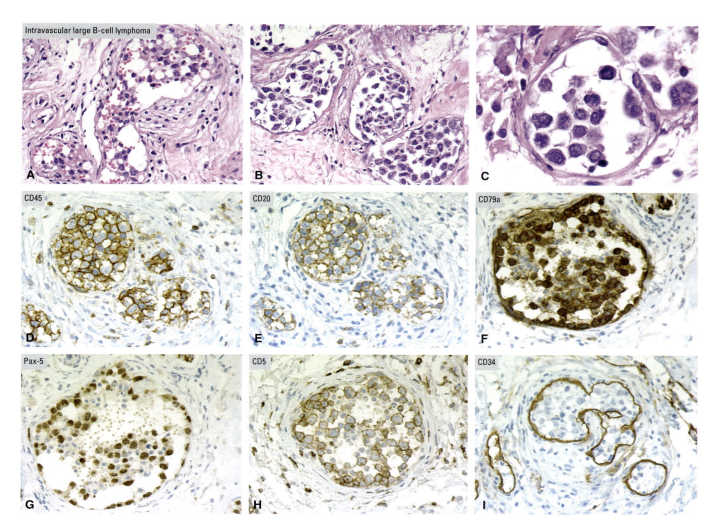

Figure 2.100   Intravascular large B-cell lymphoma (bladder). (**A**–**C**) Histology: large atypical lymphoid cells with nucleoli within vascular spaces. (**D**–**I**) Immunohistochemistry: tumor cells are positive for CD45 (**D**), CD20 (**E**), CD79a (**F**), Pax-5 (**G**) and CD5 (**H**). CD34 staining shows vessel wall (**I**)

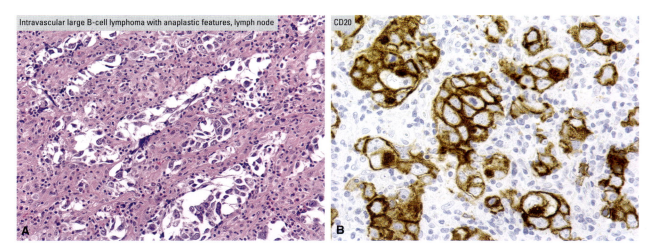

Figure 2.101   Intravascular large B-cell lymphoma. (**A**) Dilated sinuses contain large lymphomatous cells with anaplastic features. (**B**) Tumor cells exhibit strong membranous expression of CD20

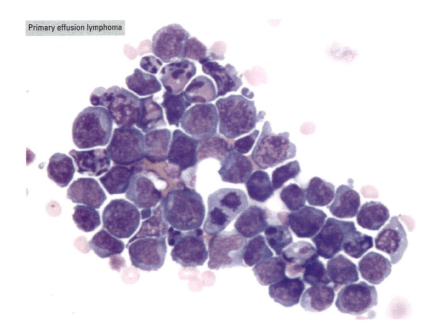

Figure 2.102   Primary effusion lymphoma – cytology (cytospin preparation). The tumor cells are large and pleomorphic with increased nuclear: cytoplasmic ratio, basophilic cytoplasm and irregular nuclei

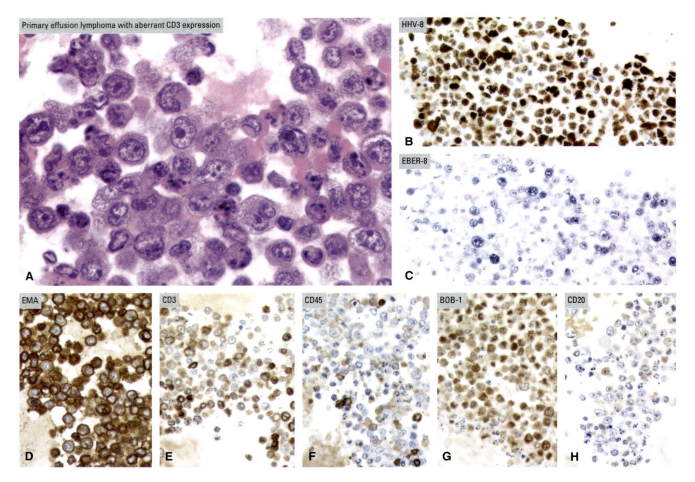

Figure 2.103   Primary effusion lymphoma with aberrant expression of CD3 – immunohistochemistry (cell block preparation) (**A**) Highly pleomorphic tumor cells have prominent nucleoli. Lymphomatous cells are positive for HHV-8 (**B**), EBER (**C**), EMA (**D**), CD3 (**E**), CD45 (**F**) and BOB-1 (**G**). CD20 is not expressed (**H**)

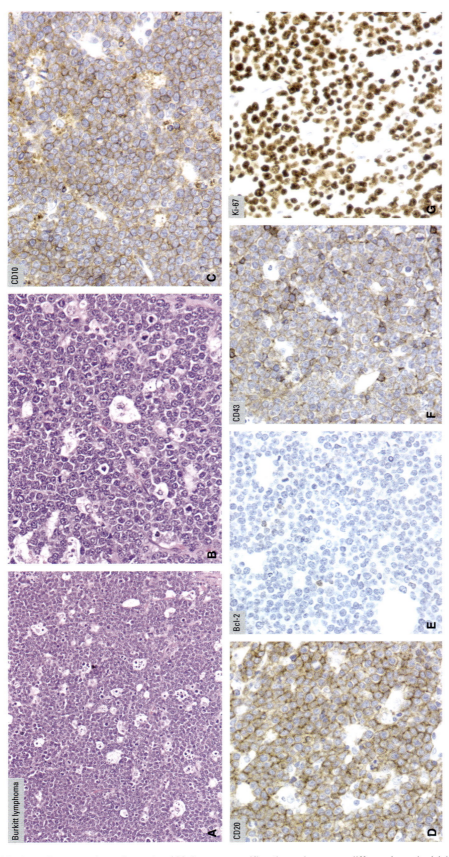

Figure 2.104   Burkitt lymphoma – lymph node. (**A**) Low magnification shows a diffuse lymphoid infiltrate with scattered histiocytes ('starry-sky' pattern). (**B**) High magnification shows medium-sized, monomorphic lymphomatous cells with increased nuclear: cytoplasmic ratio. Tingible-body macrophages are present. Immunohistochemistry reveals the classic phenotype: positive expression of CD10 (**C**), CD20 (**D**) and CD43 (**F**) and lack of staining with bcl-2 (**E**). Proliferation index as determined by staining with Ki-67 (MIB-1) approaches 100% (**G**)

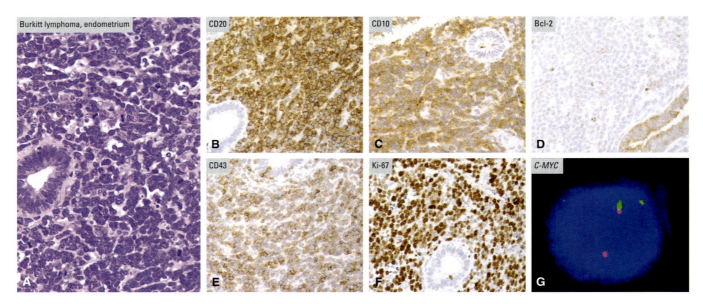

Figure 2.105 Burkitt lymphoma – endometrium. (**A**) Dense monomorphic lymphoid infiltrate with somewhat 'blastoid' appearance composed of medium-sized cells with high nuclear: cytoplasmic ratio. The tumor cells are positive for CD20 (**B**), CD10 (**C**) and CD43 (**E**) and are negative for bcl-2 (**D**). Ki-67 is strongly positive (**F**). The diagnosis of Burkitt lymphoma was confirmed by molecular studies (translocation involving c-*myc*; **G**)

The differential diagnosis of Burkitt lymphoma includes diffuse large B-cell lymphoma[96,325,326], which may resemble Burkitt lymphoma morphologically or phenotypically (Figure 2.106). DLBCL with a monomorphic lymphoid infiltrate (Figure 2.106, column A) differs from Burkitt lymphoma in lack of CD10, CD43 and positive bcl-2 expression. The proliferation fraction rarely exceeds 80%, whereas in Burkitt lymphoma it is close to 100%[96]. DLBCL which are positive for CD10, CD43 and bcl-6, and negative for bcl-2 (Figure 2.106, column C) can be differentiated from Burkitt lymphoma by cellular pleomorphism, larger cell size, and/or lower proliferation fraction. FISH/molecular studies for c-*myc*

may be needed for final interpretation, keeping in mind that c-*myc* is not 100% specific for Burkitt lymphoma[96]. Differential diagnosis also includes precursor B- and T-lymphoblastic lymphoma/leukemia[326–329]. Precursor B-lymphoblastic leukemia/lymphoma (B-ALL) can be distinguished by positive expression of blastic markers (e.g., CD34 or TdT), lack of bcl-6 and lack of the expression of surface immunoglobulins. Precursor T-lymphoblastic lymphoma/leukemia is distinguished by lack of expression of B-cell markers and presence of one or more pan-T antigens.

LYMPHOMATOID GRANULOMATOSIS

Lymphomatoid granulomatosis is an EBV-associated B-cell lymphoproliferative process with a polymorphous lymphoid infiltrate composed of a variable number of large B-cells and reactive small T-lymphocytes, characterized by an angiocentric/angiodestructive growth pattern[331–335]. Lymphomatoid granulomatosis most often involves lung, but other extranodal sites may be also involved[336,337].

Morphologically (Figure 2.107), lymphomatoid granulomatosis shows an atypical polymorphic infiltrate composed predominantly of lymphocytes in an inflammatory background (histiocytes, eosinophils, plasma cells) with vascular tropism. Prominent areas of (distal) necrosis may be present as a result of vascular compromise. Large B-cells are positive for EBV/EBER (Figure 2.107E). Depending on the number of those cells, lymphomatoid granulomatosis is divided into grades 1, 2 and 3.

Table 2.9   Immunophenotypic profile of Burkitt lymphoma

CD5	–
CD10	+
CD19	+ (moderate)
CD20	+ (moderate to bright)
CD22	+
CD23	–/+ (rare)
CD25	–
CD30	–
CD43	+
CD45	+
CD79a	+
Bcl-1	–
Bcl-2	–
Bcl-6	+
EBV/EBER	–*
Ki-67	+ (strong, approximately 100%)
Light-chain Ig (kappa/lambda)	+
Pax-5	+
TdT	–

*Burkitt lymphomas in HIV+ patients may be positive for EBV/EBER.

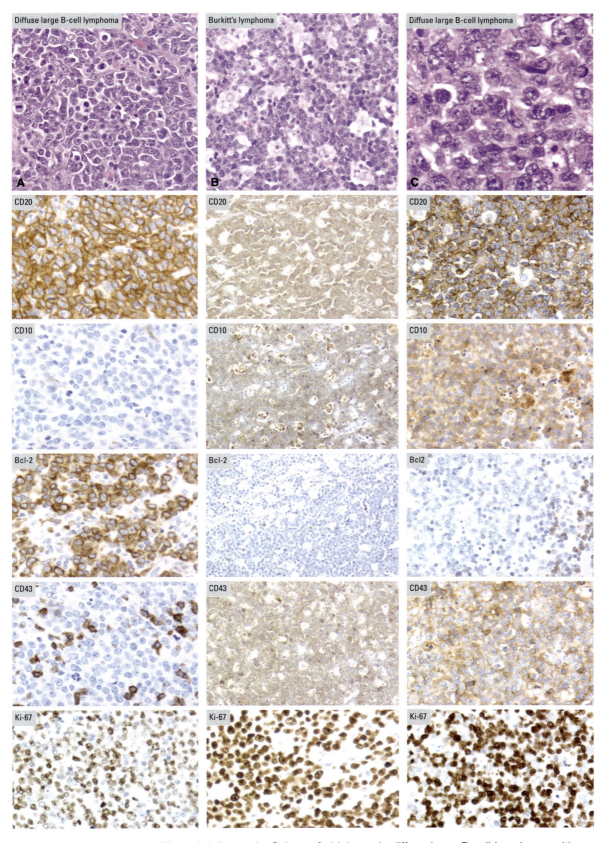

Figure 2.106   Burkitt lymphoma – differential diagnosis. Column **A**, high-grade diffuse large B-cell lymphoma with morphologic features resembling Burkitt lymphoma. Negativity for CD10 and CD43 and positive expression of bcl-2 distinguishes this from Burkitt lymphoma. Column **B**, Burkitt lymphoma with typical morphology and phenotype (CD20$^+$, CD10$^+$, bcl-2$^-$, CD43$^+$). Column **C**, diffuse large B-cell lymphoma with phenotype similar to Burkitt lymphoma (compare with column B). In contrast to Burkitt lymphoma, neoplastic cells are larger and nuclei display prominent pleomorphism. Additionally, the fraction of proliferating cells as determined by immunostaining with Ki-67 (MIB-1) is usually lower in DLBCL than in Burkitt lymphoma

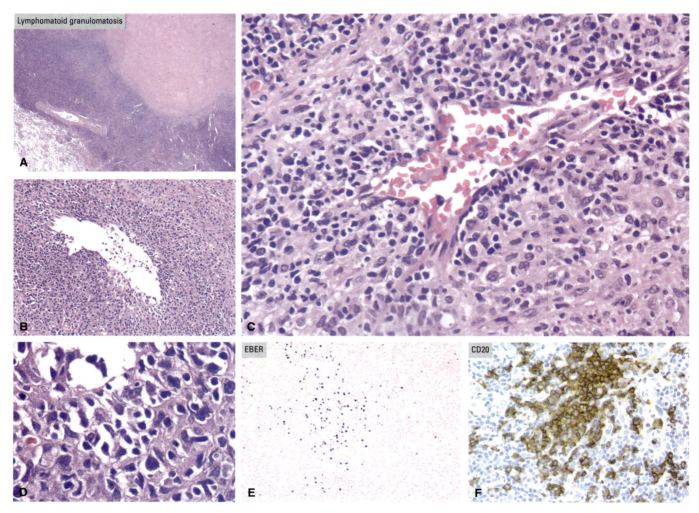

Figure 2.107   Lymphomatoid granulomatosis – lung. (**A**) Low magnification shows lung parenchyma with dense lymphoid infiltrate and infarct-like tissue necrosis. (**B–D**). Higher magnifications show a polymorphous infiltrate in and around the vascular wall. Scattered large pleomorphic cells are present. They are positive for EBER (**E**) and CD20 (**F**)

CHAPTER 3

Mature T-cell lymphoproliferative disorders

T-cell lymphoproliferative disorders are a heterogeneous and relatively uncommon group of lymphoid tumors that can present as adenopathy, hepatosplenomegaly, skin lesions, a mass involving a variety of other organs or as leukemia[338–354]. T/NK-cell lymphoproliferations show variations in incidence in different geographical regions, mostly associated with the prevalence of HTLV-I and EBV infections[355–359]. Morphologically and clinically, they can mimic both benign conditions and non-hematopoietic neoplasms. The diagnosis often requires a multimethodological approach including morphology, flow cytometry, immunohistochemistry, cytogenetics/FISH and molecular studies (PCR, Southern blot)[20,22,38,41–43,265,348,360–362]. Since all these techniques are not always precise, clinical data still play an important role in their diagnosis and subclassification. Clinically, they are usually aggressive, although some disorders respond well to treatment (e.g., ALK+ anaplastic large cell lymphoma) or have prolonged, non-progressive course (T-large granular lymphocyte leukemia). Table 3.1 presents the current WHO classification of T- and NK-cell lymphoproliferative disorders.

T-CELL PROLYMPHOCYTIC LEUKEMIA (T-PLL)

T-cell prolymphocytic leukemia (T-PLL) is a neoplastic process of small to medium-sized lymphocytes with nuclear contour irregularities and occasionally prominent nucleoli[124,363–367]. It is an aggressive disorder involving peripheral blood, bone marrow, lymph node, spleen, liver, skin and other organs[78,368]. Most patients have marked lymphocytosis, hepatosplenomegaly and adenopathy. There is no association with human T-cell lymphotropic viruses (HTLV-I/II)[369–371].

Table 3.1 Classification of peripheral (mature) T-cell and NK-cell neoplasms

T-cell prolymphocytic leukemia (T-PLL)
T-cell large granular lymphocytic leukemia (T-LGL leukemia)
Aggressive NK-cell leukemia
Adult T-cell leukemia/lymphoma
Extranodal NK/T-cell lymphoma, nasal type
Enteropathy-type T-cell lymphoma
Hepatosplenic T-cell lymphoma
Subcutaneous panniculitis-like T-cell lymphoma
Mycosis fungoides/Sezary syndrome (MF/SS)
Primary cutaneous anaplastic large cell lymphoma
Peripheral T-cell lymphoma, unspecified
Angioimmunoblastic T-cell lymphoma (AILD lymphoma)
Anaplastic large cell lymphoma (ALCL)
T-cell proliferation of uncertain malignant potential
    Lymphomatoid papulosis

In the peripheral blood film (Figure 3.1), there are numerous lymphoid cells with scanty basophilic cytoplasm and prominent nuclear irregularities. A nucleolus is usually prominent, but it may be inconspicuous, resembling B-cell chronic lymphocytic leukemia. Bone marrow (Figure 3.2) involvement is characterized by an interstitial lymphoid infiltrate, which varies from subtle to diffuse.

Immunophenotypic analysis by immunohistochemistry (Figure 3.2) or flow cytometry (Figure 3.3) shows expression of CD45 and pan-T antigens (CD2, CD3, CD5, CD7) and lack of expression of B-cell markers, HLA-DR, CD1a, TdT and CD34. Table 3.2 presents phenotypic characteristics of T-PLL. The majority of cases show moderate/bright expression of CD45 (rare cases are CD45 negative). Normal expression of pan-T antigens is present in 57% of cases, a feature rarely seen in other

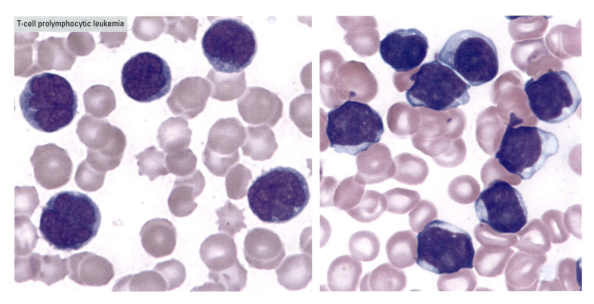

Figure 3.1   T-cell prolymphocytic leukemia (T-PLL) – peripheral blood films. Small to medium-sized lymphocytes with scanty basophilic cytoplasm and markedly irregular nuclei are seen

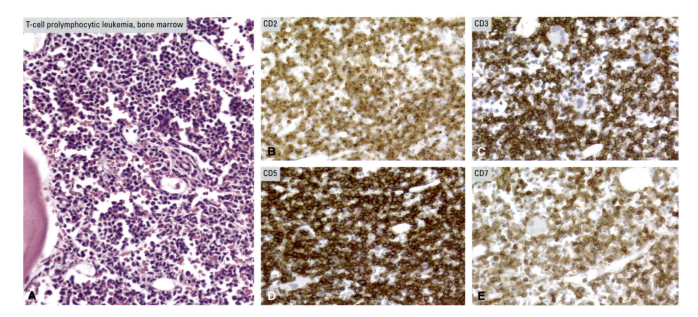

Figure 3.2   T-cell prolymphocytic leukemia (T-PLL) – bone marrow. Core biopsy shows prominent lymphocytosis of predominantly small lymphocytes (**A**) with expression of all four pan-T antigens (**B–E**). The expression of CD2 and CD7 (**B** and **E**) is slightly dimmer than that of CD3 and CD5 (**C** and **D**)

T-cell lymphoproliferations (see Table 1.6; Chapter 1). In 50% of cases, the T-PLL are CD4$^+$, in 25% they are CD8$^+$, in 14% they coexpress CD4/CD8, and in the remaining 11% they are CD4/CD8 negative. Figure 3.4 presents complex chromosomal abnormalities in T-PLL, which include inversion of chromosome 14. The latter is a characteristic feature of T-PLL.

T-PLL involvement of the lymph node (Figures 3.5 and 3.6) is usually paracortical with preserved follicles but may be diffuse with total effacement of lymph node architecture. The spleen shows dense white and red pulp infiltration, and the liver (Figure 3.7) shows dense lymphoid infiltration in portal areas and within sinusoids.

The differential diagnosis of T-PLL includes B- and T-cell disorders (Figure 3.8) composed of small to medium-sized lymphocytes. B-CLL/SLL is distinguished by expression of B-cell antigens and HLA-DR. B-CLL/PLL, except

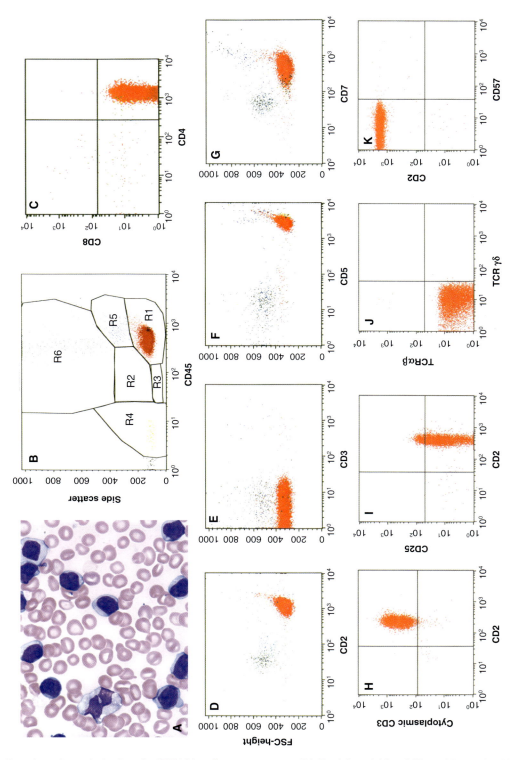

Figure 3.3 T-cell prolymphocytic leukemia (T-PLL) – flow cytometry. (**A**) Peripheral blood film with marked lymphocytosis. (**B**) Flow cytometry analysis shows predominance of lymphocytes (red). Note the paucity of granulocytes and monocytes. Lymphocytes display CD4 subset restriction (**C**) and bright expression of CD2 (**D**), CD5 (**F**) and CD7 (**G**). Surface CD3 is absent (**E**) but cytoplasmic CD3 is present (**H**). Neoplastic lymphocytes do not coexpress CD25 (**I**) or CD57 (**K**). They show lack of TCR alpha/beta and TCR gamma/delta (**J**)

for the characteristic coexpression of CD5/CD23/ CD43, may be rarely positive for other pan-T antigens and/or CD8. Other B-cell lymphoproliferations are excluded by positive expression of B-cell antigens. Adult T-cell leukemia/lymphoma (ATLL) and Sezary syndrome (SS) are predominantly CD4+ and have more pronounced nuclear

Table 3.2   Immunophenotypic profile of T-prolymphocytic leukemia

Marker	%
CD2+	96
CD3+	89
CD5+	92
CD7+	89
All pan-T antigens normally expressed	57
One pan-T antigens negative	17
Two pan-T antigens negative	7
Three pan-T antigens negative	0
Four pan-T antigens negative	0
CD4+	50
CD8+	25
CD4/CD8+	14
CD4/CD8−	11
TCRαβ+	92
TCRγδ+	0
TCR−	8
CD10+	0
CD11c+	4
CD25+	Rare
CD56+	7
CD117+	14.3*

*Expression of CD117 is restricted to CD8+ T-PLL (!).

T-PLL with inv(14)(q11.2q32), add(7)(p22), r(17), −19, −20, −22, +1,

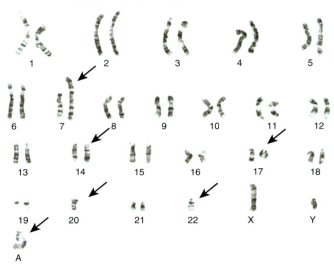

Figure 3.4   T-cell prolymphocytic leukemia (T-PLL) – cytogenetics. Complex chromosomal abnormalities, including inversion of chromosome 14, are present

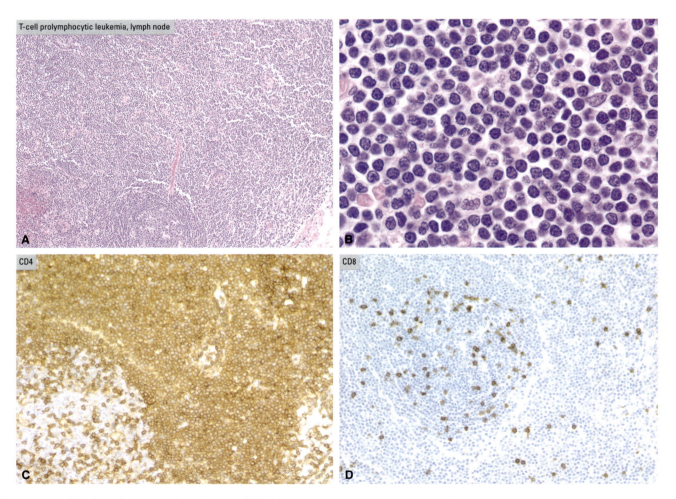

Figure 3.5   T-cell prolymphocytic leukemia (T-PLL) – lymph node. (**A**) Low magnification shows a diffuse lymphoid infiltrate sparing the follicle. (**B**) High magnification shows predominance of small, mature-appearing lymphocytes. Neoplastic cells show CD4 restriction (**C** and **D**)

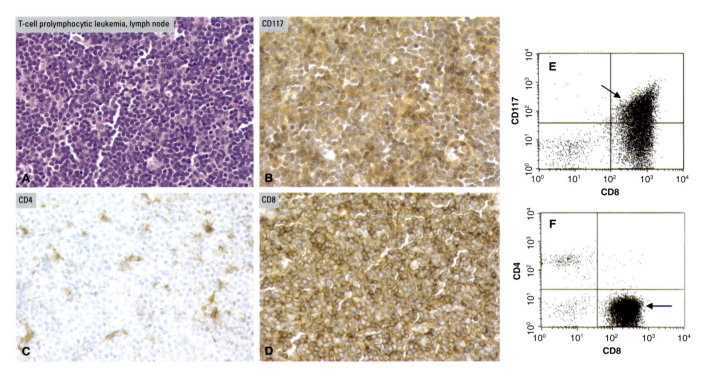

Figure 3.6   T-cell prolymphocytic leukemia (T-PLL) – lymph node. (**A**) Diffuse small lymphocytic infiltrate. Lymphomatous cells show aberrant expression of CD117 (**B**, immunohistochemistry; **E**, flow cytometry) and are CD4⁻/CD8⁺ (**C** and **D**, immunohistochemistry; **F**, flow cytometry). Aberrant expression of CD117 is seen in occasional cases of T-PLL (only in CD8⁺ cases); see Table 3.2 for details

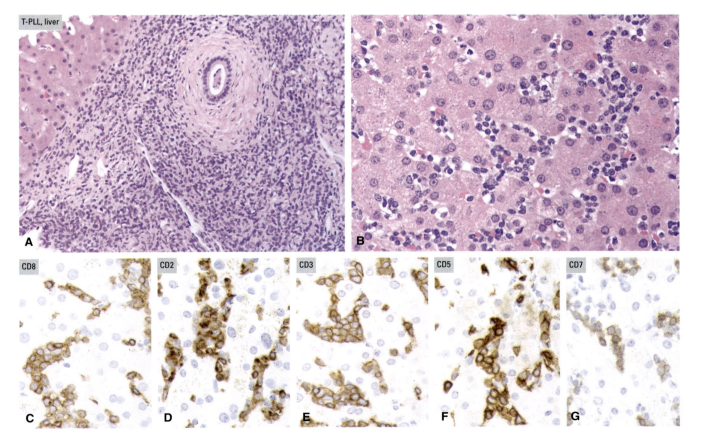

Figure 3.7   T-cell prolymphocytic leukemia (T-PLL) – liver. (**A**) Low magnification shows a dense lymphoid infiltrate within the portal area. (**B**) High magnification shows lymphocytes within sinusoidal spaces. Neoplastic cells are CD8 positive (**C**) and express all pan-T antigens (**D–G**)

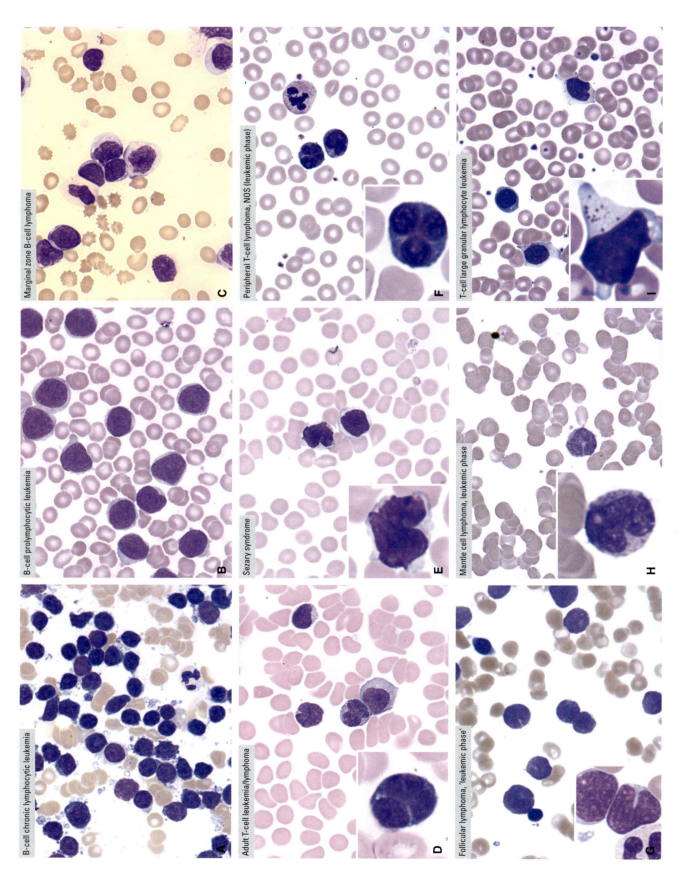

Figure 3.8   Peripheral blood with lymphocytosis – differential diagnosis of T-PLL. (**A**) B-chronic lymphocytic leukemia. (**B**) B-prolymphocytic leukemia. (**C**) Marginal zone B-cell lymphoma. (**D**) Adult T-cell leukemia/lymphoma. (**E**) Sezary syndrome. (**F**) Peripheral T-cell lymphoma, unspecified. (**G**) Leukemic phase of follicular lymphoma. (**H**) Mantle cell lymphoma. (**I**) T-cell large granular lymphocyte leukemia

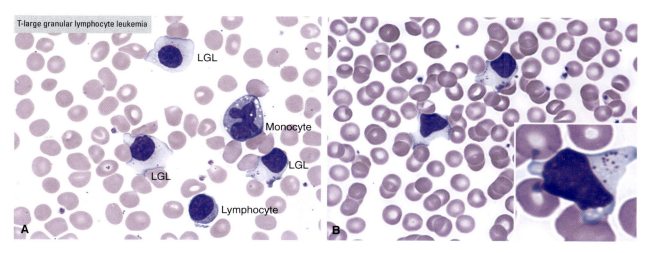

Figure 3.9   T-cell large granular lymphocyte (LGL) leukemia. Peripheral blood films (**A** and **B**) show several LGLs with prominent cytoplasmic granules. Compare with monocytes and normal small lymphocytes (**A**)

irregularities. In contrast to T-PLL, they rarely display normal expression of all four pan-T antigens (Table 1.6; Chapter 1). Clinical and laboratory data are helpful in the differential diagnosis (e.g., hypercalcemia and positive HTLV-1 favor ATLL). Peripheral T-cell lymphoma, unspecified, is generally a more pleomorphic T-cell infiltrate composed of medium-sized to large cells which display aberrant expression of pan-T antigens in more than 90% of cases. Large granular lymphocyte leukemia is distinguished by specific cytomorphology and phenotype (see below).

LARGE GRANULAR LYMPHOCYTE (LGL) LEUKEMIA

LGL leukemia is characterized by lymphoid cells with abundant cytoplasm and azurophilic MPO-negative granules (Figure 3.9). Two variants of LGL proliferations can be recognized: T-cell LGL leukemia and NK-LGL leukemia[345,358,362,372-386]. T-LGL leukemia involves the peripheral blood, bone marrow, liver and spleen. It has an indolent clinical course and may be associated with neutropenia, red cell aplasia, hypergammaglobulinemia and rheumatoid arthritis (RA). Apart from RA, T-LGL leukemia may be associated with other systemic autoimmune diseases, as well as hematologic malignancies, such as paroxysmal nocturnal hemoglobinuria, myelodysplastic syndromes, acute myeloid leukemia and B-cell lymphoproliferative disorders. Transformation of T-LGL leukemia to high-grade tumors is rare[387].

On flow cytometry analysis, T-LGL leukemia has a mature T-cell phenotype (Table 3.3) with CD8 expression and TCRαβ expression. Rare cases may be CD4+/CD8+, CD4+/CD8- or CD4-/CD8-. CD11b, CD11c and NK-cell-associated markers are variably expressed (Table 3.3).

Table 3.3   Immunophenotypic profile of large granular lymphocyte leukemia (LGL)

Marker	T-LGL (%)	NK-LGL (%)
CD2+	100	100
CD3+	100	0
CD5+	80	0
CD7+	89	100
All pan-T antigens positive	8.3	0
One pan-T antigen negative	30.5	0
Two pan-T antigens negative	0	100
Three pan-T antigens negative	0	0
Four pan-T antigens negative	0	0
CD4+	2.5	0
CD8+	87	23
CD4/CD8+	8	0
CD4/CD8-	2.5	77
TCRαβ+	78	8
TCRγδ+	22	0
TCR-	0	92
CD11c+	44	61
CD16+	34*	70*
CD56+	33*	70*
CD57+	97	61

*None of the T-LGL leukemias coexpressed CD16 and CD56, whereas 1/3 of NK-LGL leukemias coexpressed all three antigens (CD16, CD56, CD57).

Of the NK-cell-associated markers, CD57 is most frequently expressed (97%), whereas CD16 or CD56 are present in approximately one-third of cases. T-LGL leukemias generally lack CD16 and CD56 coexpression.

NK-LGL leukemias are less common and are usually classified with NK-cell disorders. They usually have a chronic, non-progressive clinical course. Patients are either asymptomatic or have a gradual increase in circulating large granular lymphocytes. These cases differ clinically from T-LGL leukemia in lack of neutropenia, anemia or rheumatoid arthritis. The phenotypic hallmark of NK-LGL leukemia is lack of CD3 and CD5 and positive

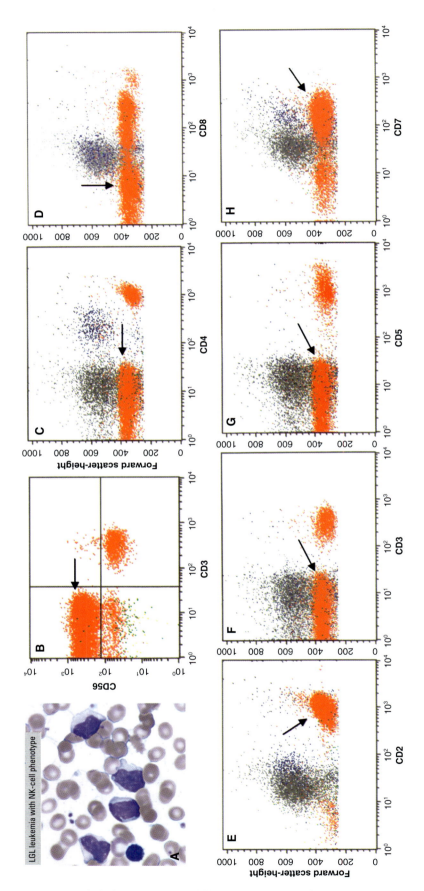

Figure 3.10   Large granular lymphocyte (LGL) leukemia with NK-cell phenotype – flow cytometry. Atypical lymphocytes (**A**) are positive for CD56 (**B**), and negative for CD4 and CD8 (**C** and **D**). Characteristically, NK-LGL cells are positive for CD2 and CD7 and lack the expression of CD3 and CD5 (**E–H**)

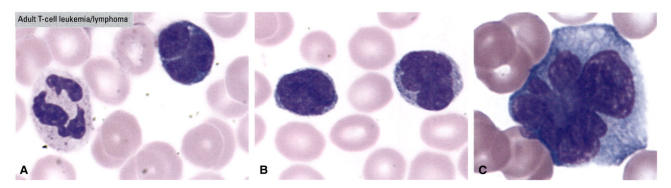

Figure 3.11 Adult T-cell leukemia/lymphoma. (**A–C**) Typical medium to large neoplastic cells with prominent nuclear pleomorphism ('flower cells')

expression of CD2 and CD7 (Figure 3.10). In contrast to T-LGL leukemias, LGL with NK-cell phenotype more often shows expression of CD16 (70%) and CD56 (70%), with 35% of cases coexpressing those two antigens (Table 3.3). CD57 is present in 60% of cases.

ADULT T-CELL LYMPHOMA/LEUKEMIA

Adult T-cell lymphoma/leukemia (ATLL) is a peripheral T-cell disorder associated with human T-cell leukemia virus type 1 (HTLV-I) infection and is characterized by highly pleomorphic lymphoid cells[358,370,388–391]. Clinically, ATLL varies in prognosis. The acute variant of ATLL presents with disseminated disease involving peripheral blood, skin, and lymph nodes, and is characterized by leukocytosis and hypercalcemia with lytic bone lesions. Generalized lymphadenopathy without peripheral blood involvement is the main feature of the lymphomatous variant. In the chronic variant, patients present with exfoliative skin lesions. In the smoldering variant, the white blood count is normal and there are only occasional atypical circulating leukemic cells. The distribution of ATLL is closely linked to the prevalence of HTLV-I infection.

In the peripheral blood (Figure 3.11), the leukemic cells are medium-sized to large with prominent nuclear contour irregularities. Many cells with polylobated nuclei ('flower-like' nuclear configuration) are present (Figure 3.11C). Bone marrow infiltrate is interstitial and patchy. Leukemic cells are positive for CD4, CD5 and CD25 and in a majority of cases also for CD2 and CD3 (Figure 3.12). Approximately one-third of cases are negative for both TCRαβ/TCRγδ, and the remaining cases express TCRαβ. ATLL is negative for CD7, NK-cell-associated antigens (CD16, CD56 and CD57), CD11b, CD11c, TIA-1 and granzyme (Table 1.7; Chapter 1).

In the lymphomatous variant (Figure 3.13), the neoplastic infiltrate is diffuse or paracortical with dilated sinuses. The tumor cells are medium-sized and pleomorphic with irregular nuclear contours and conspicuous nucleoli. Occasional cases may show scattered Reed–Sternberg-like cells. Similarly to other T-cell lymphomas, scattered eosinophils are easily identified.

EXTRANODAL NK/T-CELL LYMPHOMA, NASAL TYPE

Nasal NK/T-cell lymphoma is an aggressive, predominantly extranodal, EBV-associated neoplasm with a characteristic angiocentric growth pattern, necrosis and expression of EBV/EBER and CD56. Although the nasal cavity and nasopharynx are the most common sites of involvement, NK/T-cell lymphoma can occur in palate, skin, soft tissue, lung, spleen, breast, lymph nodes, testis and gastrointestinal tract[355,374,392–406]. The clinical presentation varies depending on the site of involvement. Nasal lesions usually present with nasal obstruction or a midfacial destructive tumor ('lethal midline granuloma'). Systemic symptoms are common and include fever, malaise and weight loss. Prognosis varies, depending on stage and response to chemotherapy. Tumors occurring outside the nasal cavity are usually highly aggressive. The lymphoid infiltrate is diffuse and pleomorphic (Figures 3.14 and 3.15), and is composed of variable proportions of small, medium-sized and large atypical lymphocytes. The latter have irregular large and hyperchromatic nuclei with pale to clear cytoplasm. Inflammatory cells (eosinophils, histiocytes and plasma cells) are often present. A characteristic feature of NK/T-cell lymphoma is its angiocentric growth pattern (Figure 3.15A), which may lead to prominent distal necrosis.

Most cases display a NK-cell phenotype: CD2⁺, surface CD3⁻ (flow cytometry), cytoplasmic CD3⁺ (flow cytometry and immunohistochemistry), CD5⁻, CD7⁺/⁻, CD4⁻, CD8⁻, TCRαβ/TCRγδ⁻, CD16⁻, CD56⁺ and CD57⁻.

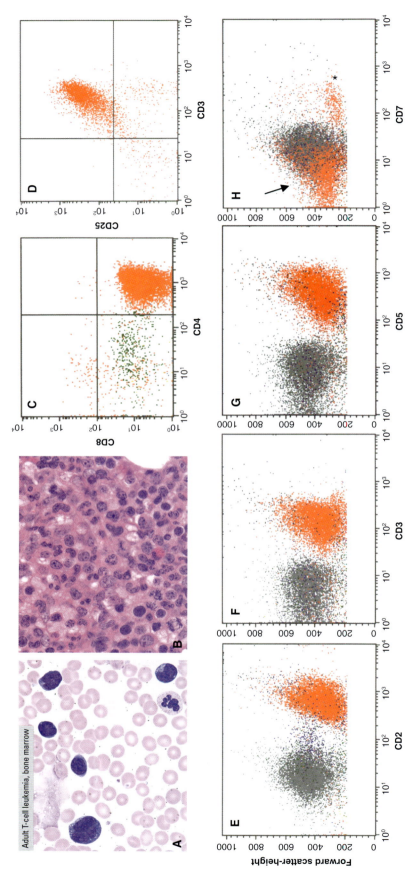

Figure 3.12   Adult T-cell leukemia/lymphoma – flow cytometry of the bone marrow. Bone marrow aspirate (**A**) and core biopsy (**B**) show an atypical lymphoid infiltrate. Leukemic cells show CD4 subset restriction (**C**) and typical CD25 expression (**D**). Of all pan-T antigens, only CD7 is absent (**E–H**)

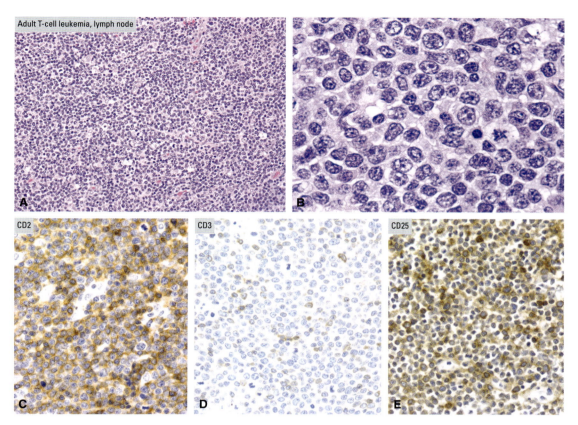

Figure 3.13 Adult T-cell leukemia/lymphoma – lymph node. Diffuse infiltrate (**A**) of small to medium-sized lymphocytes with nuclear irregularities (**B**). Neoplastic T-cells (CD2⁺, **C**) display aberrant lack of CD3 (**D**) and coexpress CD25 (**E**)

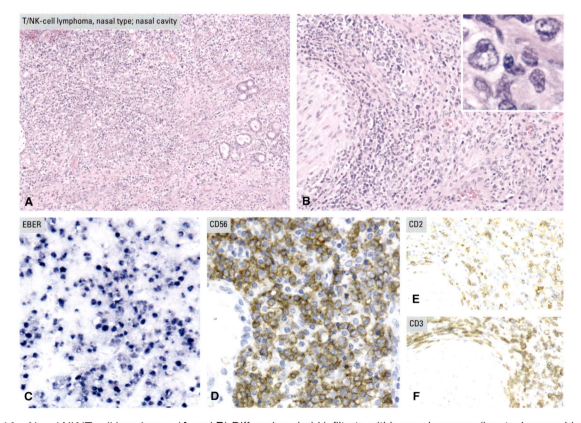

Figure 3.14 Nasal NK/T-cell lymphoma. (**A** and **B**) Diffuse lymphoid infiltrate within nasal mucosa (inset: pleomorphic lymphoid cells). Lymphomatous cells are positive for EBER (**C**), CD56 (**D**) and T-cell antigens CD2 and CD3 (**E** and **F**)

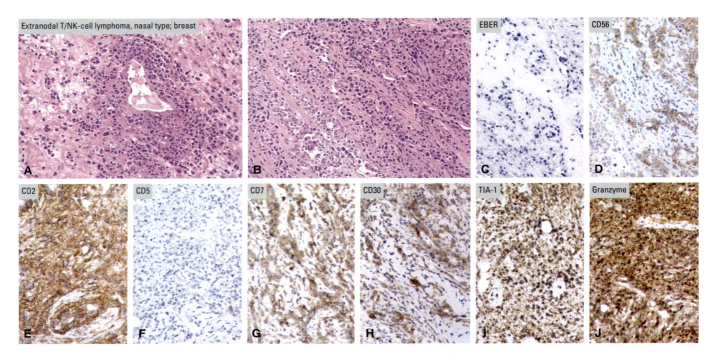

Figure 3.15   Extranodal NK/T-cell lymphoma, nasal type – breast. (**A**) Atypical angiocentric lymphomatous infiltrate. (**B**) Other areas contain a highly pleomorphic diffuse lymphoid infiltrate with necrosis. Neoplastic cells are positive for EBER (**C**), CD56 (**D**), CD2 (**E**), CD7 (**G**), CD30 (**H**), TIA-1 (**I**) and granzyme (**J**). CD5 is absent (**F**)

Cytotoxic granule-associated antigens (granzyme, TIA-1) are most often positive (Figure 3.15I and J). All cases express EBV/EBER (Figures 3.14C and 3.15C). Occasional cases are positive for CD30 (Figure 3.15H) and S100[407]. The presence of necrosis is a helpful diagnostic clue. Evaluation of phenotypic markers under high magnification usually shows cells with an aberrant phenotype: positive expression of EBV/EBER, CD56 and lack of CD5, CD4 and CD8.

Apart from T/NK-cell lymphoma, nasal type, another major type of T/NK-cell neoplasm is aggressive NK-cell leukemia/lymphoma[78,384,395,401,408]. The latter is characterized by generalized lymphadenopathy, hepatosplenomegaly and circulating neoplastic cells. The phenotype is similar to nasal T/NK-cell lymphoma: CD2[+], CD3[−] CD8[−] and CD56[+].

The differential diagnosis of extranodal NK/T-cell lymphoma includes reactive inflammatory infiltrates, plasma cell tumors, plasmablastic lymphoma, nasopharyngeal carcinoma, large B-cell lymphoma (especially in the setting of HIV infection, immunosuppression or elderly individuals with concomitant EBV/EBER expression), peripheral T-cell lymphoma, NOS, malignant melanoma, lymphomatoid granulomatosis and other small blue cell tumors (e.g., PNET, sarcoma, etc.)[392,396,397,404,409–413]. Plasma cell neoplasms (Figure 3.16A) generally show more monomorphic and diffuse infiltrate without

angiocentricity or prominent necrosis. Positive monotypic expression of light- and heavy-chain immunoglobulins and lack of EBV/EBER, CD2, TIA-1 and granzyme differentiate plasma cell neoplasia from extranodal NK/T-cell lymphoma. Plasmablastic lymphoma (Figure 3.16B) may be confused with extranodal NK/T-cell lymphoma because of its extranodal location and coexpression of CD56 and EBV/EBER. Plasmablastic lymphoma differs from extranodal NK/T-cell lymphoma by diffuse infiltration predominantly of large cells which lack CD2, CD43, TIA-1 and granzyme, and may be positive for Pax-5, bcl-1 and CD10. Poorly differentiated carcinoma (Figure 3.16C) and melanoma are distinguished by expression of keratins and S100/HMB-45, respectively. Variants of diffuse large B-cell lymphoma (Figure 3.16D) are usually distinguished by positive expression of at least one B-cell associated marker (CD19, CD20, CD22, CD79a, Pax-5) and lack of CD2.

ENTEROPATHY-TYPE T-CELL LYMPHOMA

Enteropathy-type T-cell lymphoma is a large cell lymphoma with cytotoxic T-cell phenotype occurring most commonly in the small intestine[44,343,344,360,414–419]. Patients either have history of celiac disease or present with the symptoms of celiac disease at the time of diagnosis.

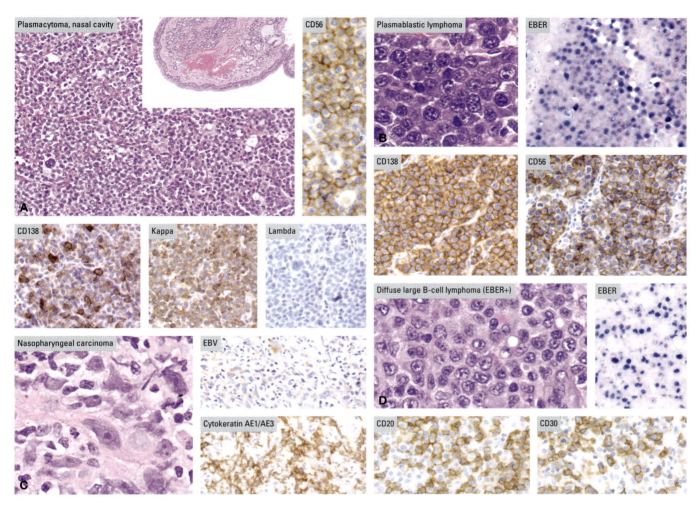

Figure 3.16 Differential diagnosis of extranodal NK/T-cell lymphoma, nasal type. (**A**) Plasmacytoma. Atypical diffuse plasma cell infiltrate within nasal cavity may suggest NK-cell lymphoma. Expression of light-chain immunoglobulins and lack of EBER expression helps in distinguishing a plasma cell neoplasm. (**B**) Plasmablastic lymphoma. Positive expression of EBER and CD56 is common for both plasmablastic lymphoma and NK-cell lymphoma. Lack of angiocentrism and lack of expression of pan-T antigens (e.g., CD2) and cytotoxic granule-associated proteins (granzyme, TIA-1) distinguish these two neoplasms. (**C**) Poorly differentiated nasopharyngeal carcinoma. Pleomorphic infiltrate with expression of EBV in nasopharyngeal carcinoma may be confused with nasal NK-cell lymphoma. Expression of cytokeratin establishes the correct diagnosis. (**D**) Diffuse large B-cell lymphoma (DLBCL). EBV-associated DLBCL (e.g., in immunocompromised or elderly patients) may be mistaken for nasal NK-cell lymphoma

Involvement of sites other than the jejunum or ileum, including liver, stomach, duodenum or bone marrow, is rare. Intestinal perforation is a common complication. The clinical course is aggressive. Clonal rearrangements of the T-cell receptor are present and often they are similar to those found in an adjacent mucosa[414,418]. The tumor infiltrates the intestinal wall with areas of ulceration and necrosis, or forms large polypoid masses. The lymphomatous cells display a spectrum of morphologic features with either a pleomorphic infiltrate (Figure 3.17) with occasional large, multinucleated (Reed–Sternberg-like) cells or a monomorphic infiltrate of medium-sized to large cells (Figure 3.18). There is often a reactive infiltrate of eosinophils, small lymphocytes, histiocytes and plasma cells.

The neoplastic cells have the following phenotypes: CD45$^+$, CD2$^{+/-}$, CD3$^+$, CD5$^-$, CD7$^+$, CD11c$^+$, CD43$^+$, CD30$^+$, CD56$^{+/-}$, CD103$^+$ (Figures 3.17 and 3.18). The expression of CD103 is a characteristic flow cytometric immunophenotypic feature (Figure 3.18C). Expression of CD30 is seen in most cases, and is usually more pronounced in large pleomorphic cells (Figure 3.17I). Most cases are CD8$^+$, but a subset of tumors is CD4/CD8$^-$.

The differential diagnosis includes other peripheral T-cell neoplasms, classical Hodgkin lymphoma, diffuse

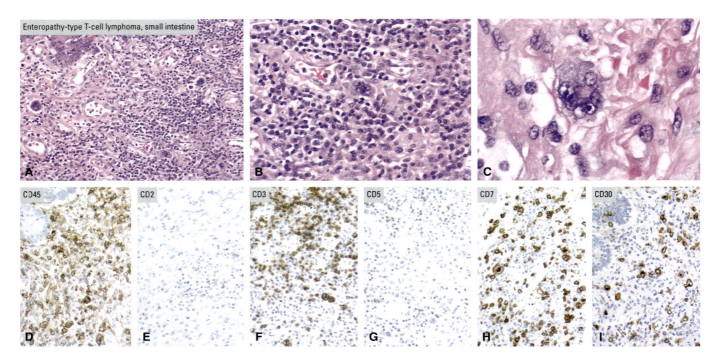

Figure 3.17   Enteropathy-type T-cell lymphoma – small intestine. (**A**) Low magnification shows a dense lymphoid infiltrate within mucosa and submucosa. (**B** and **C**) Higher magnifications show scattered pleomorphic multinucleated cells, which may mimic Reed–Sternberg cells. Neoplastic cells are positive for CD45 (**D**), CD3 (**F**), CD7 (**H**) and CD30 (**I**). They show aberrant loss of two of pan-T antigens: CD2 and CD5 antigens (**E** and **G**)

large B-cell lymphoma, inflammatory disorders, and atypical reactive processes[175,284,286,420–424].

HEPATOSPLENIC T-CELL LYMPHOMA

Hepatosplenic T-cell lymphoma is an aggressive tumor of cytotoxic T-cells involving the liver, spleen and bone marrow[424–432]. It is characterized by an intrasinusoidal distribution of tumor cells. Patients present with hepatosplenomegaly and pancytopenia. Isochromosome 7q [i(7q)] represents the primary, non-random cytogenetic abnormality in hepatosplenic gamma/delta T-cell lymphoma, and plays a role in its pathogenesis[425]. Morphologic examination reveals distended splenic or hepatic sinusoids with monomorphic medium-sized lymphoid cells with scanty cytoplasm and irregular nuclei (Figures 3.19 and 3.20). In contrast to other T-cell lymphoproliferations, the portal triads are usually not involved.

The tumor cells are positive for CD3, CD45 and TCRγδ, but rare cases of hepatosplenic T-cell lymphoma that are TCRαβ+ have been reported[430,432,434,435]. The majority of cases are dual CD4/CD8− and are negative for CD5 (rare cases display dim expression of CD5). Most cases are positive for CD2, CD7 and TIA-1, and display dual negative expression of CD4/CD8 (only rare tumors may be CD8+). NK-cell-associated antigens are variably expressed: CD16 is positive in approximately 25% of cases, CD56 is positive in majority of cases and CD57 is negative. Figure 3.21 presents flow cytometry analysis of hepatosplenic T-cell lymphoma.

Bone marrow shows prominent intrasinusoidal involvement (Figure 3.22). Minimal involvement or early phase of the disease may be difficult to recognize in routine HE sections. Immunohistochemical staining for CD3 (Figure 3.22D) and/or CD56 is very helpful in confirming bone marrow involvement.

The differential diagnosis of hepatosplenic T-cell lymphoma includes B- and T-cell lymphoproliferative disorders and reactive lymphoid infiltrates[128,153,154,156,159,161,270,343,344,400,436–438]. Intrasinusoidal involvement of the bone marrow is not specific for hepatosplenic T-cell lymphoma, and is displayed by other types of lymphoma such as anaplastic large cell lymphoma (ALCL), splenic lymphoma with villous lymphocytes, T-LGL leukemia, MCL and intravascular large B-cell lymphoma[12,13].

SUBCUTANEOUS PANNICULITIS-LIKE T-CELL LYMPHOMA

Subcutaneous panniculitis-like T-cell lymphoma is a rare tumor of primary cutaneous origin with variable, often

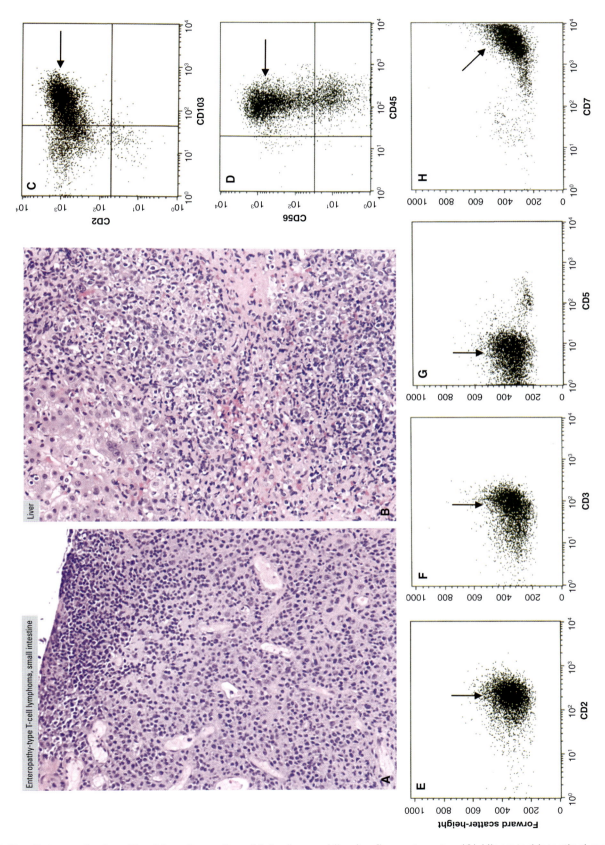

Figure 3.18 Enteropathy-type T-cell lymphoma (small intestine and liver) – flow cytometry. (**A**) Ulcerated intestinal mucosa with dense, rather monomorphic lymphoid infiltrate. (**B**) Tissue section from liver contains a prominent lymphoid infiltrate. Flow cytometry (**C–H**) displays the following phenotype of lymphomatous cells: CD103+ (**C**), CD56+ (**D**), CD2+ (**E**), CD3+ (**F**), CD5– (**G**) and aberrantly bright CD7+ (**H**)

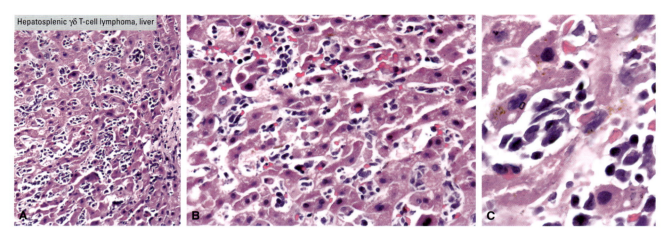

Figure 3.19   Hepatosplenic T-cell lymphoma – liver. (**A** and **B**) Liver sinusoids are distended by an atypical lymphoid infiltrate. (**C**) High magnification shows lymphoid cells within sinusoids

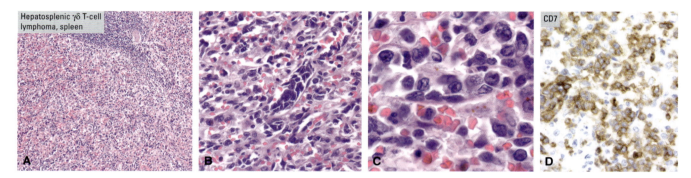

Figure 3.20   Hepatosplenic T-cell lymphoma – spleen. (**A**) Low magnification shows red pulp with increased numbers of lymphocytes. (**B** and **C**) Higher magnification shows sinusoids distended by atypical lymphoid cells, highlighted by CD7 immunostaining (**D**)

aggressive clinical course[343,344,431,439–443]. It represents one of the three major categories of extranodal T/NK-cell tumors (the other two being extranodal T/NK-cell lymphoma, nasal type and enteropathy-type T-cell lymphoma)[357,400]. It involves subcutaneous tissue with characteristic rimming of individual fat spaces by tumor cells. Clinical features are related to mass effect, but some patients have fever, pancytopenia and hemophagocytic syndrome[442].

Morphologically, tumors are confined to the subcutaneous tissue with sparing of the dermis and epidermis (Figure 3.23). The neoplastic infiltrate is lobular and diffuse with necrosis and karyorrhexis. Neoplastic cells range in size, but many large atypical cells with hyperchromatic nuclei are present. Characteristic rimming of the neoplastic cells surrounding fat cells can be accentuated by immunohistochemical staining (Figure 3.24). Tumor cells are positive for CD45, CD56, cytotoxic molecules (granzyme and TIA-1) and one or more of the pan-T antigens (Figure 3.24). Most tumors have a CD4$^-$/CD8$^+$ phenotype[441,443,444]. Most cases express the αβ

T-cell receptor protein, but approximately 25% of cases may be γδ positive[78,343,344,440,441,443–445]. Subcutaneous panniculitis-like T-cell lymphoma with γδ phenotype is double CD4/CD8 negative[343,440]. EBV is closely linked to nasal T/NK-cell lymphoma, and is usually negative in subcutaneous panniculitis-like T-cell lymphoma, although there may be geographic and racial variations in EBV expression[439,440,443].

The differential diagnosis of subcutaneous panniculitis-like T-cell lymphoma includes other peripheral T-cell lymphomas, which preferentially involve skin, extranodal T/NK-cell lymphoma, nasal type, large B-cell lymphoma, blastic NK-cell lymphoma, metastatic tumors and extramedullary myeloid tumors[357,401,446–450]. A majority of peripheral T-cell disorders involving skin have a predilection for the papillary dermis with epidermotropism. They are most often CD4$^+$ and rarely express CD56. Blastic NK-cell lymphoma is CD4$^+$/CD8$^-$, and CD56$^+$. The infiltrate is not confined to the subcutaneous tissue. Other neoplasms are distinguished by specific phenotypic profile.

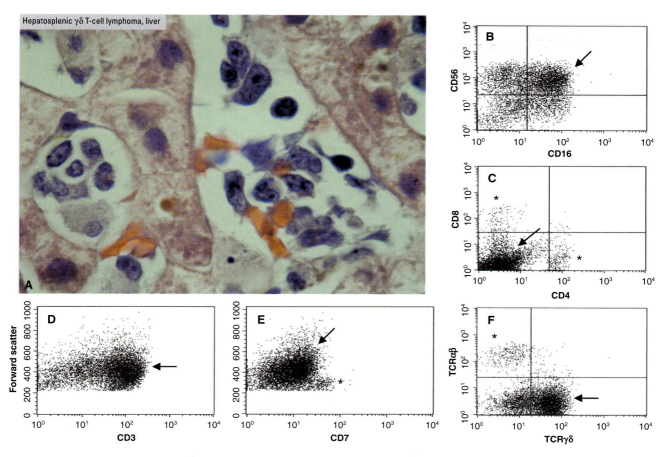

Figure 3.21   Hepatosplenic T-cell lymphoma (liver) – flow cytometry. (**A**) The neoplastic cells infiltrate the hepatic sinusoids. (**B–F**) Flow cytometry analysis shows the following phenotype of atypical T-cells: CD16+/CD56+ (**B**), CD4−/CD8− (**C**), CD3+ (**D**), CD7− (**E**) and TCR gamma/delta+ (**F**). Rare normal T-cells (*) are present

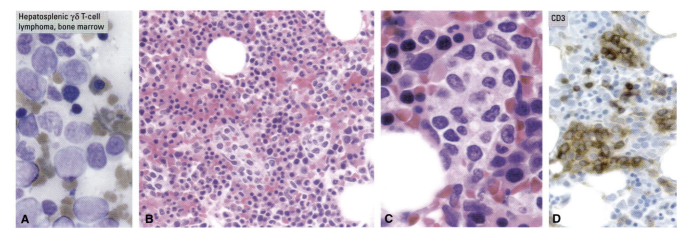

Figure 3.22   Hepatosplenic T-cell lymphoma – bone marrow. (**A**) Bone marrow aspirate shows atypical lymphoid cells. (**B**) Hypercellular bone marrow with neoplastic cells within sinusoids. (**C**) High magnification shows sinusoids packed with atypical cells, easily identified with immunohistochemical staining for CD3 (**D**)

MYCOSIS FUNGOIDES (MF) AND SEZARY SYNDROME

MF is a peripheral T-cell lymphoma involving the skin, characterized by lymphocytes with irregular nuclear borders (cerebriform nuclei) and clusters of cells within epithelium (Pautrier microabscesses)[451–460]. The course of MF is indolent except when transformation to a large cell lymphoma occurs[454,461].

MF is the most common type of primary cutaneous lymphoma. The early lesions are characterized by skin

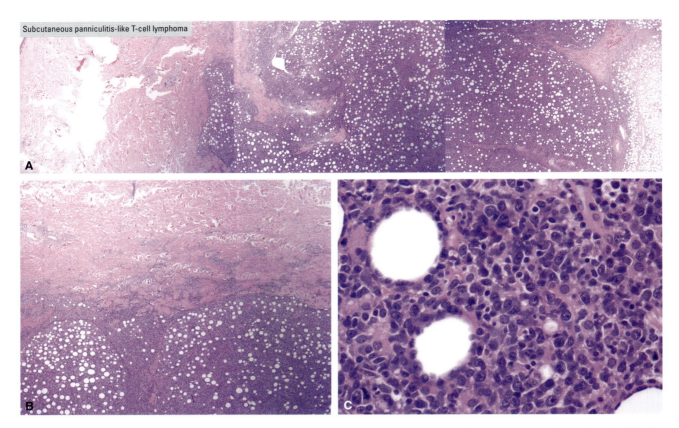

Figure 3.23   Subcutaneous panniculitis-like T-cell lymphoma. **(A)** Composite illustration showing a dense lymphoid infiltrate confined to the subcutaneous tissue without involvement of the epidermis or dermis (left side). **(B)** Another area with diffuse infiltrate within adipose tissue (lobular panniculitis). The dermis is not involved. **(C)** High magnification shows atypical lymphoid cells with irregular hyperchromatic nuclei and rimming of the individual fat lobules by neoplastic cells

patches and plaques, most often affecting the trunk. After an initial indolent and protracted course, MF usually progresses with generalized erythroderma and involvement of peripheral blood, lymph node, liver and spleen (Sezary syndrome)[453–455,457,458,462,463].

The morphologic pattern depends on the stage of the disease. In early skin involvement (Figure 3.25), there is a patchy lymphoid infiltrate in the upper dermis with epidermotropism and single-cell exocytosis, or, less commonly, aggregates of atypical lymphocytes within the epidermis (Pautrier microabscesses). The lymphoid cells are small to medium-sized and have irregular hyperchromatic nuclei. Occasional large lymphocytes may be also present, as well as reactive small lymphocytes and eosinophils. The early stages of MF are difficult to diagnose solely by cytomorphologic features[451,464,465]. The presence of prominent epidermotropism, cytologic atypia and aberrant pan-T antigen expression (e.g., lack of CD2, CD3 and/or CD5) and CD4 restriction helps differentiate MF from benign conditions. Presence of lymphocytes with extremely convoluted nuclei (cerebriform cells) within the epidermis or in small clusters within the dermis is the single most

reliable histomorphologic feature of early MF. Correlation with clinical data and molecular studies is often required for definite diagnosis of early MF. Tumor lesions of MF (Figure 3.26) show prominent lymphoid infiltrate in the papillary dermis with epidermotropism, cytologic atypia and often aberrant pan-T antigen expression. MF usually is CD4+ and TCRαβ+. Of the pan-T antigens, CD7 is most frequently lost.

Sezary syndrome in peripheral blood is characterized by the presence of atypical lymphocytes with irregular convoluted nuclei (Figure 3.27A and B). Flow cytometry immunophenotyping demonstrates the predominance of CD4+ T-cells (Figure 3.27D) with aberrant loss of CD7 in a majority of cases.

Lymph nodes show variable histologic patterns depending on the stage of the disease. Cases without lymph node involvement (category I) often show dermatopathic changes and paracortical hyperplasia. Scattered rare atypical lymphocytes may be present. In early involvement (category II), there is a paracortical expansion with focal/partial effacement of the architecture and sheets of atypical lymphocytes with irregular nuclear contours

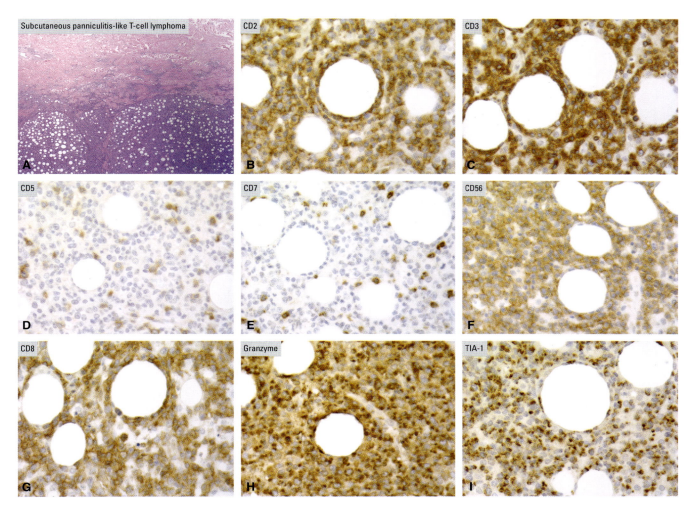

Figure 3.24   Subcutaneous panniculitis-like T-cell lymphoma – immunohistochemistry. Neoplastic cells are positive for CD2 (**B**), CD3 (**C**), CD56 (**F**), CD8 (**G**), granzyme (**H**) and TIA-1 (**I**). Two pan-T antigens (CD5 and CD7) are aberrantly absent (**D** and **E**)

(Figure 3.28). In cases with massive involvement (category III), there is complete replacement of lymph node architecture by a diffuse atypical lymphoid infiltrate.

The differential diagnosis of MF includes reactive skin disorders with lymphoid infiltrate, primary and secondary B- and T-cell lymphomas, and non-hematopoietic tumors with prominent reactive lymphoid infiltrate (see also Chapter 15)[46,91,169,170,239,273,336,364,368,440,446,448,466–472].

PRIMARY CUTANEOUS ANAPLASTIC LARGE CELL LYMPHOMA

Anaplastic large cell lymphoma is divided into two categories: (systemic) anaplastic large cell lymphoma (ALCL) and primary cutaneous ALCL[78,440,444,446,450,466,471,473]. Both types are characterized by diffuse large cell CD30+ infiltrate with pleomorphic, often horseshoe-shaped nuclei ('hallmark cells'). Primary cutaneous ALCL differs from systemic ALCL and secondary (CD30+) peripheral T-cell lymphomas involving skin by being limited to the skin at

the time of diagnosis and by lack (in most cases) of ALK expression and/or t(2;5) translocation[466,467,471,473,474]. Most patients with primary cutaneous ALCL have limited disease but multicentric involvement may occur. Although partial or complete spontaneous regression may occur, frequent relapses and dissemination may occur.

The morphologic features of primary cutaneous ALCL are similar to its systemic counterpart. There is either a diffuse monomorphic large cell infiltrate (Figure 3.29) or a highly pleomorphic infiltrate with numerous multinucleated giant cells resembling Reed–Sternberg cells (Figure 3.30). The latter variant is more common. The tumor involves upper and lower dermis, but both epidermotropism and subcutis involvement is uncommon. Phenotypically, tumor cells are positive for CD45, CD43 and CD30 and display aberrant expression of pan-T antigens. Most tumors are CD4+. Primary CD30+ cutaneous T-cell lymphomas frequently express cytotoxic proteins[445]. In contrast to secondary skin involvement by systemic

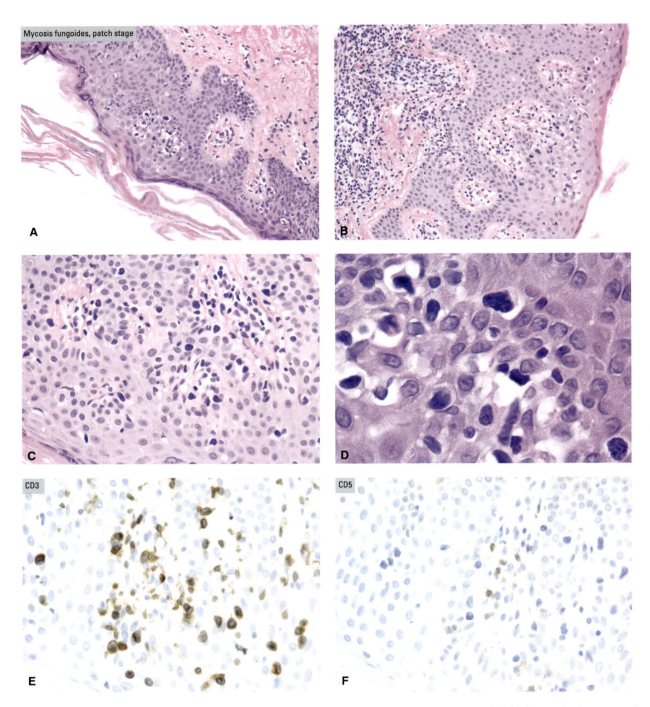

Figure 3.25   Mycosis fungoides – patch stage. (**A–D**) Histologic sections show atypical lymphoid infiltrate in the upper dermis with epidermotropism. Lymphoid cells have irregular nuclei (**D**). Intraepidermal T-cells are CD3⁺ (**E**) and lack CD5 (**F**)

ALCL (Figure 3.31), primary cutaneous ALCL do not express ALK and EMA (Figures 3.29F and 3.30G).

PERIPHERAL T-CELL LYMPHOMA, UNSPECIFIED

Peripheral T-cell lymphoma, unspecified is a mature T-cell lymphoma which does not fulfill morphologic, phenotypic or genetic criteria for any distinctive mature T-cell lymphoma

category, hence the designation 'unspecified' (or 'not otherwise specified', NOS)[78,338–343,348–352,354,359,360,456,467,475–480]. The distinction from other, specific peripheral T-cell disorders is based on clinical, morphologic, phenotypic and genetic data, but is not always clear, especially at the time of initial diagnosis. The main entities from which peripheral T-cell lymphoma, unspecified has to be differentiated include nodal involvement by T-cell prolymphocytic leukemia (T-PLL), lymphomatous variant of adult T-cell

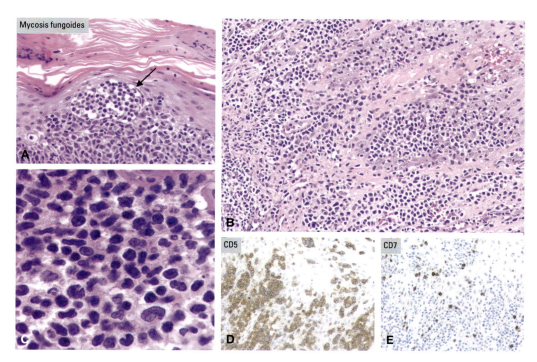

Figure 3.26 Mycosis fungoides – tumor stage. (**A**) Neoplastic cells form Pautrier microabscesses within the epidermis (arrow). (**B**) Tumor cells diffusely infiltrate the dermis. (**C**) High magnification shows nuclear atypia with irregular nuclear contours and occasional nucleoli. (**D** and **E**) The lymphomatous cells show expression of CD5 (**D**) and aberrant loss of CD7 (**E**)

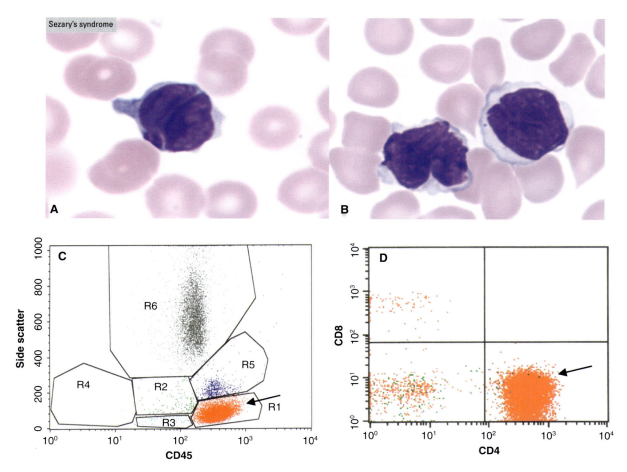

Figure 3.27 Sezary syndrome. (**A** and **B**) Peripheral blood films with atypical lymphocytes with cerebriform nuclei. Flow cytometry (**C** and **D**) shows T-cells with CD4 restriction (arrow)

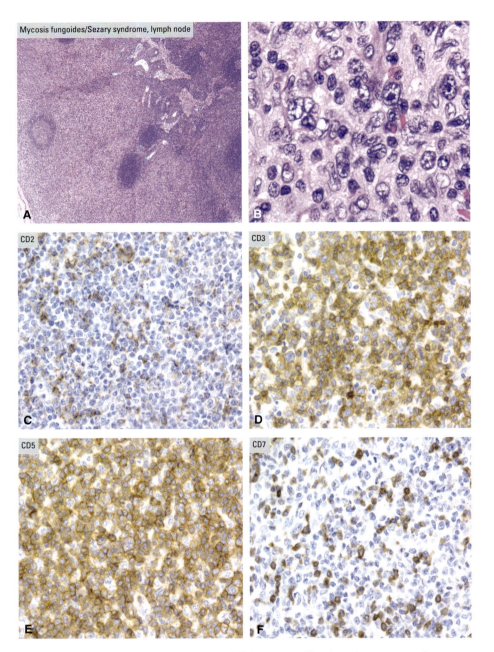

Figure 3.28   Mycosis fungoides – lymph node involvement. (**A**) Low magnification shows a prominent paracortical/interfollicular infiltrate. (**B**) High magnification shows medium-sized to large lymphoid cells with nuclear pleomorphism and nucleoli. Neoplastic cells show lack of CD2 and CD7 expression (**C** and **F**). CD3 and CD5 are positive (**D** and **E**)

leukemia/lymphoma (ATLL), anaplastic large cell lymphoma (ALCL), angioimmunoblastic T-cell lymphoma and reactive T-cell infiltrates in benign processes (such as Kikuchi lymphadenitis) or accompanying B-cell lymphomas (e.g., T-cell rich large B-cell lymphoma). The distinction between peripheral T-cell lymphoma, unspecified and anaplastic large cell lymphoma is problematic since both disorders may share cytomorphologic and phenotypic characteristics. Tumors positive for ALK protein and/or t(2;5), regardless of morphology, are classified as systemic ALCL. Tumors composed of large pleomorphic cells with

classic anaplastic cytologic features, which are strongly positive for CD30 but not for ALK, are usually classified as ALCL category. However, since the prognosis of ALK-negative ALCL is similar to that of peripheral T-cell lymphoma, unspecified (e.g., unfavorable) they might represent the latter rather than ALCL.

Peripheral T-cell lymphoma, unspecified occurs at any age, usually in older patients (range: 19–92 years old, average 66 years; IMPATH material). It is most often a nodal disease but any other site in the body (including peripheral blood, bone marrow, bone, omentum, skin,

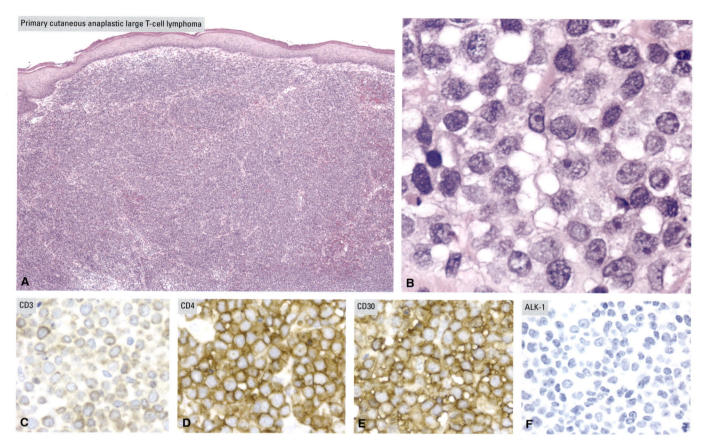

Figure 3.29   Primary cutaneous anaplastic large cell lymphoma. (**A**) Extensive diffuse lymphoid infiltrate without epidermotropism. (**B**) High magnification shows large cells with indistinct pale cytoplasm and nucleoli. Neoplastic cells display dim expression of CD3 (**C**), and strong membranous staining with CD4 and CD30 (**D** and **E**). ALK-1 is negative (**F**)

CSF, soft tissues, gastrointestinal tract, spleen, liver, lung) may be involved.

Histologic examination shows either a prominent paracortical infiltrate (T-zone variant; Figure 3.32) or diffuse infiltration with effacement of the normal lymph node architecture. Although the cell size and cytologic features may vary, medium-sized or large cell infiltrates predominate. Nuclei are irregular and pleomorphic (Figure 3.32C) with unevenly distributed coarse chromatin and nucleoli. Scattered large multilobated Reed–Sternberg-like cells may be present, or an inflammatory cell infiltrate of small lymphocytes, eosinophils, histiocytes and/or plasma cells. Many cases have increased numbers of small blood vessels (high endothelial venules) and clusters of epithelioid histiocytes which may form granulomas.

Phenotyping (Figure 3.33) by either flow cytometry or immunohistochemistry plays an important role in the diagnosis of peripheral T-cell lymphoma, unspecified[20–22,38,41]. The expression of CD45 is usually normal (~88%), but some cases show either dim (~10%) or negative (~2%) CD45. Although normal expression of all four pan-T antigens is occasionally seen (Figure 3.34A), most cases show aberrant expression of one or more of the pan-T antigens (Figure 3.34B–D; see also Table 3.4). Among pan-T antigens, CD7 is most frequently lost (56%) and CD2 is least frequently lost (13%). Dim expression of CD2, CD3, CD5 and CD7 is noted in 4.4%, 11.8%, 17.6% and 8.8% of cases, respectively. Approximately 8% of cases do not reveal any loss or diminution of pan-T antigens. Although CD4+ lymphomas predominate (60%), dual negative expression of CD4/CD8 is observed on significant proportions of tumors (22%). Of additional markers, CD10, CD11c, CD15, CD25, CD30, CD56, CD57, CD117, EMA and HLA-DR are occasionally expressed (see Table 3.4 for details)[20–22,481].

Some peripheral T-cell lymphomas show numerous clusters of clear cells or signet-ring cell features (Figure 3.35). A variant of peripheral T-cell lymphoma with numerous aggregates of epithelioid cells is designated as Lennert's lymphoma (lymphoepithelioid cell variant of peripheral T-cell lymphoma) (Figure 3.36).

The differential diagnosis of (nodal) peripheral T-cell lymphoma, unspecified, includes a wide variety of malignant and reactive lesions which either show T-zone

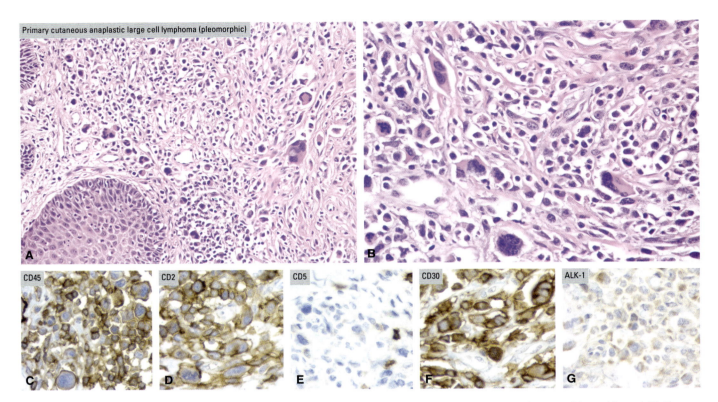

Figure 3.30   Primary cutaneous anaplastic large cell lymphoma with prominent nuclear pleomorphism. (**A** and **B**) Dense lymphoid infiltrate within the papillary dermis with marked nuclear pleomorphism. Multinucleated, Reed–Sternberg-like cells are present. Neoplastic cells are positive for CD45 (**C**), CD2 (**D**) and CD30 (**F**). CD5 is aberrantly missing (**E**). ALK-1 is negative (**G**)

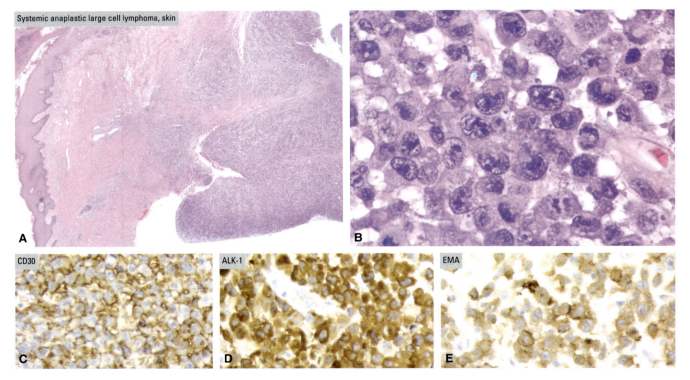

Figure 3.31   Systemic anaplastic large cell lymphoma involving skin. (**A**) Low magnification shows a deep dense lymphoid infiltrate with areas of necrosis. (**B**) High magnification shows large neoplastic cells with hyperchromatic nuclei and prominent nucleoli. Tumor cells are positive for CD30 (**C**), ALK-1 (**D**) and EMA (**E**)

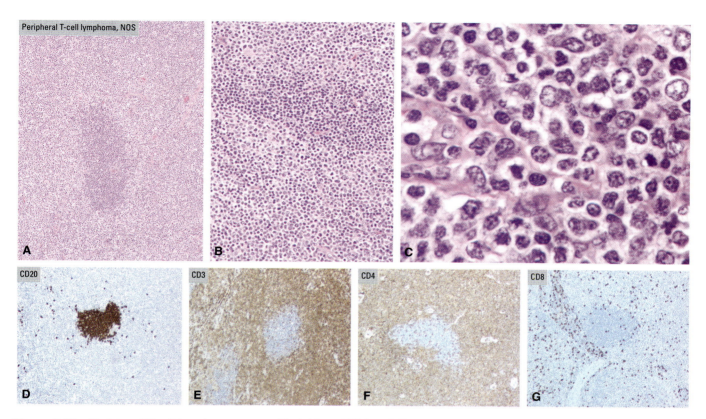

Figure 3.32   Peripheral T-cell lymphoma, unspecified. (**A** and **B**) Interfollicular pattern of involvement (T-zone variant). (**C**) High magnification shows pleomorphic lymphomatous cells with irregular nuclear outlines. CD20 staining shows preserved B-cell areas (**D**). Neoplastic cells are positive for CD3 (**E**) and CD4 (**F**). Only rare CD8⁺ small T-cells are present (**G**)

pattern of lymph node involvement or display cytomorphologic features that may be confused with peripheral T-cell lymphoma. This includes diffuse B-cell lymphoma, classical Hodgkin lymphoma, ALCL, specific T-cell lymphoproliferations involving lymph node (T-PLL, adult T-cell leukemia/lymphoma, MF/Sezary syndrome), extramedullary myeloid tumor, blastic NK-cell lymphoma, histiocytic neoplasms, reactive paracortical hyperplasia, dermatopathic lymphadenitis and Kikuchi lymphadenitis. T-cell lymphoma with numerous granulomas may be confused with infections or sarcoidosis.

Extramedullary myeloid tumor (granulocytic sarcoma) (Figure 3.37A) may display a prominent T-zone pattern of involvement. Some cases show very subtle changes, which may be confused with reactive paracortical hyperplasia. Careful comparison of staining with CD3 and CD43 in those cases usually reveals a CD3⁻/CD43⁺ population, which represents myeloid cells. Extramedullary myeloid tumors (EMT) are usually positive for one or more of the pan-myeloid markers (MPO, muramidase), CD68, and CD34 and/or CD117. Many cases are also positive for TdT. However, blastic EMT may only be CD43⁺. ALCL (Figure 3.37B) can be easily distinguished by positive expression of ALK protein. The differential diagnosis of

ALK-negative ALCL is more problematic. The WHO classification recognizes ALK-negative ALCL, but since the prognosis and clinical behavior of those tumors is similar to peripheral T-cell lymphoma, they most likely represent the latter entity with 'anaplastic features'. In problematic cases, confirmation of T-cell clonality by molecular tests (PCR) or recognition of specific chromosomal changes by cytogenetic and/or FISH studies helps to establish a diagnosis of lymphoma. Dermatopathic lymphadenitis (Figure 3.37C) is a reactive condition of the lymph node associated with skin lesions, leading to proliferation of histiocytes, interdigitating reticulum cells and Langerhans cells in the paracortical area, some of which contain phagocytosed melanin pigment. Langerhans cells can be identified with immunohistochemical staining with S100 and CD1a.

There are no specific features to differentiate between B- and T-cell processes solely on morphologic grounds. Some diffuse large B-cell lymphomas may display a prominent T-zone pattern of involvement (Figure 3.37D), anaplastic features with Reed–Sternberg-like cells and an inflammatory background, or a predominance of small T-cells and histiocytes with scattered large atypical cells.

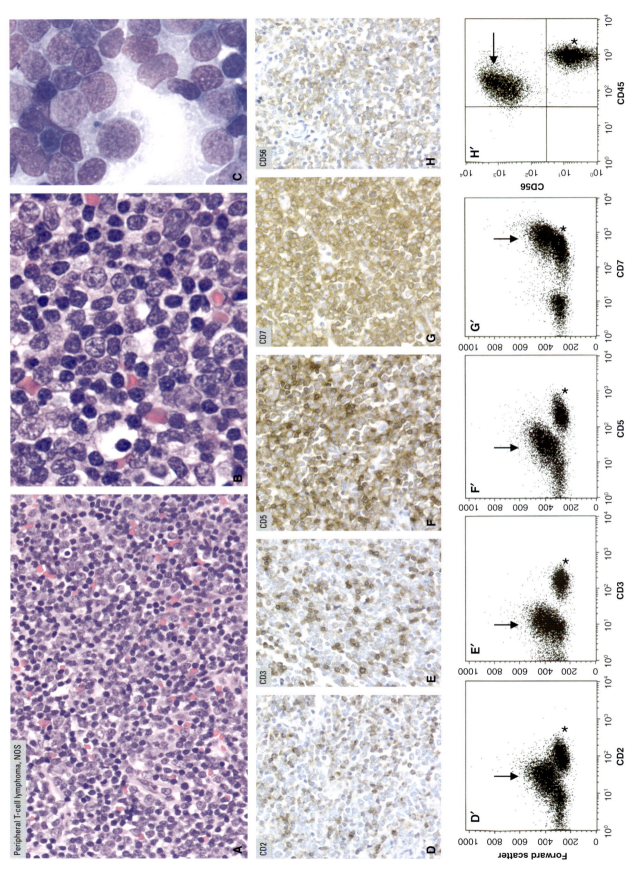

Figure 3.33   Peripheral T-cell lymphoma, unspecified – comparison of immunohistochemistry (middle row) and flow cytometry (lower row). (**A** and **B**) Tissue section shows diffuse lymphoid infiltrate. (**C**) Touch smear shows medium-sized lymphoid cells with inconspicuous nucleoli. Neoplastic cells are negative for CD2 (**D**, immunohistochemistry; **D'**, flow cytometry), negative for CD3 (**E** and **E'**), dimly positive for CD5 (**F** and **F'**), positive for CD7 (**G** and **G'**) and positive for CD56 (**H** and **H'**)

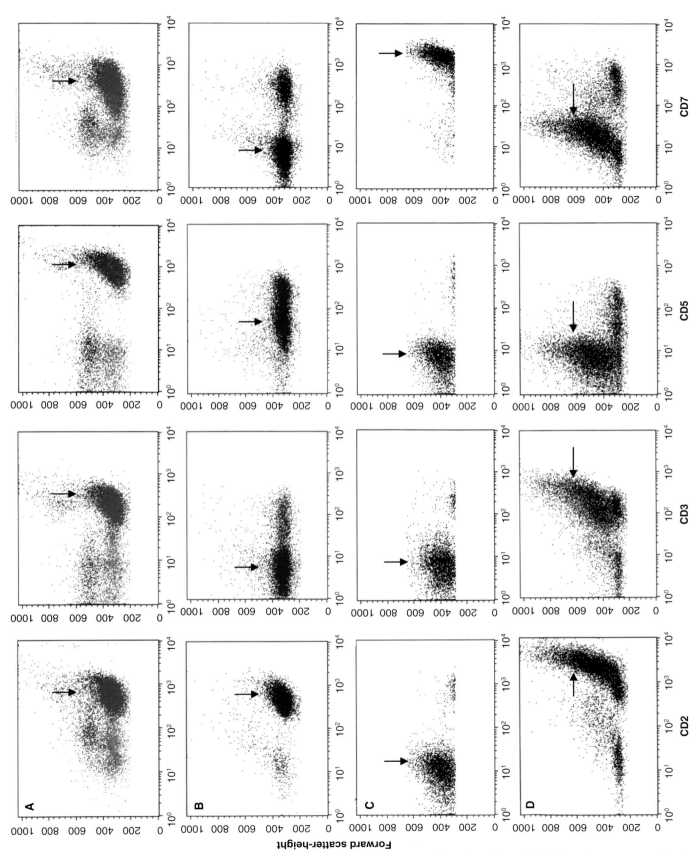

Figure 3.34 Peripheral T-cell lymphoma – flow cytometry. Four different examples of peripheral T-cell lymphoma, unspecified, analyzed by flow cytometry. (**A**) Peripheral T-cell lymphoma with normal expression of all four pan-T markers (no loss or aberrant dim expression of CD2, CD3, CD5 and CD7). (**B**) Peripheral T-cell lymphoma with loss of CD3 and dim expression of CD5. (**C**) Peripheral T-cell lymphoma with loss of all pan-T antigens except CD7 (arrow). (**D**) Peripheral T-cell lymphoma with increased forward scatter (arrow), aberrant bright expression of CD2, normal expression of CD3, and aberrant loss of both CD5 and CD7

Table 3.4 Immunophenotypic profile of peripheral T-cell lymphoma, unspecified

Marker	%
CD2+	88
CD3+	60
CD5+	87
CD7+	45
All pan-T antigens positive	7.5
One pan-T antigens negative	49.2
Two pan-T antigens negative	25.4
Three pan-T antigens negative	7.5
Four pan-T antigens negative	0
CD4+	60
CD8+	12
CD4/CD8+	6
CD4/CD8−	22
TCRαβ+	76
TCRγδ+	0
TCR−	24
CD10+	7
CD11c+	12
CD25+	15
CD30+	8
CD56+	13
CD117+	0

Hodgkin lymphoma is distinguished from peripheral T-cell lymphoma by recognition of classic Reed–Sternberg cells and its variants in the background of small lymphocytes and inflammatory cells. T-cell lymphomas more often display a spectrum of atypical cells, from small normal-looking lymphocytes to medium-sized and large ones. The latter may resemble Reed–Sternberg cells by both cytology and CD30 expression, but are positive for CD45, pan-T markers, CD45 and CD43. Neoplastic Hodgkin cells and true Reed–Sternberg cells, apart from CD30 expression, are positive for Pax-5 (B-cell-associated marker), often express bcl-6, CD15 and EBV/EBER, and are negative for CD45 (Figure 3.37E). One has to keep in mind that there is overlap of phenotypic features between peripheral T-cell lymphoma, ALCL and classical Hodgkin lymphoma; e.g., some T-cell lymphomas are CD15+ and CD45−, whereas rare cases of classical Hodgkin lymphoma may display CD2 expression by Reed–Sternberg cells.

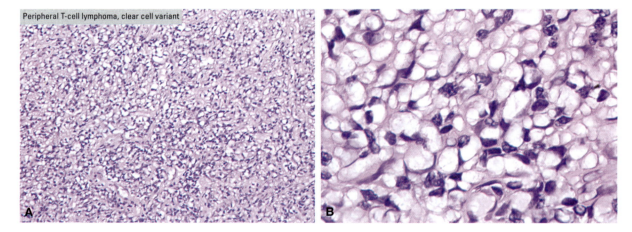

Figure 3.35 Peripheral T-cell lymphoma – clear cell variant. Neoplastic cells have abundant clear cytoplasm, which displaces nuclei to the periphery (**A** and **B**, low and high magnification)

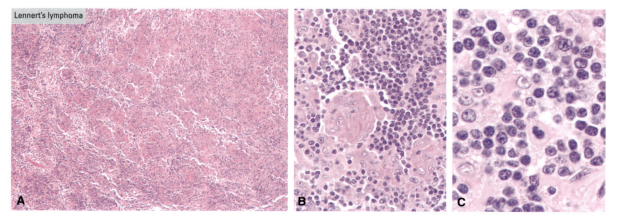

Figure 3.36 Lennert's lymphoma (peripheral T-cell lymphoma of the lymphoepithelioid variant). (**A**) Clusters of epithelioid histiocytes occupy most of the lymph node. (**B** and **C**) Atypical lymphoid cells admixed with epithelioid clusters

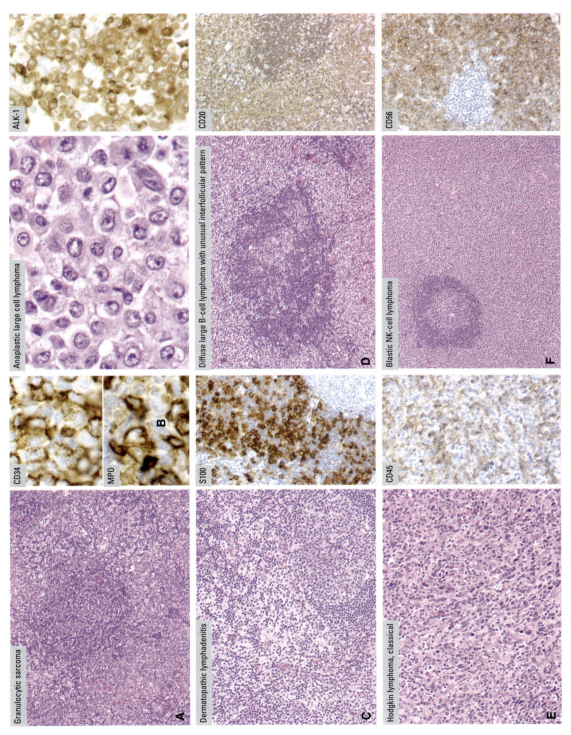

Figure 3.37 Peripheral T-cell lymphoma, unspecified – differential diagnosis (lymph node). (**A**) Granulocytic sarcoma. Extramedullary myeloid tumor (granulocytic sarcoma) usually is tropic to the interfollicular area (T-zone) and therefore has a similar low-power appearance to peripheral T-cell lymphomas. Lack of pan-T antigens and positivity for CD34, CD43, and one or more pan-myeloid antigens (MPO, muramidase, CD68) leads to the diagnosis. (**B**) Anaplastic large cell lymphoma (ALCL). Classic cytomorphologic features (e.g., large cells with horseshoe nuclei) and positive expression of ALK-1 differentiates ALCL from peripheral T-cell lymphoma. (**C**) Dermatopathic lymphadenitis. It is characterized by the presence of pigmented cells and clusters of S100⁺ interdigitating reticulum cells. (**D**) Diffuse large B-cell lymphoma with unusual interfollicular distribution. Expression of B-cell antigens and lack of pan-T antigens distinguishes DLBCL from a T-cell process. (**E**) Hodgkin lymphoma (classical). Neoplastic cells in Hodgkin lymphoma are negative for CD45 and pan-T cell markers, CD4/CD8. They often express B-cell antigens (CD20, Pax-5) and bcl-6. (**F**) Blastic NK-cell lymphoma. This rare tumor is (by definition) positive for CD56 and CD4. It often expresses CD7. Other pan-T antigens are negative. (**G**) Kikuchi lymphadenitis. Prominent histiocytic infiltrate with necrosis and karyorrhectic nuclear debris without neutrophils

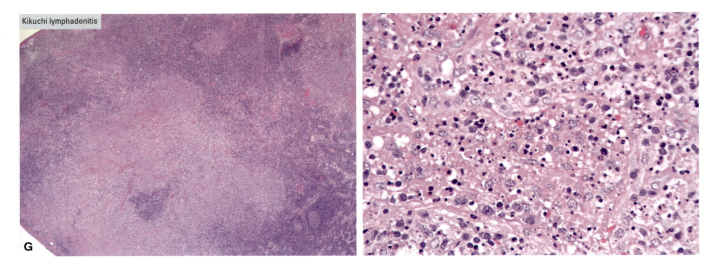

Kikuchi lymphadenitis

G

Figure 3.37   *(Continued)*

Blastic NK-cell lymphoma (Figure 3.37F) is distinguished from peripheral T-cell lymphoma by blastic morphology of tumor cells, lack of expression of CD3 and CD5, and positive expression of CD56 and HLA-DR. Peripheral T-cell lymphomas are rarely positive for CD56 and are most often HLA-DR negative.

Kikuchi lymphadenitis (Figure 3.37G), also known as histiocytic necrotizing lymphadenitis[482,483], is a benign disorder presenting with fever and adenopathy (most often cervical). Morphologically, it shows a polymorphic cellular infiltrate composed of lymphoid cells, crescentic histiocytes and necrotic foci surrounded by clusters of histiocytes, scattered atypical lymphoid cells and much extracellular and intracellular karyorrhectic (apoptotic) debris without neutrophils. Staining with CD68 and T-cell markers is useful in confirming histiocytic infiltrate.

ANGIOIMMUNOBLASTIC T-CELL LYMPHOMA

Angioimmunoblastic T-cell lymphoma is a mature T-cell lymphoproliferative process characterized by systemic symptoms, (reactive) polyclonal hypergammaglobulinemia and generalized lymphadenopathy with a polymorphous lymphoid infiltrate and numerous arborizing blood vessels[19,484–489]. Common clinical symptoms include skin rash, arthritis and edema with pleural and/or peritoneal effusions.

Morphology (Figure 3.38A) shows variable degrees of effacement of the lymph node architecture with polymorphous infiltrate composed of small reactive lymphocytes, histiocytes, eosinophils, plasma cells and clusters of atypical medium-sized or large T-cells with clear to pale cytoplasm. The atypical cells have a tendency to cluster or have prominent perivascular distribution. Majority of B-cells are displaced towards the periphery of the lymph node (Figure 3.38G). There is expansion of follicular dendritic cell meshwork (Figure 3.38I) and prominent arborizing small blood vessels (Figure 3.38B). Large B-cells with immunoblastic features are scattered through the lymph node. They are positive for EBER (Figure 3.38H).

Immunophenotyping reveals predominance of T-cells. Both CD4 and CD8 positive T-lymphocytes are present; the latter usually predominate. Clusters of atypical T-cells usually display aberrant expression of pan-T markers, most often loss of CD3 and/or CD7. The expression of T-markers may be much dimmer than in residual small (benign) T-cells. The majority of cases of angioimmunoblastic T-cell lymphomas display coexpression of CD10 by neoplastic T-cells[484]. The number of CD10+ tumor cells in each tumor may vary significantly[490]. Approximately 50% of cases show expression of CD10 by a majority of neoplastic cells. Bcl-6 is positive in T-cells in approximately one-third of cases (bcl-6 may be also positive in ALCL)[475]. Staining with CD21 or CD23 shows expansion of follicular dendritic cell meshwork in the majority of cases (Figure 3.38I).

Although general adenopathy is the main presenting sign, many patients have evidence of extranodal involvement at the time of diagnosis[490]. The most frequently involved extranodal sites include the bone marrow, spleen, skin and lungs[490]. Bone marrow involved by angioimmunoblastic T-cell lymphoma shows either large interstitial lymphoid aggregates or diffuse infiltrate with

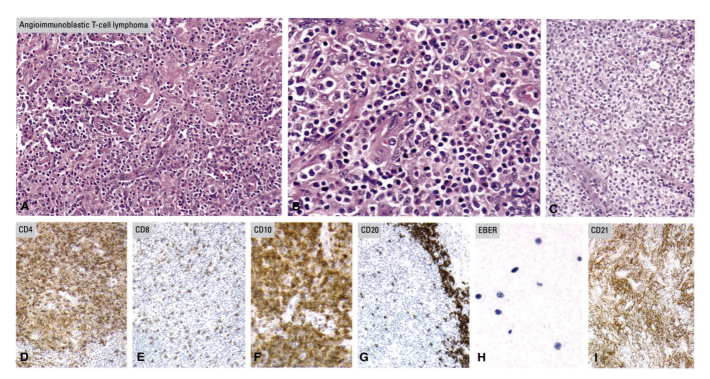

Figure 3.38   Angioimmunoblastic T-cell lymphoma. (**A**) Low power shows effacement of the architecture by a polymorphous lymphovascular infiltrate. (**B**) Higher magnification shows a mixture of small and medium-sized lymphocytes, plasma cells, eosinophils and blood vessels. (**C**) Another area shows clusters of atypical lymphocytes with clear cytoplasm. (**D**) CD4⁺ T-cells predominate. (**E**) Only rare CD8⁺ T-cells are present. (**F**) T-cells display aberrant expression of CD10. (**G**) B-cells are sparse and tend to be displaced to the periphery of the lymph node. (**H**) Scattered B-immunoblasts are expressing EBER. (**I**) Staining for CD21 highlights the expansion of follicular dendritic cells

paratrabecular component (Figure 3.39). The infiltrate shows mixed population of small, medium-sized and large lymphocytes with focal atypia and irregular nuclear outlines. The background, which may be focally myxoid, shows eosinophils, plasma cells and histiocytes, increased reticulin fibers, and small blood vessels.

The differential diagnosis includes reactive processes, classical Hodgkin lymphoma and T-cell lymphomas other than angioimmunoblastic T-cell lymphoma[359,478].

ANAPLASTIC LARGE CELL LYMPHOMA (ALCL)

ALCL is a T-cell lymphoma composed of large pleomorphic cells, that have irregular kidney-shaped nuclei ('hallmark cells') and are positive for CD30, and in the majority of cases ALK (anaplastic lymphoma kinase protein)[59,267,491–512]. ALCL involves lymph nodes and extranodal sites, such as skin, soft tissues, lung, and bone and less often the gastrointestinal tract. ALCL occurs at any age including childhood, but ALK-positive cases are more common in young adults. The prognosis of ALK-positive ALCL is favorable,

except for cases with peripheral blood involvement, which are aggressive[496,509,510,512–517]. Patients with ALK-negative tumors have a poor prognosis, similar to peripheral T-cell lymphoma, unspecified[496,498,509,517]. It is controversial but likely that ALK-negative lymphomas with anaplastic features represent a variant of CD30⁺ peripheral T-cell lymphoma.

ALK-positive ALCL displays a broad range of morphologic features with the presence of large neoplastic cells with characteristic horseshoe- or kidney-shaped nuclei (hallmark cells), prominent nucleoli and abundant cytoplasm (Figure 3.40A). Some of the tumor cells have prominent invagination of the nuclear membrane, creating 'doughnut'-like cells (Figure 3.40; arrow), whereas other cells resemble Reed–Sternberg cells. The pattern of lymph node involvement may be diffuse, perifollicular/T-zone or focal with characteristic intrasinusoidal distribution of tumor cells, mimicking metastatic tumor (Figure 3.40B and C). Several variants of ALCL have been recognized based on histomorphologic features: common variant, lymphohistiocytic variant, monomorphic variant and small cell variant[78,267,498,502,503,507,513,518]. The common variant of ALCL (Figure 3.40) comprises the majority of cases of ALCL. The

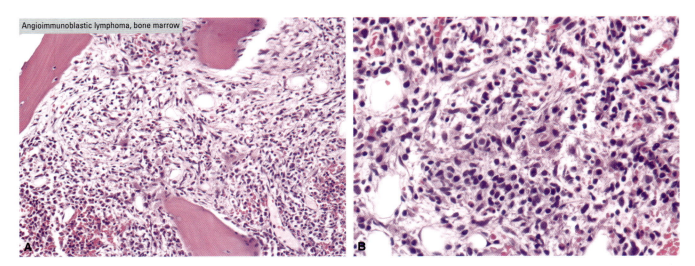

Figure 3.39   Angioimmunoblastic T-cell lymphoma – bone marrow. Polymorphic lymphoid infiltrate accompanied by fibrosis (**A**). Higher magnification shows atypical lymphoid cells mixed with eosinophils, plasma cells and histiocytes (**B**)

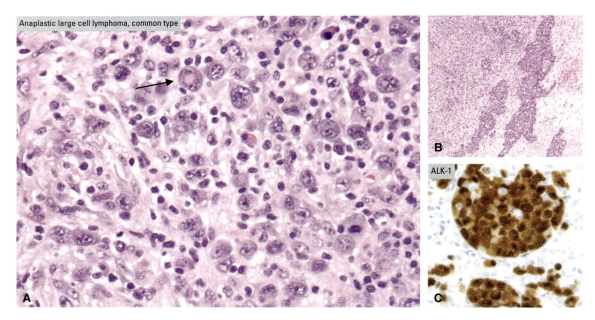

Figure 3.40   Anaplastic large cell lymphoma (ALCL) – common variant. (**A**) Pleomorphic large cell lymphoid infiltrate. Many nuclei are irregular with a horseshoe shape, so-called hallmark cells. (**B**) Low power shows a focal intrasinusoidal distribution of tumor cells. (**C**) Intrasinusoidal clusters of tumor cells show strong nuclear and cytoplasmic expression of ALK-1

lymphohistiocytic variant (Figure 3.41) is characterized by a mixture of typical tumor cells and a large number of histiocytes. The monomorphic variant (Figure 3.42) contains a diffuse infiltrate of large monomorphic cells with predominantly round nuclei and prominent nucleoli, resembling immunoblastic lymphoma. The small cell variant has a predominance of small to medium-sized lymphocytes with scattered large hallmark cells (Figure 3.43). Expression of ALK puts this variant into the ALCL category, despite small cell size and lack of overt anaplastic features[498].

The neoplastic cells are positive for CD30 with strong membrane and Golgi area staining. The majority of cases are

positive for CD45, CD43 and EMA. Pan-T antigens are often aberrantly expressed (only about 10% of ALCL are positive for all four pan-T antigens). CD7 is most frequently and CD2 is least frequently absent. The majority of cases are CD4+ (~70%), but CD8+, CD4+/8+ or CD4−/8− cases also occur (see Table 1.7; Chapter 1). Most cases are TCRαβ+ (~70%), and the remaining cases do not express TCR. A subset of ALCL may be CD56+.

The most frequent chromosomal abnormality in ALCL is t(2;5)(p23;35), which involves the *ALK* gene on chromosome 2 and the nucleophosmin gene *(NPM)* on chromosome 5. Variant translocations involving ALK and

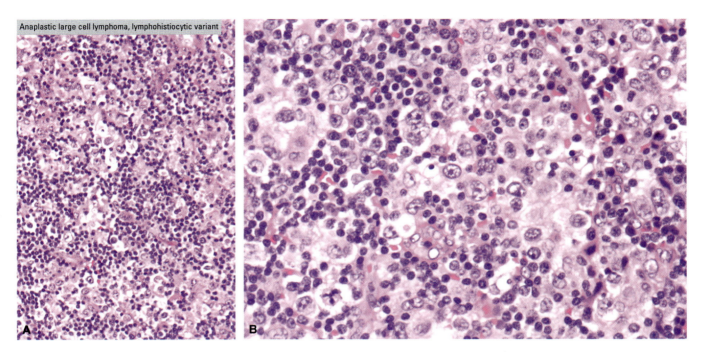

Figure 3.41 Anaplastic large cell lymphoma (ALCL) – lymphohistiocytic variant. Pleomorphic tumor cells are admixed with histiocytes and small lymphocytes (**A**, low magnification; **B**, high magnification)

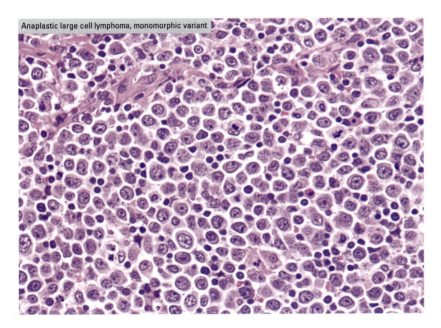

Figure 3.42 Anaplastic large cell lymphoma (ALCL) – monomorphic variant. Atypical large lymphoid cells show little difference in size and shape

other partner genes can also be detected in ALCL. In contrast to t(2;5), which is associated with both nuclear and cytoplasmic staining for ALK protein (Figure 3.44A), the variant translocations are associated with cytoplasmic-only staining with ALK protein by immunohistochemistry (Figure 3.44B)[59,519–521].

The ALK-negative variant (Figure 3.45) comprises 20–40% of ALCL. As mentioned above, the diagnosis of ALK-negative ALCL is controversial. It is likely a variant of peripheral T-cell lymphoma with anaplastic features.

A small subset of ALCL may express CD15 (Figure 3.46), and therefore display some overlapping phenotypic features with classical Hodgkin lymphoma. Expression of CD45, CD43, pan-T markers, CD4 and EMA, and lack of expression of CD20, Pax-5 and EBV/EBER favor ALCL. Figure 3.47 shows examples of extranodal ALK⁺ ALCL.

The differential diagnosis of ALCL depends on the location of the tumor and includes large cell hemato-lymphoid and non-hematopoietic tumors

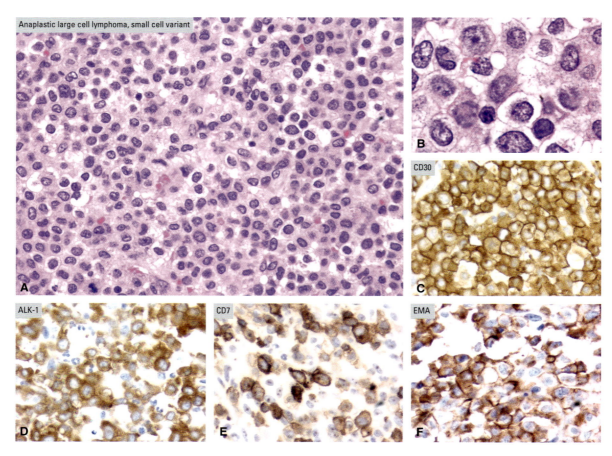

Figure 3.43   Anaplastic large cell lymphoma (ALCL) – small cell variant. (**A**) Diffuse lymphoid infiltrate of predominantly small cells with irregular nuclei (**B**, high magnification). Tumor cells are positive for CD30 (**C**), ALK-1 (**D**), CD7 (**E**) and EMA (**F**)

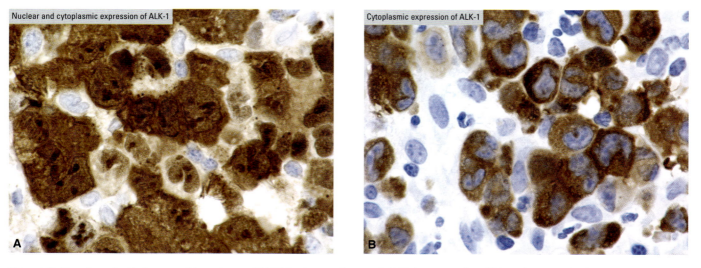

Figure 3.44   Anaplastic large cell lymphoma (ALCL) – two patterns of ALK-1 expression: (**A**) nuclear, nucleolar and cytoplasmic staining; (**B**) cytoplasmic staining

(Figure 3.48)[261–264,266,275,276,320,354,498,520,522–524]. Classical Hodgkin lymphoma differs in lack of CD45 and (dim) expression of Pax-5. In contrast to Pax-5 expression, which favors HL, positive staining with bcl-6 does not distinguish between HL and ALCL. Bcl-6 may be dimly expressed in ALCL and is often positive in HL. CD15 expression, although typical for HL, may be occasionally seen in ALK+ ALCL[481].

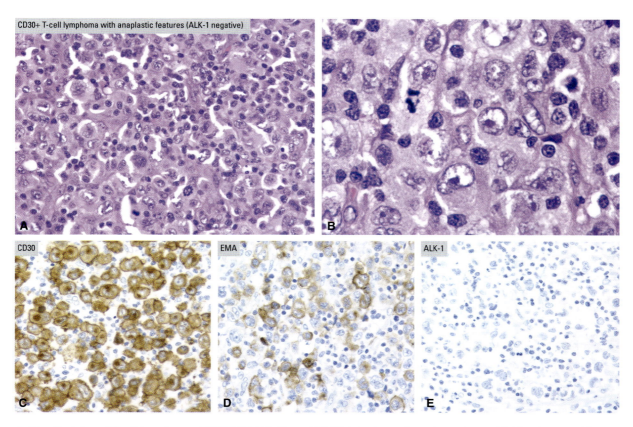

Figure 3.45   Peripheral T-cell lymphoma (CD30$^+$/ALK$^-$). (**A** and **B**) Histologic section shows large, highly pleomorphic tumor cells with prominent nucleoli. Tumor cells are strongly positive for CD30 (**C**) and express EMA (**D**), but ALK-1 is not expressed (**E**). It is controversial whether an ALK-negative tumor with morphologic features of ALCL should be considered a more aggressive variant of ALCL or a subtype of peripheral T-cell lymphoma

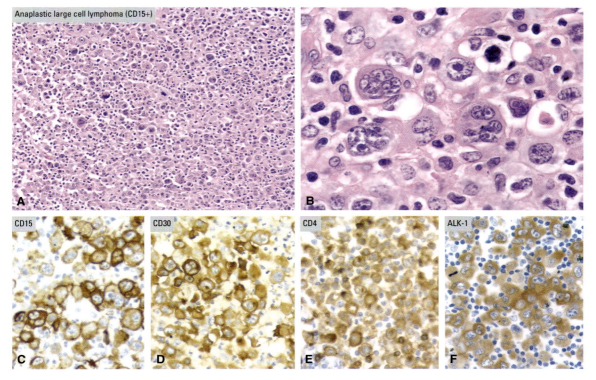

Figure 3.46   Anaplastic large cell lymphoma (ALCL) with aberrant expression of CD15. (**A**) Low magnification shows a polymorphous lymphoid infiltrate. (**B**) High magnification shows large, multinucleated cells resembling Reed–Sternberg cells. Tumor cells are positive for CD15 (**C**), CD30 (**D**), CD4 (**E**) and ALK-1 (**F**, cytoplasmic staining)

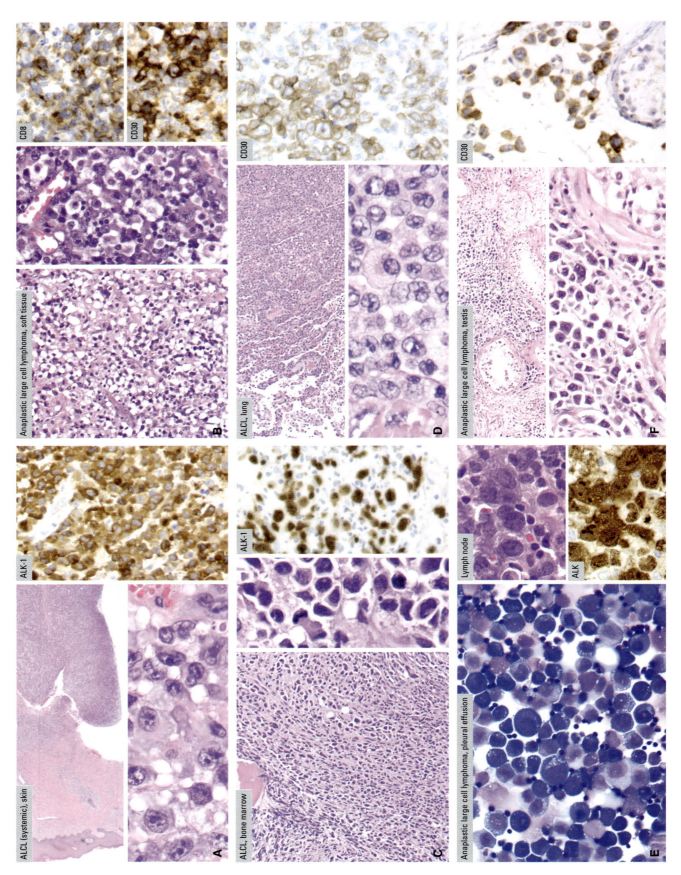

Figure 3.47   Extranodal anaplastic large cell lymphoma (ALCL). (**A**) Skin. (**B**) Soft tissue. (**C**) Bone marrow. (**D**) Lung. (**E**) Pleural effusion. (**F**) Testis

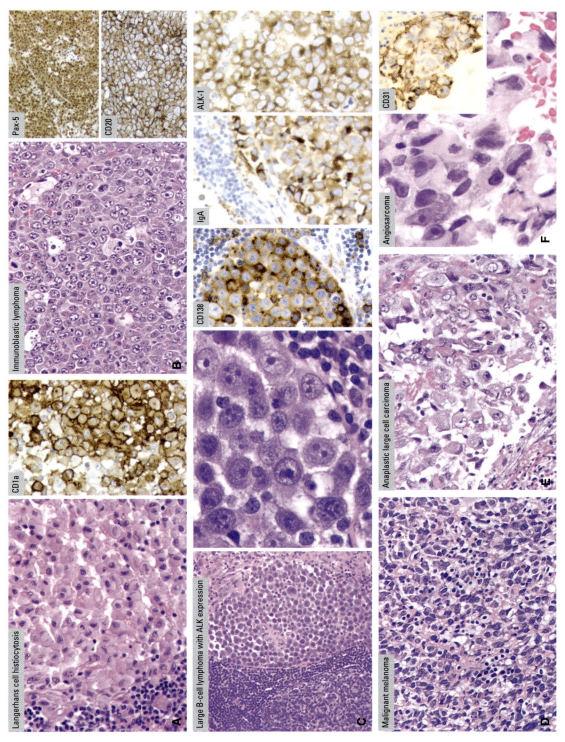

Figure 3.48   Anaplastic large cell lymphoma (ALCL) – differential diagnosis. (**A**) Langerhans cell histiocytosis. Tumor cells have abundant cytoplasm and characteristic nuclear features (grooves) and are positive for CD1a and S100. (**B**) Immunoblastic lymphoma. It may resemble the monomorphic subtype of ALCL, but it expresses B-cell markers. (**C**) Large B-cell lymphoma with ALK expression. This unusual variant of DLBCL is negative for CD20 and expresses CD138, IgA and ALK (cytoplasmic). (**D**) Malignant melanoma. (**E**) Anaplastic large cell carcinoma. (**F**) Angiosarcoma. (**G**) Classical Hodgkin lymphoma (lymphocyte-depleted variant). Distinction between ALCL and HL may be difficult. Both entities may show overlapping morphologic and phenotypic features. Intrasinusoidal distribution, rarity of diagnostic Reed–Sternberg cells, lack of CD15 and B-cell markers, and positive staining with CD45, EMA and T-cell markers favor ALCL. (**H**) Histiocytic sarcoma. The neoplastic cells lack reactivity with pan-T antigens and B-cell markers and show variable staining with CD68 and CD15. (**I**) Classical Hodgkin lymphoma with aberrant expression of CD2. (**J**) Follicular dendritic cell sarcoma. Tumor cells are positive for CD21. (**K**) Anaplastic variant of plasma cell myeloma. (**L**) Diffuse large B-cell lymphoma with anaplastic features

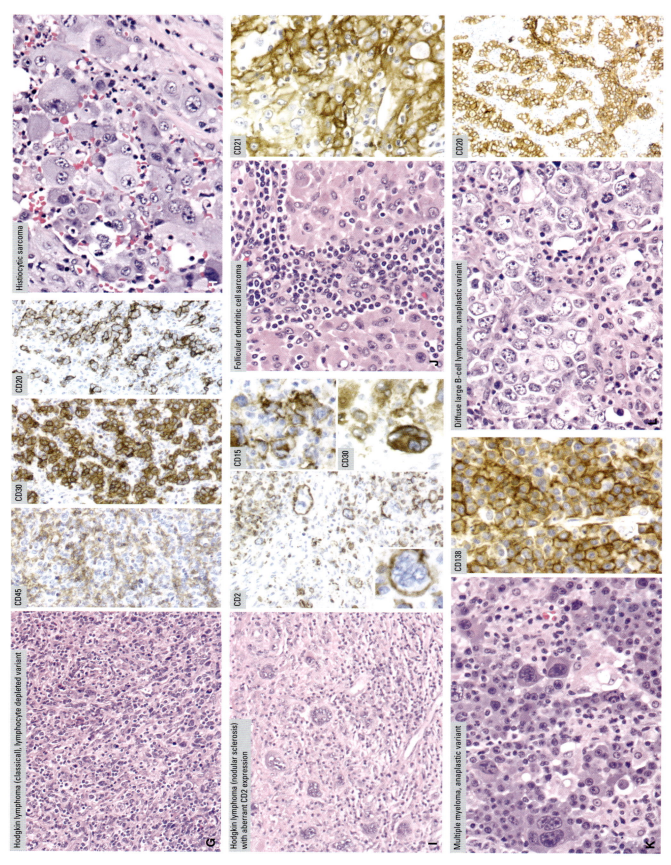

Figure 3.48   (*Continued*)

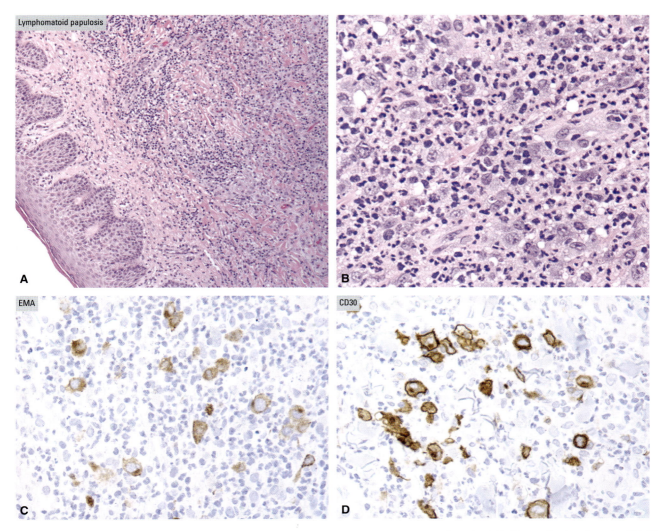

Figure 3.49   Lymphomatoid papulosis. (**A**) Low magnification shows pleomorphic lymphoid infiltrate in the dermis. (**B**) High magnification shows large neoplastic cells mixed with inflammatory cells. Tumor cells express EMA (**C**) and CD30 (**D**)

LYMPHOMATOID PAPULOSIS

Lymphomatoid papulosis (Figure 3.49) is an atypical lymphoproliferative process associated with recurrent skin lesions (papules), which often regress and recur[236,331–335,337,446,474,525]. Morphologically, two types of lymphomatoid papulosis are recognized: type A shows predominance of small lymphocytes and scattered large atypical cells resembling Reed–Sternberg cells, and type B shows numerous lymphoid cells with cerebriform nuclei. The distinction between primary cutaneous ALCL and type A is based on the relative predominance of CD30+ atypical large cells, and there is a degree of histologic overlap.

CHAPTER 4

Hodgkin lymphoma

CLASSIFICATION OF HODGKIN LYMPHOMA

Hodgkin lymphoma (HL) is a B-cell neoplasm characterized by distinctive morphologic features with a paucity of large neoplastic cells and the predominance of an inflammatory (reactive) background with small lymphocytes, eosinophils, histiocytes and plasma cells[70,78,284,286,287,437,521,525–539]. Two major categories of HL are recognized (Figure 4.1): nodular lymphocyte-predominant HL (NLPHL) and classical HL. Classical HL differs from non-HL by its bimodal age distribution, including young adulthood, contiguous nodal spread, predilection for cervical and mediastinal presentation, and relative lack of extranodal involvement. The nodular sclerosis type of HL frequently is mediastinal in location, whereas abdominal lymph node and splenic involvement are more often seen in the mixed cellularity subtype. NLPHL generally occurs in young adulthood and presents with stage I peripheral nodal involvement. Diagnostic cells of NLPHL ('popcorn cells' or L&H cells) are positive for B-cell markers (CD20, CD79a, Pax-5), CD45 (LCA) and EMA, and are negative for CD30, CD15 and EBV/EBER (Figure 4.1G–I). Diagnostic cells of classical HL (Reed–Sternberg cells, Hodgkin cells and variants) are positive for CD30 and CD15 (Figure 4.1C and D), often positive for EBV/EBER and are negative for CD45. Based on the number of neoplastic cells, growth pattern, presence of sclerosis and clinical presentation, classical HL is further divided into four subtypes: nodular sclerosis, lymphocyte-rich, mixed cellularity and lymphocyte-depleted (Table 4.1).

NODULAR LYMPHOCYTE-PREDOMINANT HL

NLPHL is a B-cell neoplasm characterized by the presence of scattered large atypical 'popcorn cells' or L&H cells (lymphocyte and histiocyte cell) and a distinct nodular pattern on low magnification

Table 4.1 Classification of Hodgkin lymphoma

Nodular lymphocyte-predominant Hodgkin lymphoma (NLPHL)
Classical Hodgkin lymphoma (HL)
    Nodular sclerosis Hodgkin lymphoma
    Lymphocyte-rich classical Hodgkin lymphoma
    Mixed cellularity Hodgkin lymphoma
    Lymphocyte-depleted Hodgkin lymphoma

(Figure 4.1F)[293,294,526–528,534,535,538,539,541]. There is an association between NLPHL and progressively transformed germinal centers (PTGC); however, they are not synonymous, since PTGC is reactive phenomenon. PTGC may be seen simultaneously with or may proceed NLPHL. Therefore, patients with PTGC but without typical L&H cells should be closely followed since they have a slightly higher risk of developing NLPHL[542]. The prognosis of NLPHL is usually favorable, especially in early-stage disease. NLPHL may progress to diffuse large B-cell lymphoma.

The most characteristic morphologic feature of NLPHL is the distinct nodular pattern of the lymph node under low magnification (Figure 4.2A). Nodules are often ill defined and vague and are usually larger than those of follicular lymphoma, follicular hyperplasia or nodular mantle cell lymphoma. The nodules are studded with histiocytes, which may give the nodules a pseudo-starry-sky appearance by low magnification. The nodular pattern is easily visualized by staining with either CD20 or CD21 (Figure 4.2B and C). There are no fibrous septa separating individual nodules, as seen in nodular sclerosis HL. Tumor cells are large with multilobated or folded nuclei, prominent nucleoli and pale vesicular chromatin (Figure 4.3). Because of their cytologic features, they are called 'popcorn cells' or L&H cells. 'Popcorn cells' differ morphologically from Reed–Sternberg cells by smaller size, less pronounced lobation, smaller nucleoli and scantier cytoplasm. Phenotypically, 'popcorn cells' are positive for

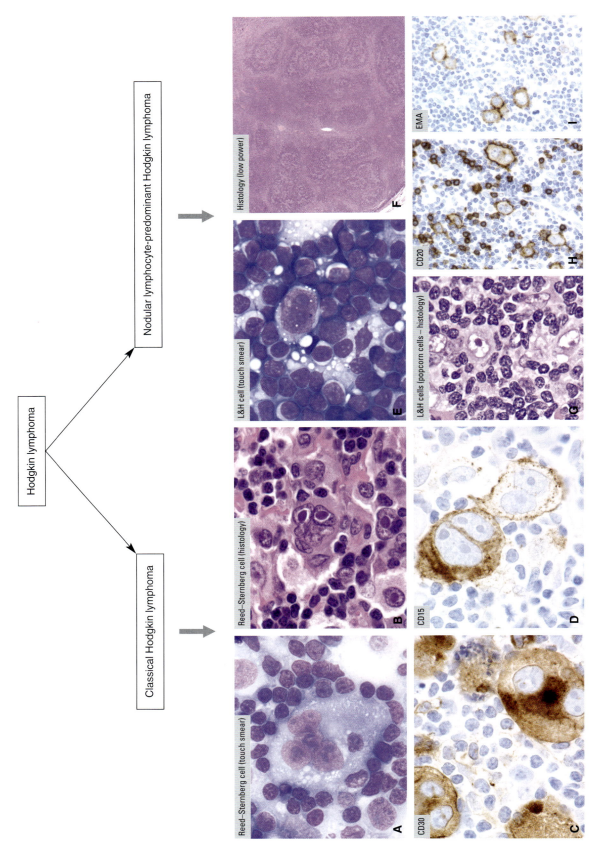

Figure 4.1   Classification of Hodgkin lymphoma. (**A–D**) classical Hodgkin lymphoma: (**A**) touch imprint with Reed–Sternberg cells, (**B**) histologic section with typical multinucleated R–S cell, (**C**) expression of CD30, (**D**) expression of CD15. (**E–I**) Nodular lymphocyte-predominant Hodgkin lymphoma: (**E**) touch imprint showing an atypical cell with large nucleus, (**F**) low magnification of the lymph node showing nodular pattern, (**G**) high magnification showing typical 'popcorn' cells, (**H**) expression of CD20, (**I**) expression of EMA

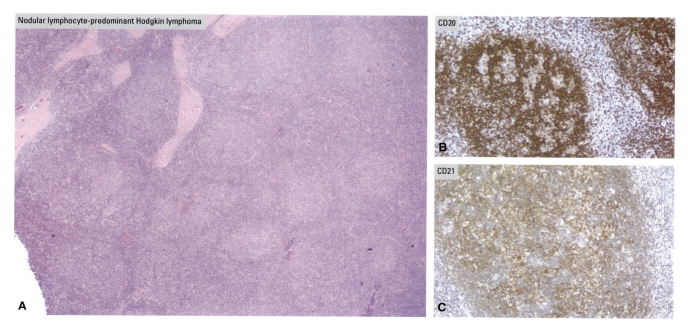

Figure 4.2   Nodular lymphocyte-predominant Hodgkin lymphoma. Low magnification of the lymph node (**A**) shows typical nodular architecture. Nodular architecture is best visualized with the staining for CD20 (**B**) or CD21 (**C**)

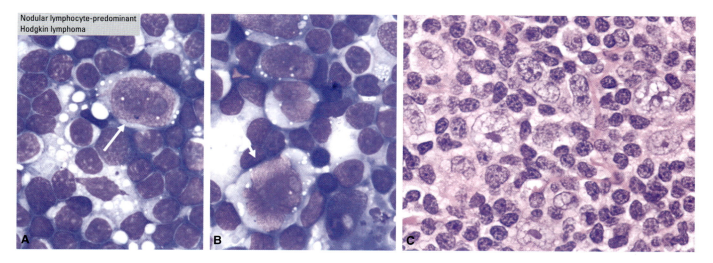

Figure 4.3   Nodular lymphocyte-predominant Hodgkin lymphoma – cytologic features of neoplastic cells (popcorn cells/L&H cells). (**A** and **B**) Touch imprint preparations. (**C**) Histologic section (high magnification)

CD45, B-cell markers (CD20, CD22, CD79a, Pax-5, BOB-1, OCT-2), bcl-6 and often epithelial membrane antigen (Figure 4.4). Bcl-2 is usually negative[539]. Most often, the expression of Pax-5 is dimmer than in surrounding benign small B-cells and the expression of OCT-2 is stronger (compare Figure 4.4H and I). A majority of cases of NLPHL do not express CD30, CD15, pan-T markers, CD43 and EBV/EBER. Tumor cells are surrounded by a single layer of small benign T/NK-cells expressing CD57 (Figure 4.5). The remaining cells comprising the major constituent of nodules in NLPHL are small B-lymphocytes. This differs from classical HL, where the majority of background cells are small T-cells. Apart from the most common and most characteristic nodular 'B-cell-rich' pattern, several other distinct immunoarchitectural patterns have been identified in NLPHL: nodular T-cell-rich pattern, nodular pattern with prominent extranodular L&H cells and T-cell-rich B-cell lymphoma-like pattern. Figure 4.6 depicts partial lymph node involvement by NLPHL. Rare cases of

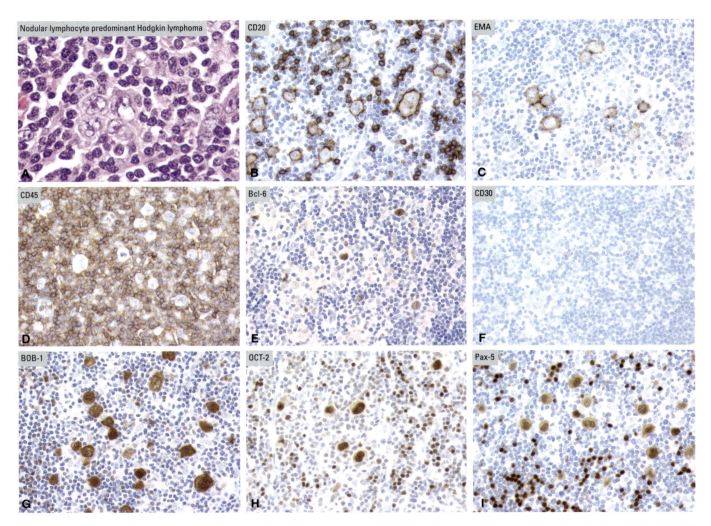

Figure 4.4   Nodular lymphocyte-predominant Hodgkin lymphoma (NLPHL) – immunohistochemistry. Neoplastic cells in NLPHL (popcorn cells or L&H cells, see **A**), are positive for CD20 (**B**), EMA (**C**), CD45 (**D**), bcl-6 (**E**), BOB-1 (**G**), OCT-2 (**H**) and Pax-5 (**I**). Note typical membranous staining with CD20 and EMA (**B** and **C**). The nuclear expression of BOB-1 and OCT-2 is stronger than in normal small B-cells (**G** and **H**). The nuclear staining with Pax-5 is weaker than in normal small B-cells (**I**). CD30 is negative (**F**), which distinguishes popcorn cells from classical Reed–Sternberg cells

NLPHL display expression of CD15 by L&H cells (Figure 4.7).

The unique morphologic and immunophenotypic features of NLPHL are preserved in extranodal sites (liver, spleen, tonsil, salivary gland, soft tissue, bone marrow)[292].

The differential diagnosis of NLPHL includes both reactive and neoplastic conditions (Figure 4.8)[286,294,538,541–544]. Reactive conditions (Figure 4.8A) with scattered large atypical cells are distinguished by the lack of typical for NLPHL low-power characteristics. Activated cells may be of B- and T-lineage but they do not coexpress EMA and may be positive for EBV markers. Follicular lymphoma (FL) (Figure 4.8B) usually occurs in older patients than does NLPHL. FL displays effacement of the lymph node architecture by nodules, which are usually smaller than in NLPHL and show predominance of atypical cells, rather

than small B-cells and large atypical cells as seen in NLPHL. There are no CD57+ rosettes around large cells. NLPHL, especially cases with only partial lymph node involvement, have to be distinguished from PTGC[541]. PTGC (Figure 4.8C) is a reactive transformation of a follicle in which the mantle zones of the follicle expands, and the follicle is large and ill defined, with obscure borders between the germinal center and mantle/marginal zone. PTGC are scattered throughout the lymph node with florid follicular hyperplasia. Higher magnification does not reveal typical 'popcorn cells' or EMA+ large B-cells.

Classical HL may mimic NLPHL by showing vague nodularity or presence of large multilobated cells dispersed in the background of small lymphocytes (e.g., lymphocyte-rich HL). Some L&H cells may have prominent nucleoli and multinucleation and resemble Reed–Sternberg

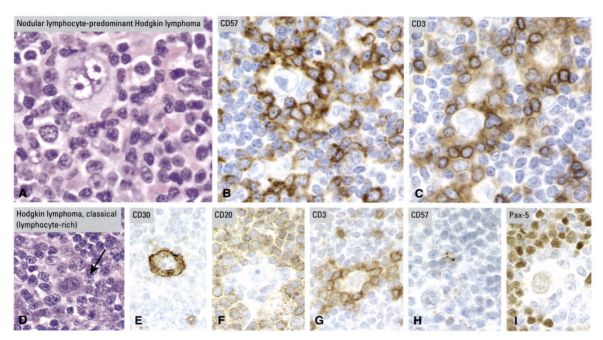

Figure 4.5 Nodular lymphocyte-predominant Hodgkin lymphoma (NLPHL **A–C**) – differential diagnosis with lymphocyte-rich classical Hodgkin lymphoma (**D–I**). Typical popcorn cells of NLPHL are surrounded by small T/NK-lymphocytes in a rosette-like pattern (**A**); expression of CD57 (**B**) and CD3 (**C**). Neoplastic cells in lymphocyte-rich classical HL are CD30$^+$ (**E**), CD20$^-$ (**F**) and are dimly positive for Pax-5 (**I**). They are surrounded by small CD3$^+$ T-cells (**G**), which do not co-express CD57 (**H**)

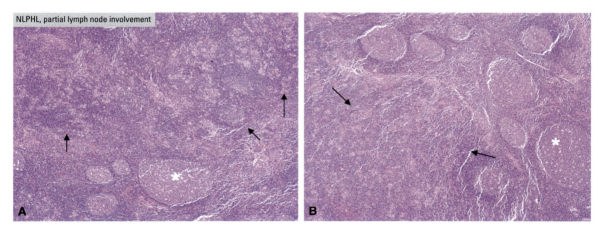

Figure 4.6 Nodular lymphocyte-predominant Hodgkin lymphoma (NLPHL) – partial lymph node involvement. (**A** and **B**) Low magnification of two different areas of the lymph node partially involved by NLPHL (arrow). Reactive follicles (*) surround neoplastic area

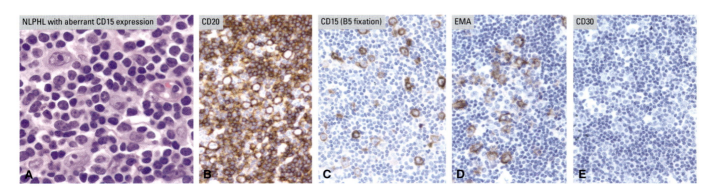

Figure 4.7 Nodular lymphocyte-predominant Hodgkin lymphoma (NLPHL) with unusual expression of CD15 (B5 fixation). Typical popcorn cells (**A**) are positive for CD20 (**B**), CD15 (**C**), EMA (**D**) and are negative for CD30 (**E**)

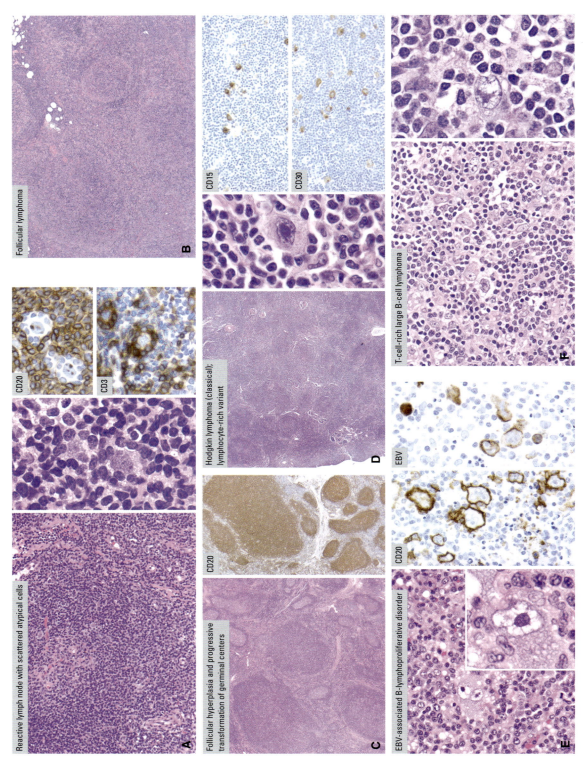

Figure 4.8   Differential diagnosis of NLPHL. (**A**) Reactive lymph node with scattered large immunoblasts (activated cells). Low magnification shows vague nodularity. High magnification shows large cells surrounded by rosettes of small lymphocytes. Atypical large cells, which are negative with CD20, are surrounded by small lymphocytes labeled with CD3. (**B**) Follicular lymphoma. Although low magnification may resemble NLPHL, high magnification does not reveal popcorn cells. There is no EMA expression or CD57⁺ rosettes. (**C**) Follicular hyperplasia with progressive transformation of germinal centers (PTGC). Low magnification shows lymph node with hyperplastic follicles and several PTGC. Both reactive follicles and PTGC are staining with CD20. (**D**) Classical Hodgkin lymphoma – lymphocyte-rich variant. Scattered large neoplastic cells are positive for CD30 and CD15 and do not express EMA. (**E**) EBV-associated lymphoproliferative disorder compatible with large B-cell lymphoma. Neoplastic large B-cells are positive for CD20 and EBV. (**F**) T-cell rich large B-cell lymphoma. There are no nodules with typical features of NLPHL

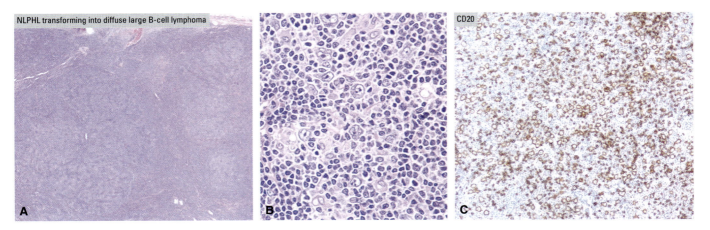

Figure 4.9   NLPHL transforming into large B-cell lymphoma. (**A**) Low power shows typical features of NLPHL. (**B** and **C**) High magnification and CD20 staining show numerous large B-cells with relatively few small B-lymphocytes

(R–S) cells. On the other hand, some R–S cells, especially lacunar variants, may have less prominent nucleoli and scanty (retracted) cytoplasm and therefore imitate popcorn cells. Also, the phenotype in occasional cases may overlap between classical HL and NLPHL[284]. Some cases (especially if tissue was fixed in B5) may express CD15 by L&H cells (Figure 4.7). Low-power histology of the lymph node and evaluation of the cytology and phenotype of the neoplastic and background cells differentiate classical HL from NLPHL. Popcorn cells are generally smaller and have less prominent nucleoli than R–S cells. The nuclear membrane is thinner and the cytoplasm less abundant. The phenotype of R–S and Hodgkin cells is different (Figure 4.8D). Although neoplastic cells in classical HL are Pax-5[+] and may be CD20[+], they display expression of CD30, often CD15, and EBV/EBER, and are negative for CD45, which differentiates them from NLPHL. The presence of a distinct rim of small T/NK-cells with strong coexpression of CD57 favors NLPHL[294]. Classical R–S cells are surrounded by small T-cells, but they rarely express CD57. In contrast to NLPHL, the majority of small lymphocytes in classical HL are T-cells. Nodules of NLPHL are mainly composed of small B-cells (except for the rosette of T/NK-cells directly apposing the neoplastic large cells).

Reactive lymph nodes under chronic immune stimulation may contain scattered individual large atypical cells, suggesting NLPHL or classical HL. The large cells are perifollicular or interfollicular in distribution, and may express CD30 and represent B-immunoblasts or, less often, CD4[+] or CD8[+] T-immunoblasts. Reactive processes (Figure 4.8A and E) lack the vague nodularity typical for NLPHL. Large cells in reactive conditions do not express EMA and are not rimmed by CD57[+] T/NK-cells. Cases related to EBV infection show positive EBV/EBER expression by large atypical cells (Figure 4.8E).

FL (Figure 4.8D) most often occurs in older age group than NLPHL. Lymph nodes in FL show effacement of the architecture by nodules, which are usually smaller than in NLPHL and display a back-to-back arrangement with less intervening paracortex. The cellular composition of both processes is also different. FL, regardless of the grade, is composed of small and large centrocytes with twisted, irregular nuclear contours and variable numbers of centroblasts with vesicular nuclei and multiple nucleoli. Large cells do not express EMA and are not rimmed by CD57[+] cells.

NLPHL may present with an increased number of L&H cells, or may undergo transformation into diffuse large B-cell lymphoma (Figure 4.9). Transformation into DLBCL is heralded by spillover of large B-cells outside the PTGCs, with a loss of small B-cells. The differential diagnosis between NLPHL with increased large cells, DLBCL transformed from NLPHL, and T-cell/histiocyte-rich, large B-cell lymphoma (TCRLBCL) (Figure 4.8F) is often difficult[294,527,528,544]. A subset of TCRBCL may have an increased number of bcl-6[+] large cells and CD57[+] small cells[294]. Diffuse effacement of the lymph node architecture with haphazardly distributed large atypical cells forming occasional clusters, and absence of even focal nodularity favors TCRLBCL or DLBCL[526]. Cases with an overall pattern of DLBCL, but with focal nodular areas compatible with NLPHL or with expanded dendritic meshwork typical of PTGC with atypical large cells within, may be regarded as DLBCL, having transformed from NLPHL. NLPHL and TCRLBCL may occur concurrently or subsequently in the same patients[544].

CLASSICAL HL

Classical HL is a B-cell neoplasm characterized by the presence of R–S cells and an accompanying polymorphic inflammatory infiltrate with eosinophils, histiocytes, small lymphocytes and plasma cells caused by cytokine production by the neoplastic cells[70,285,287,288,438,522,529–533,536–538,540]. Neoplastic cells in HL are positive for CD30, Pax-5 and, in many cases, CD15 and EBV/EBER (Figure 4.10). CD45 is negative and a majority of cases are CD20⁻. A subset of HL expresses CD20 and/or bcl-6. Based on the proportion of neoplastic cells (R–S cells and Hodgkin cells), the inflammatory background and the amount of fibrosis, HL is subdivided into four types: nodular sclerosis, lymphocyte-rich, mixed cellularity and lymphocyte-depleted (Figure 4.11). EBV has been implicated in the etiology of HL. Rare cases of HL follow EBV-associated histologic changes (Figure 4.12).

Nodular sclerosis HL (NS HL)

NS HL is the most common subtype of classical HL. It is characterized by a thickened lymph node capsule, and prominent bands of collagen springing from the capsule, dividing the lymph node into variably sized nodules (Figure 4.13A and B). Even early faint collagenous bands, which are birefringent under polarized light, qualify for categorization as NS HL. The neoplastic cells occur in variable proportions. They have multiple or multilobated nuclei (Figure 4.13B and C) with prominent macronucleoli. In formalin-fixed tissue, R–S cells often display contraction of the cytoplasm, creating 'empty' space around large tumor cell (Figure 4.13D); hence, the term 'lacunar cells'. The syncytial variant of NS HL (Figure 4.14) contains increased numbers of neoplastic cells, which form sheets and large clusters. The lacunar variant of R–S cells and all other variants in this type of HL have a classic

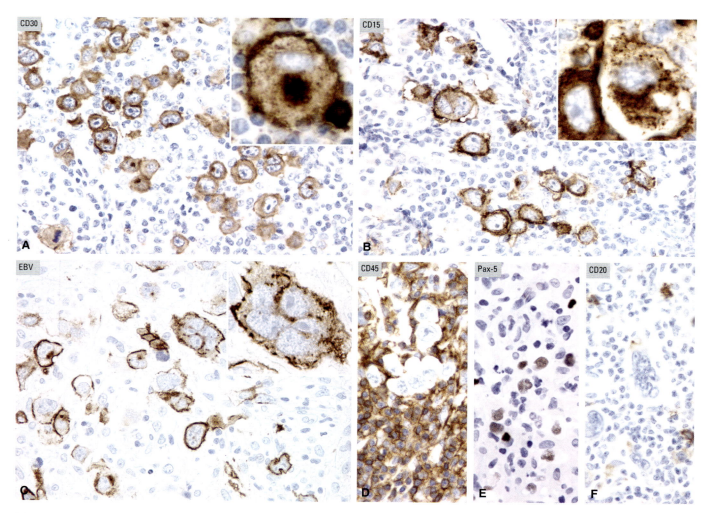

Figure 4.10   Hodgkin lymphoma (classical) – immunohistochemistry. (**A**) Expression of CD30. (**B**) Expression of CD15. (**C**) Expression of EBV. (**D**) Lack of expression of CD45. (**E**) Expression of Pax-5. (**F**) Lack of expression of CD20

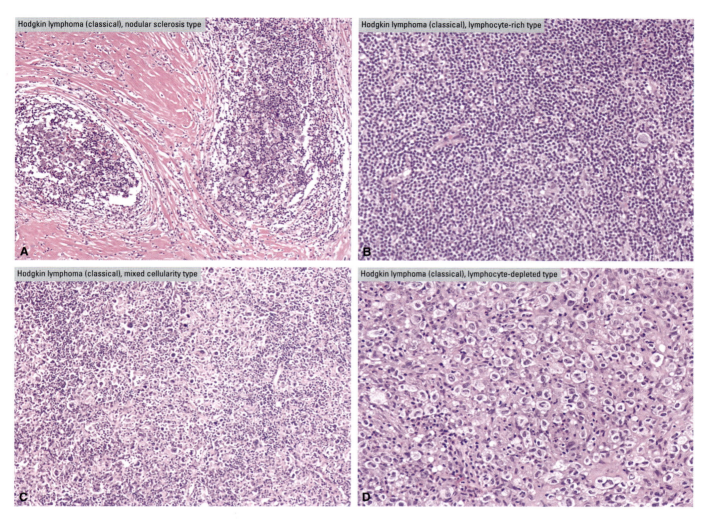

Figure 4.11 Hodgkin lymphoma (classical) – major histologic types. (**A**) Nodular sclerosis. (**B**) Lymphocyte-rich type. (**C**) Mixed cellularity type. (**D**) Lymphocyte-depleted type

phenotype (CD30$^+$. CD15$^{+/-}$, CD20$^{-/+}$, CD45$-$, EBV/EBER$^{-/+}$, Pax-5$^+$). The expression of Pax-5 is dimmer than in benign small B-cells. Although NS HL is a well-defined category, it is still very heterogeneous in its histologic appearance and survival[545]. It is suggested that the grading of NS HL based on the eosinophilia, lymphocyte depletion and atypia of the Hodgkin/R–S cells may indicate a prognosis in intermediate and advanced stages of HL[546].

Lymphocyte-rich classical HL

Lymphocyte-rich classical HL is a rare subtype of HL with a vaguely nodular pattern of small B-cells and scattered rare large neoplastic cells with the classic morphology of R–S cells (Figure 4.15), which are present within the B-cell zones, often at the periphery of the nodules. Inflammatory cells (eosinophils, neutrophils, histiocytes)

are not present or are very rare. Occasional cases may lack nodularity but have a similar cellular composition. Although low-power architecture and cytomorphology of large neoplastic cells may mimic NLPHL, the neoplastic cells have the same immunophenotype as other classical HL: positive CD30, CD15, negative CD20 (most cases), dim Pax-5 and negative CD45 and EBV/EBER.

Mixed cellularity HL

Mixed cellularity HL (Figure 4.16) is a subtype of classical HL with an increased number of large neoplastic cells and numerous polymorphic inflammatory cells (eosinophils, histiocytes, plasma cells and neutrophils) without broad bands of fibrosis, a thickened capsule and nodular architecture. Lacunar cells are infrequent. Occasional cases show prominent clusters of epithelioid histiocytes, mimicking an inflammatory process. The phenotype of neoplastic cells

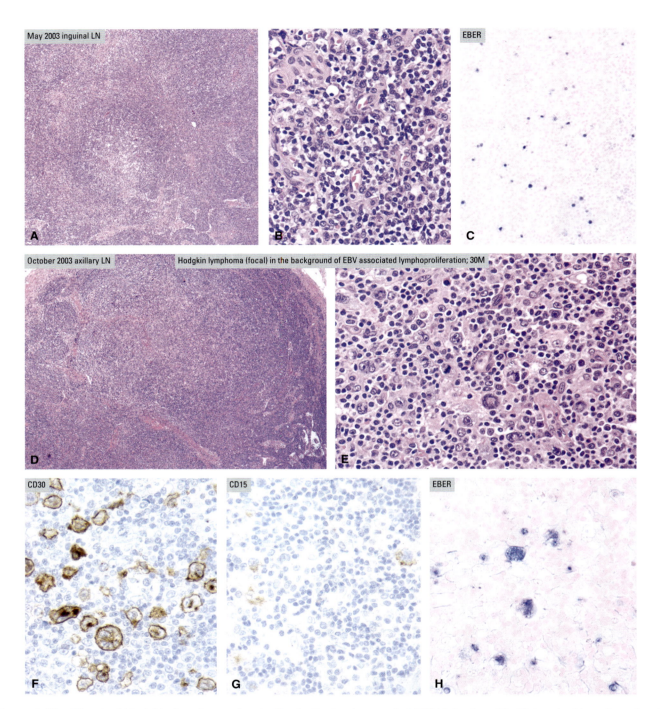

Figure 4.12   Classical Hodgkin lymphoma developing in the background of EBV infection. (**A–C**) Inguinal lymph node with scattered EBER+ cells (**C**). No diagnostic Reed–Sternberg cells were present. (**D–H**) After several months the patients developed Hodgkin lymphoma in an axillary lymph node. Neoplastic cells were labeled with CD30 (**F**), CD15 (**G**) and EBER (**H**). Note difference in the size of EBER+ nuclei in reactive (**C**) and neoplastic (**H**) process

is typical for HL; EBV/EBER positivity is more frequent than in NS HL.

Lymphocyte-depleted HL

Lymphocyte-depleted HL (Figure 4.17) is a rare form of HL with diffuse pattern and predominance of large neoplastic cells. It has a predilection for abdominal organs and retroperitoneal lymph nodes, occurs more often in elderly patients and is usually associated with advanced stage. Morphologic examination shows numerous large atypical neoplastic cells with prominent pleomorphism, suggesting ALCL. Tumor cells are positive for CD30 and may be positive for CD15 and EBV/EBER. CD45, EMA, CD43 and ALK-1 are not expressed, differentiating it from ALCL. Lack of CD45, CD22

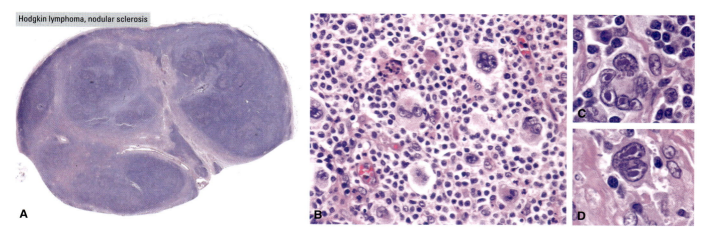

Figure 4.13 Nodular sclerosis subtype of classical Hodgkin lymphoma. (**A**) Nodular pattern caused by collagen bands is evident. (**B**) Higher magnification shows a polymorphic infiltrate with scattered large multilobated lacunar cells. (**C** and **D**) Cytologic features of R–S cells with an eosinophilic inclusion-like macronucleolus surrounded by a pale zone

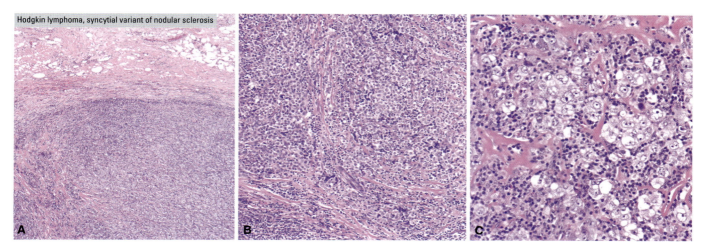

Figure 4.14 Syncytial variant of nodular sclerosis classical Hodgkin lymphoma. (**A**) Collagenous bands divide the lymph node into nodules. (**B**) Intermediate magnification shows nodules composed of numerous large cells. (**C**) High magnification shows numerous lacunar cells

and CD79a distinguishes it from diffuse large B-cell lymphoma with anaplastic features; however, many investigators think that it should be classified as DLBCL, if CD20 positive.

Extranodal involvement of classical HL

The presence of typical R–S cells in the appropriate cellular background is diagnostic for extranodal involvement of HL. In the bone marrow, the infiltrate may be subtle, with rare atypical large cells, few eosinophils and focal fibrosis. Evaluation of several levels of a trephine core biopsy, with additional immunophenotypic analysis

for CD30, Pax-5, EBV/EBER and CD20, helps to identify R–S cells. Figure 4.18 depicts two patterns of prominent bone marrow involvement: diffuse (Figure 4.18A) and nodular (Figure 4.18B).

Other organs (Figure 4.19) including the liver, spleen, lung, thymus, large intestine, urinary bladder and Waldeyer's ring may be occasionally involved, most often in advanced-stage disease, but rarely as the primary site. Skin involvement is exceedingly rare.

The differential diagnosis of HL (Figure 4.20) includes DLBCL, T-cell-rich large B-cell lymphoma, NLPHL, ALCL and non-hematopoietic tumors[69,125,271,283–286,288–291,489,523,538,547,548].

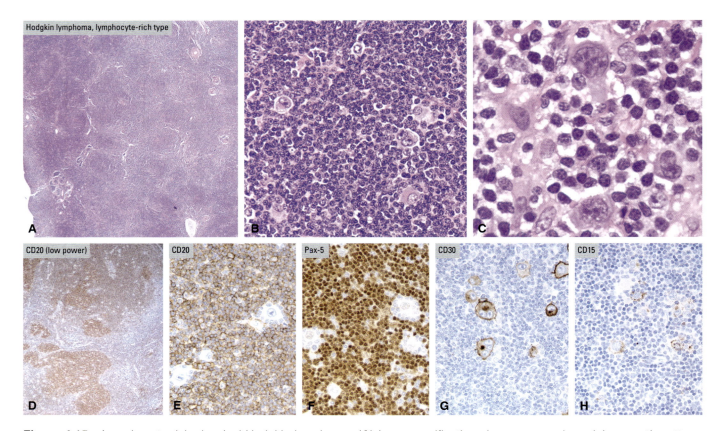

Figure 4.15   Lymphocyte-rich classical Hodgkin lymphoma. (**A**) Low magnification shows a vaguely nodular growth pattern. (**B**) Intermediate magnification shows predominance of small lymphocytes. (**C**) High magnification shows scattered large multi-lobated cells with prominent nucleoli. These are located within the nodular B-cell zones, often in the periphery. (**D**) CD20 staining (low magnification) highlights the nodular pattern. Reed–Sternberg cells are negative for CD20 (**E**) and are positive for Pax-5 (**F**, dim nuclear staining). Note rosettes of small T-cells around R–S cell, CD30 (**G**) and CD15 (**H**)

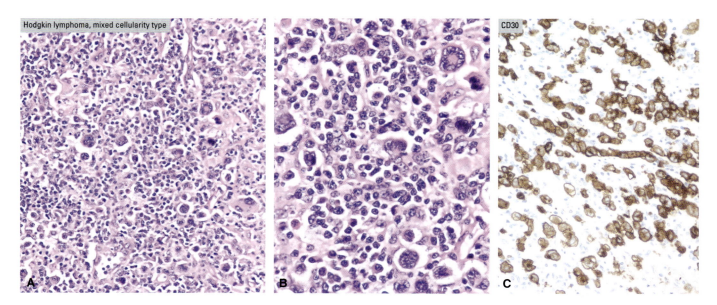

Figure 4.16   Mixed cellularity classical Hodgkin lymphoma. (**A**) Low magnification shows a polymorphic infiltrate without bands of fibrocollagen. (**B**) High magnification shows numerous multilobated large cells mixed with small lymphocytes, histiocytes and eosinophils. (**C**) Expression of CD30

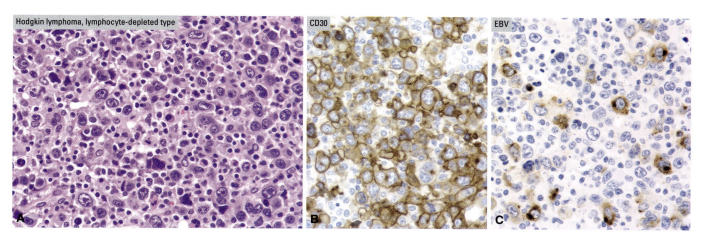

Figure 4.17 Lymphocyte-depleted classical Hodgkin lymphoma. (**A**) Large atypical cells predominate. Neoplastic cells are positive for CD30 (**B**) and EBV (**C**)

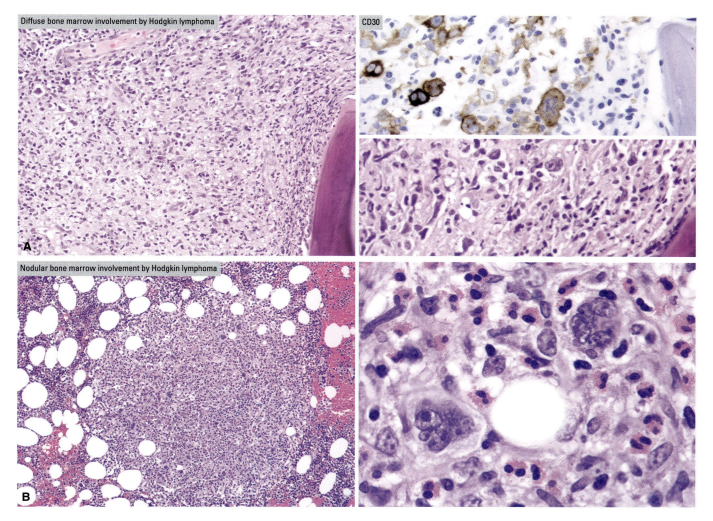

Figure 4.18 Classical Hodgkin lymphoma – bone marrow involvement characterized by a fibrohistiocytic infiltrate with/without true granuloma formation. (**A**) Diffuse bone marrow involvement by Hodgkin lymphoma. Neoplastic cells are highlighted by CD30 staining. High magnification shows atypical multilobated cells. (**B**) Nodular bone marrow involvement by Hodgkin lymphoma. Large interstitial aggregates are composed of a mixed inflammatory cell infiltrate containing eosinophils and typical Reed–Sternberg cells

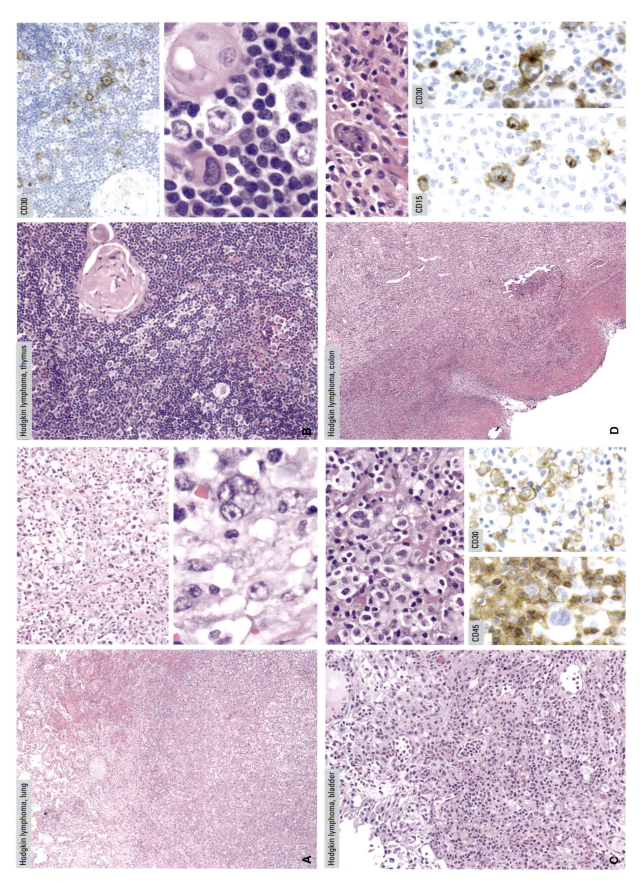

Figure 4.19   Classical Hodgkin lymphoma – extranodal. (**A**) Lung. (**B**) Thymus. (**C**) Urinary bladder. (**D**) Large intestine. (**E**) Liver. (**F**) Spleen

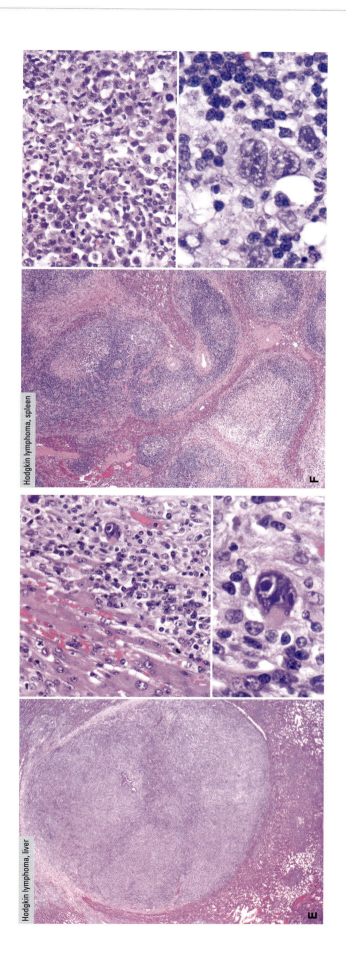

Figure 4.19   *(Continued)*

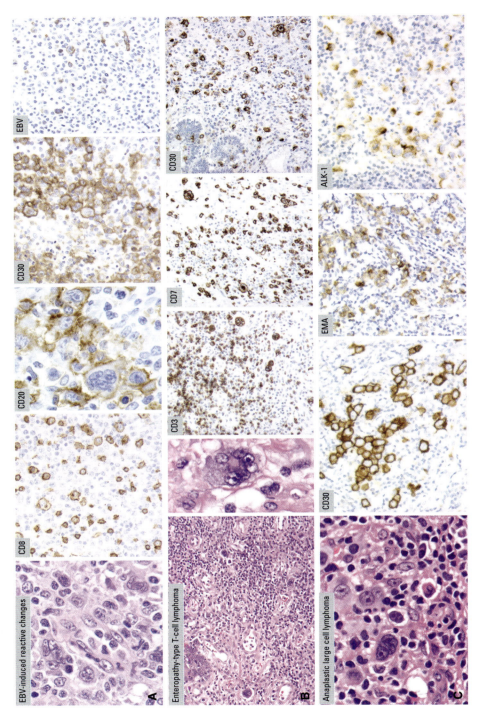

Figure 4.20 Classical Hodgkin lymphoma – differential diagnosis. (**A**) EBV-induced changes. Atypical large cells represent both CD8⁺ T-cells and large B-cells. They are positive for CD30 and EBV. (**B**) Enteropathy-type T-cell lymphoma. This T-cell process is characterized by a polymorphic lymphoid infiltrate with scattered cells resembling (R–S) cells. Atypical T-cells are positive for CD3, CD7 and CD30. (**C**) Anaplastic large cell lymphoma (ALCL). Large multinucleated cells resemble R–S cells. They are positive for CD30, EMA and ALK-1. Expression of CD45, one or more pan-T antigens, and ALK-1, and lack of expression of EBV/EBER help to differentiate ALCL from HL. (**D**) EBV-associated diffuse large B-cell lymphoma. EBV-associated B-cell lymphoproliferative disorders may be polymorphic or monomorphic. The former may be confused with Hodgkin lymphoma, especially when R–S-like cells are present. (**E**) Diffuse large B-cell lymphoma infiltrating skeletal muscle. Degenerated muscle cells may be confused with R–S cells on HE. Lack of expression of CD30 and expression of myoid (desmin, myogenin, myoglobin) are helpful in excluding HL. (**F**) T-cell-rich large B-cell lymphoma (TCRLBCL). Neoplastic cells in TCRLBCL are usually positive for CD45, CD20, CD22, and CD79a, and are negative for CD15 and EBV/EBER. (**G**) Kimura disease. Location of large atypical cells within follicles, cytomorphologic features of the polykaryocytes and lack of expression of CD30 differentiate Kimura disease from HL. (**H**) Cytomegalovirus (CMV)-associated lymphadenitis. Large cells with eosinophilic intranuclear inclusions which mimic macronucleoli of R–S cells are positive for CMV by immunohistochemistry

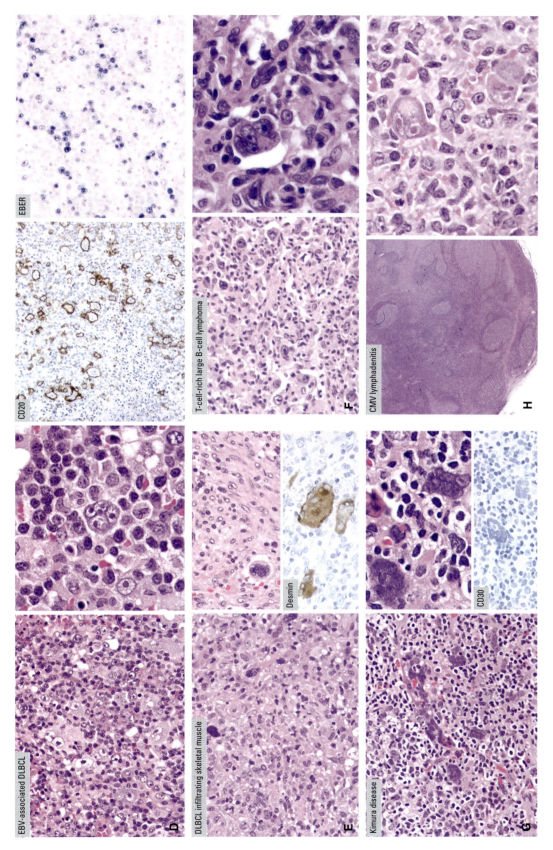

Figure 4.20   *(Continued)*

CHAPTER 5

Chronic myeloproliferative disorders

The chronic myeloproliferative disorders (CMPD) are clonal hematopoietic stem cell disorders characterized by autonomous proliferation of one or more of the myeloid lineages (granulocytic, erythroid and megakaryocytic) with effective hematopoiesis with full maturation early in the course of the disease, leading to peripheral cytoses (leukocytosis and/or polycythemia and/or thrombocytosis)[8,9,11,549–570]. There is a variable potential for bone marrow fibrosis, ineffective hematopoiesis and risk of transformation into acute leukemia. CMPD generally differ by which myeloid cell lineage dominates hematopoiesis and include chronic myeloid leukemia (CML), chronic eosinophilic leukemia, polycythemia vera (PV), essential thrombocythemia (ET) and chronic idiopathic myelofibrosis (Table 5.1). With the exception of CML, which is characterized by t(9;22)(q34;q11) (Philadelphia chromosome), leading to the active chimeric *bcr-abl* tyrosine kinase, the diagnosis of CMPD is largely clinicopathologic and to some degree relies on exclusion of reactive conditions. Given the overlap in morphology among non-CML disorders, correlation with clinical, molecular and cytogenetic findings is indicated for precise subclassification[3,4,11,551,558,563,565,566,569–577].

CLASSIFICATION AND GENERAL DIAGNOSTIC CRITERIA OF CMPD

Morphology

There is significant overlap of morphologic and laboratory features in CMPD[3,4,11,549,551,558,563,565,566,569–582]. General morphologic features are presented in Figures 5.1 and 5.18. Peripheral blood shows thrombocytosis (Figure 5.1A), neutrophilia (Figure 5.1B), eosinophilia, basophilia and/or leukoerythroblastosis. The bone marrow aspirate is often hypercellular with increased

Table 5.1 Classification of chronic myeloproliferative disorders

Chronic myelogenous leukemia (CML)
Chronic neutrophilic leukemia
Chronic eosinophilic leukemia/hypereosinophilic syndrome
Polycythemia vera (PV)
Chronic idiopathic myelofibrosis (CIMF)
Essential thrombocythemia (ET)
Chronic myeloproliferative disease, unclassifiable

megakaryocytes (Figure 5.1C). Bone marrow cellularity is usually increased (Figure 5.1D) with either panmyelosis or hyperplasia of one or two myeloid lineages. Myeloid hyperplasia may be accompanied by a leftward shift and accentuated paratrabecular myeloid immaturity. Megakaryocytes are increased and display atypia and often clustering (Figure 5.1E). Megakaryocytic clustering generally correlates with an increase in reticulin fibers. Hypolobated micromegakaryocytes are more typical for CML, whereas giant and bizarre forms of megakaryocytes are more often seen in chronic idiopathic myelofibrosis and other non-CML chronic myeloproliferative disorders. Reticulin fibers are variably increased. Fibrosis is most pronounced in chronic idiopathic myelofibrosis and in the later (fibrotic) stages of other CMPD. Sinuses may be dilated with intravascular hematopoiesis (Figure 5.1F) and accompanying extramedullary hematopoiesis.

Cytogenetics/molecular tests

Philadelphia chromosome/*BCR-ABL* fusion gene in conjunction with typical clinical and morphologic findings is diagnostic of CML. Philadelphia chromosome is not the only cytogenetic abnormality found in patients with CML. Approximately 20% of patients with CML have deletions of chromosomal material of varying size on the abnormal 9q$^+$ chromosome[556]. Atypical CML includes

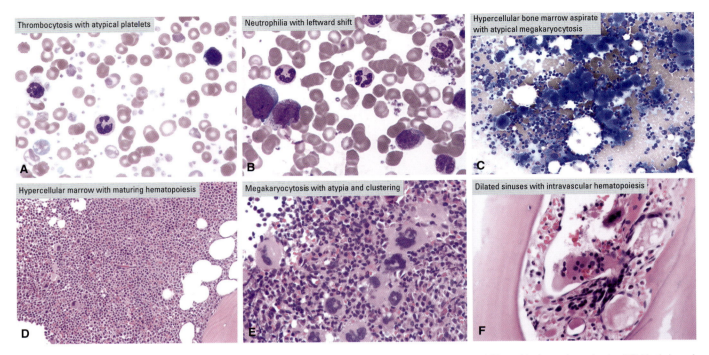

Figure 5.1   General features of chronic myeloproliferative disorders. (**A**) Peripheral blood film with thrombocytosis. (**B**) Peripheral blood film with neutrophilia with leftward shift. (**C**) Bone marrow aspirate with prominent megakaryocytosis with atypia. (**D**) Bone marrow core biopsy showing hypercellular marrow with myeloid hyperplasia and atypical hypolobated megakaryocytes. (**E**) Bone marrow core biopsy with atypical megakaryocytic clustering. (**F**) Dilated sinuses with intravascular hematopoiesis

t(8;22)(p11;q11), t(9;12)(q34;p13), t(9;22)(p24;q11) and t(4;22)(q12;q11)[556]. Philadelphia chromosome is also present on a subset of acute lymphoblastic leukemia.

There is no specific clonal marker for non-CML CMPD. *PRV-1* gene is overexpressed in granulocytes from patients with PV and essential thrombocythemia, helping to discriminate them from secondary erythrocytosis or thrombocytosis[67,570,583–585].

Hypereosinophilic syndrome/chronic eosinophilic leukemia shows del(4)(q12), and occasional myeloproliferative syndromes show translocations involving chromosomes 8 and either 6, 9, 13 or 19.

Immunophenotyping

Flow cytometry (FC) immunophenotyping has a limited role in the diagnosis of chronic myeloproliferative disorders (CMPD). FC can determine the number and phenotype of blasts, and thus help to quantify CMPD in accelerated phase or blast crisis. Additionally, there are subtle phenotypic abnormalities displayed by granulocytes in the chronic phase of the myeloproliferative process (Figure 5.2). These include slightly increased number of blasts (Figure 5.2A), decreased side scatter of granulocytes (Figure 5.2B), downregulation of CD16 (Figure 5.2C; compare with normal expression presented

on panel D), upregulation of CD56 (Figure 5.2E; compare with normal expression depicted on panel F), and aberrant expression of CD10, CD11b, CD15, CD117 and HLA-DR. These abnormalities, however, are not diagnostic per se of CMPD.

CHRONIC MYELOGENOUS LEUKEMIA (CML)

CML is a chronic myeloproliferative process, which results from clonal expansion of a single pluripotent hematopoietic stem cell containing the Philadelphia chromosome/*BCR-ABL* fusion gene[9,53,556,561,562,572,586–599]. CML cells gradually replace normal bone marrow elements, partly through increased proliferation but mostly as a result of defective apoptotic response giving the leukemic cells surviving benefit over normal (benign) marrow elements[600,601]. The *BCR-ABL* gene on the Ph chromosome is expressed in all patients with CML[556,572,586]. A subset of patients with otherwise typical clinical features of CML lack the *BCR-ABL* fusion gene and show translocations between chromosomes 9 and 12 or 22 (p24;q11) or between chromosomes 22 and 8[53,556,572,586,599].

The Ph-positive clone has an increased susceptibility to the additional molecular changes that underlie disease progression[52,591,602–604]. Most patients are diagnosed in the

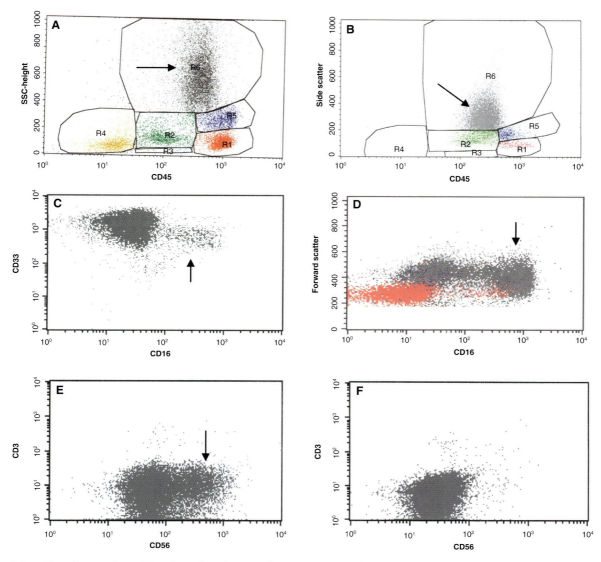

Figure 5.2 Chronic myeloproliferative disorders – flow cytometry. Granulocytes may display decreased side scatter (**B**), downregulation of CD16 (**C**) and/or upregulation of CD56 (**E**). A majority of CML cases, however, do not display overt antigenic abnormalities (**A**, **D** and **F**)

chronic phase, but an initial indolent course is followed by an accelerated phase or acute leukemia (blast crisis). This is often associated with extramedullary expansion of the leukemic infiltrate to lymph nodes, soft tissue, skin, liver, central nervous system and other tissues.

CML, chronic phase

Peripheral blood (Figure 5.3) shows leukocytosis with predominance of neutrophils, absolute basophilia and eosinophilia. Granulocytic cells show a leftward shift with a 'non-symmetrical' distribution (myelocytes > metamyelocytes). Blasts do not exceed 2%. Platelets may be slightly increased or normal. The bone marrow aspirate (Figure 5.4) is hypercellular with an increased M:E ratio

due to both myeloid hyperplasia and erythroid hypoplasia. Granulocytic cells show full maturation to segmented forms with a leftward shift and a peak ('myelocyte bulge') in the percentage of myelocytes (Figure 5.4C). Erythroid and granulocytic series do not exhibit overt dyspoiesis. Megakaryocytes may be increased in number and display atypia, most characteristically in the form of small megakaryocytes with hypolobated nuclei (Figure 5.4B and D). Blasts do not exceed 5% of the marrow cells. Eosinophils and basophils are increased in number. Scattered sea-blue histiocytes may be present. Histologic examination of the bone marrow core biopsy (Figure 5.5) reveals hypercellular bone marrow with myeloid and often megakaryocytic hyperplasia, and myeloid leftward shift without increased number of blasts, and often with

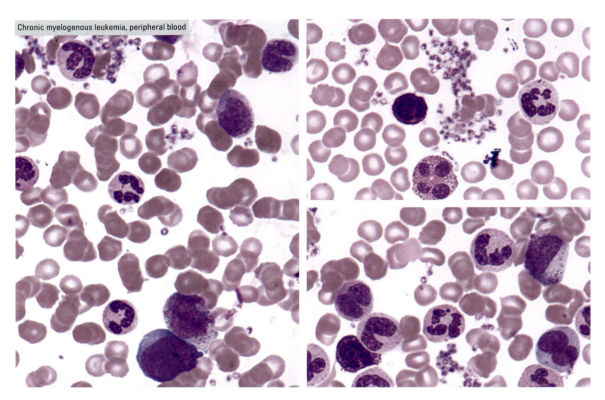

Figure 5.3 Chronic myelogenous leukemia – peripheral blood. Neutrophilia with leftward shift and eosinophilia and basophilia are present

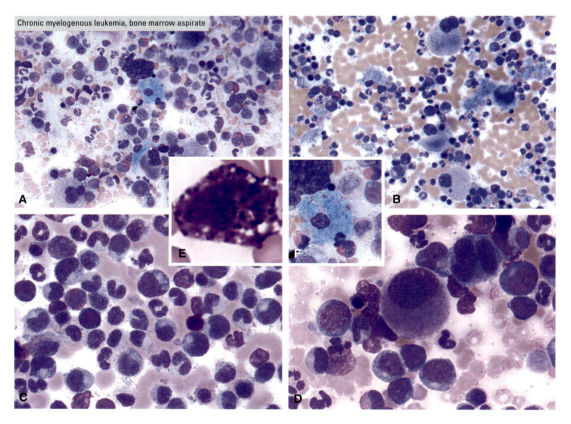

Figure 5.4 Chronic myelogenous leukemia – bone marrow aspirate. Bone marrow aspirate is hypercellular (**A**) with clusters of megakaryocytes (**A**). Many megakaryocytes have hypolobated nuclei (**B** and **D**). There is prominent myeloid hyperplasia with leftward shift (**C**). Basophils (**E**) and sea-blue histiocytes (**F**) are present

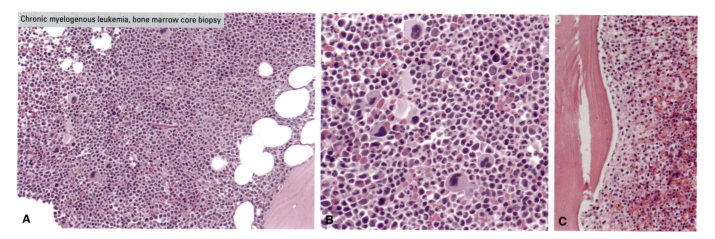

Figure 5.5   Chronic myelogenous leukemia – bone marrow core biopsy. The bone marrow is markedly hypercellular (**A**) with myeloid hyperplasia and leftward shift. Higher magnification (**B**) shows atypical hypolobated megakaryocytes. (**C**) Increased number of immature cells around trabeculae

accentuated paratrabecular immaturity (Figure 5.5C)[561,562]. Megakaryocytes are small and have hypolobated nuclei. Bizarre forms of megakaryocytes, typical for non-CML chronic myeloproliferative processes, are usually absent. Eosinophils and basophils are increased in number. Figure 5.6 depicts the karyotype from a patient with chronic phase CML (Philadelphia chromosome). Figures 5.7 and 5.8 depict the *BCR-ABL* fusion gene visualized by fluorescence *in situ* hybridization and PCR, respectively.

CML, accelerated phase

The accelerated phase of CML is defined by the presence of at least one of the following: (i) 10–19% blasts, (ii) peripheral blood basophils ≥ 20%, (iii) persistent thrombocytopenia (< 100 k/μl) or persistent thrombocytosis (> 1000 k/μl), (iv) increasing spleen size and increasing white blood cell count not responsive to therapy, and (v) clonal evolution by cytogenetic/FISH studies. Patients in the accelerated phase have symptoms of progressive bone

CML: Philadelphia chromosome t(9;22) with inversion 3

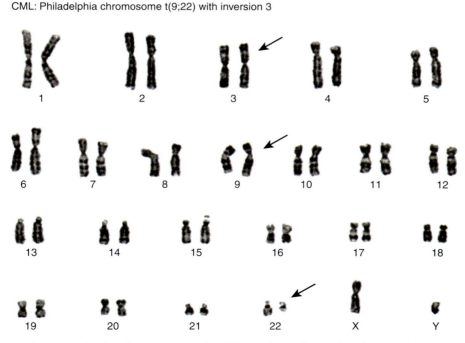

Figure 5.6   Chronic myelogenous leukemia – cytogenetics. The reciprocal translocation involving chromosomes 9 and 22 is evident. The der(22) chromosome is the Philadelphia chromosome

CML: BCR/ABL dual color dual fusion probe

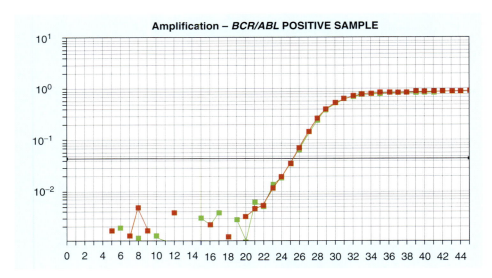

Figure 5.7 Chronic myelogenous leukemia – fluorescent *in situ* hybridization (FISH) showing the *BCR/ABL* (left, metaphase chromosomes; right, interphase cell)

Figure 5.8 Chronic myelogenous leukemia – PCR studies

marrow failure with worsening anemia and/or thrombocytopenia. The bone marrow (Figure 5.9) is hypercellular with increased number of blasts and increased number of small megakaryocytes. The reticulin fibers may be increased, especially in perivascular loci. With disease progression, diffuse reticulin fibrosis ensues. FC reveals increased number of blasts (most often myeloblasts, but lymphoblastic transformation may be also seen).

CML, blast crisis

The blast crisis of CML is defined by (i) 20% or more blasts, (ii) extramedullary blast proliferation, (iii) large foci or clusters of blasts in the bone marrow. The transformation into acute leukemia may be abrupt or may follow the accelerated phase. Occasional cases of CML are detected in blast crisis without a prior diagnosis of CML.

The majority of cases show features of acute myeloid leukemia (Figure 5.10), with either granulocytic, monocytic, erythroid or megakaryocytic differentiation. The remaining cases (~20%) show lymphoblastic differentiation or bilineage acute leukemia[595,602,603,605,606]. Figure 5.11 depicts extramedullary blast proliferation in the spleen. Extramedullary acute leukemic infiltrate may involve any part of the body, most commonly the skin, spleen, lymph node and brain. The immunophenotypic features of CML in blast crisis correspond to those of *de novo* acute leukemias, and are determined by FC and/or immunohistochemistry and cytochemical staining for NSE and MPO.

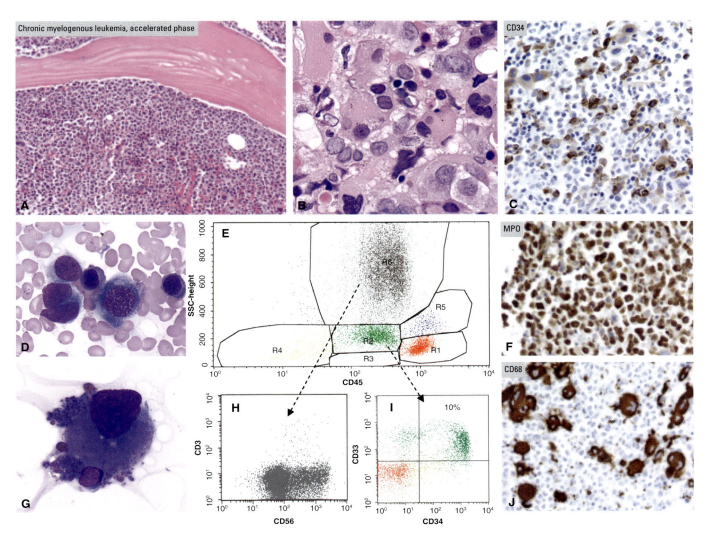

Figure 5.9   Chronic myelogenous leukemia – accelerated phase. The core biopsy is hypercellular (**A**) with increased blasts (**B** and **C**), myeloid hyperplasia (**F**) and megakaryocytosis (**J**). Aspirate smear shows blasts (**D**) and atypical megakaryocytes (**G**). Flow cytometry analysis revealed increased blasts (**E, I**, green) and dysmaturation of granulocytes (**E, H**, gray) with aberrant expression of CD56 (**H**)

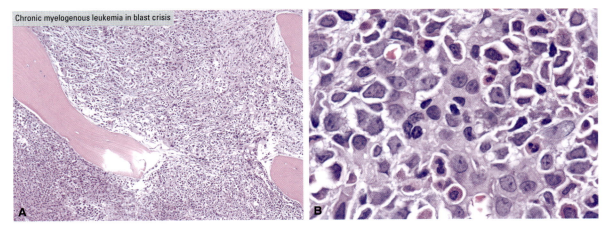

Figure 5.10   Chronic myelogenous leukemia in myeloid blast crisis (**A**, low magnification; **B**, high magnification)

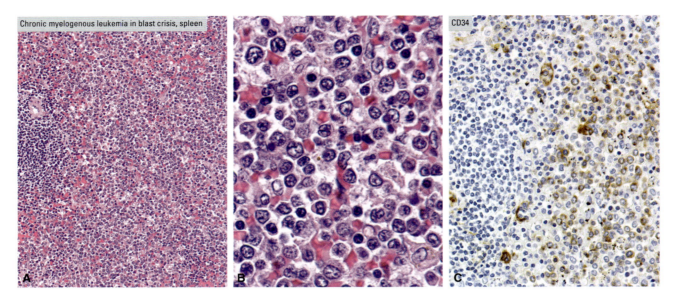

Figure 5.11 Chronic myelogenous leukemia in myeloid blast crisis – spleen. (**A** and **B**) Histologic section shows increased number of immature, blast-like cells within the red pulp. (**C**) Immunohistochemical staining with CD34 confirms the predominance of blasts

CHRONIC EOSINOPHILIC LEUKEMIA/ HYPEREOSINOPHILIC SYNDROME

Chronic eosinophilic leukemia is a multisystem disorder defined by a clonal proliferation of eosinophils with or without an increased number of blasts. The diagnosis is based on determination of clonality of eosinophils and exclusion of secondary causes for eosinophilia[479,593,607–612]. The latter include reactive eosinophilia (allergy, parasitic infestation and collagen vascular disease), reactive eosinophilia in neoplastic disorders such as Hodgkin lymphoma, mastocytosis and T-cell lymphoproliferations, or neoplastic disorders in which eosinophils are part of a neoplastic process (CML, acute myelomonocytic leukemia with eosinophilia and CMPD). Presence of a recurring karyotypic abnormality, such as +8, inv(17q) or t(5;12)(q33;p13), indicates chronic eosinophilic leukemia rather than hypereosinophilic syndrome. Apart from t(5;12)(q33;p13), chronic eosinophilic leukemia may be associated with t(8;13)(p11;q12) and other translocations involving 8p11. Cases with no demonstrable disease that may cause eosinophilia, without an increase in blasts (2%), and proven clonality of myeloid cells are termed 'idiopathic' hypereosinophilic syndrome.

Peripheral blood in chronic eosinophilic leukemia/ hypereosinophilic syndrome shows a markedly increased number of eosinophils at different stages of maturation. Nuclear and cytoplasmic abnormalities in the form of hyposegmentation, vacuolation or hypogranularity are often present. The bone marrow (Figure 5.12) is markedly hypercellular with predominance of mature eosinophils. Myeloid and erythroid precursors display normal maturation. Cases with slightly increased number of blasts or reticulin fibrosis may overlap with myelodysplastic syndromes and chronic myeloproliferative process.

POLYCYTHEMIA VERA (PV)

PV is a clonal myeloid stem cell disorder characterized by increased and autonomous production of red cells, and to lesser degree other myeloid cells[67,550,558,563–565,570,576,577,583, 584,613–615]. There is an initial proliferative polycythemic phase, which after a period of stable clinical and morphologic findings usually progresses to a 'spent' phase with myeloid metaplasia, bone marrow failure and fibrosis, and extramedullary hematopoiesis. The diagnosis of PV requires exclusion of secondary erythrocytosis (hypoxia, high oxygen affinity hemoglobin, and inappropriate erythropoietin production). The clinical symptoms are related to increased red cell mass and include hypertension, headache, pruritus due to hyperhistaminemia, dizziness, splenomegaly, hemorrhage and episodes of venous or arterial thrombosis with attendant complications[615,616]. Laboratory and morphologic findings depend on the stage of the disease. In the initial polycythemic stage, the red cell indices are increased: red blood cells more than 25% above mean normal predicted value, and hemoglobin over 18.5 g/dl (men) or over 16.5 g/dl (women). Splenomegaly is present. A minority of cases progress to acute leukemia.

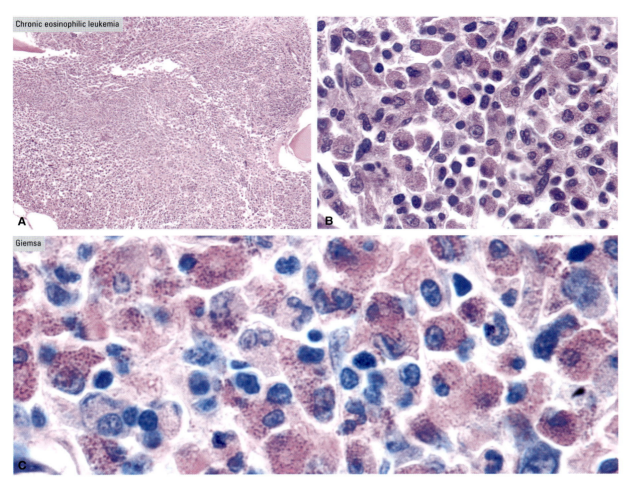

Figure 5.12 Chronic eosinophilic leukemia. (**A–C**) Hypercellular bone marrow with predominance of mature-appearing eosinophils

The polycythemic stage is characterized by a markedly hypercellular bone marrow (Figure 5.13) due to panmyelosis. Megakaryocytes are increased in number and display prominent atypia with clustering. Focal reticulin fibrosis is present. The spent phase is characterized by diffuse reticulin fibrosis and marrow hypocellularity with clusters of bizarre megakaryocytes. Without an antecedent history of PV, the marrow picture is identical to chronic idiopathic myelofibrosis.

CHRONIC IDIOPATHIC MYELOFIBROSIS (CIMF)

CIMF is a clonal stem cell disorder characterized by the autonomous proliferation of myeloid and granulocytic elements with panmyelosis, marked and diffuse bone marrow fibrosis (due to cytokine-induced non-neoplastic fibroblast proliferation) and extramedullary hematopoiesis[4,11,549,551–553,560,571,578,579,617,618]. Patients usually present with symptoms of bone marrow failure (fatigue, bleeding,

and dyspnea), and have prominent splenomegaly. Progression to acute leukemia is rare. Morbidity and mortality are associated with marrow failure with its complications. Patients in the proliferative and prefibrotic stage of CIMF have mild anemia, thrombocytosis and mild leukocytosis. The bone marrow is hypercullar with panmyelosis and atypical megakaryocytic clustering.

In the fibrotic stage of CIMF, the peripheral blood picture is that of leukoerythroblastosis, prominent red blood cell anisocytosis, poilkilocytosis and dacrocytosis. The bone marrow (Figure 5.14) is variably cellular with osteosclerosis, diffuse reticulin and often collagen fibrosis, and dilated sinuses. The latter show intrasinusoidal hematopoiesis (Figure 5.15). Megakaryocytes are atypical with many bizarre hyperchromatic forms. Clusters or even sheets of megakaryocytes are present. As fibrosis progress, marrow elements may be patchy or markedly decreased with predominance of dense reticulin and collagen fibers. Extramedullary hematopoiesis is common in CIMF. The most common sites include spleen, liver and

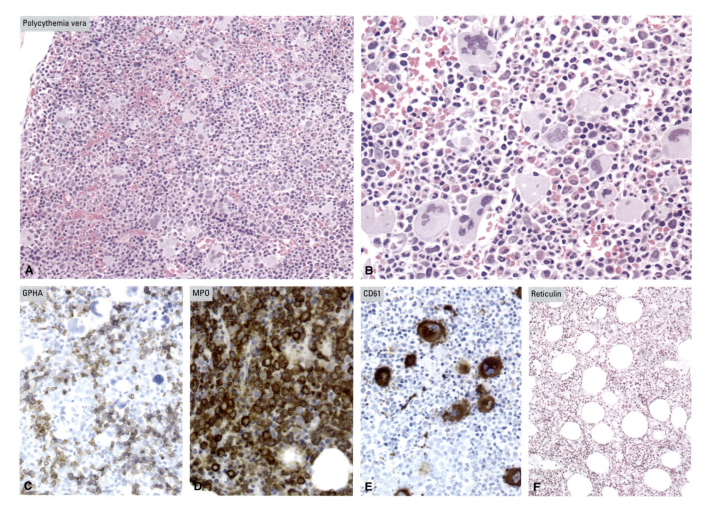

Figure 5.13 Polycythemia vera. (**A**) Bone marrow core biopsy shows panmyelosis with increased M:E ratio and megakaryocytosis. (**B**) High magnification displays numerous atypical megakaryocytes. (**C–E**) Immunohistochemical staining shows scattered red cell precursors (**C**), myeloid hyperplasia (**D**) and megakaryocytosis (**E**). Reticulin fibrosis is mildly increased (**F**)

lymph nodes. The spleen (Figure 5.16) shows expansion of the red pulp by myeloid and erythroid precursors and megakaryocytes. The latter often predominate and display marked atypia (Figure 5.16B).

ESSENTIAL THROMBOCYTHEMIA (ET)

ET is a clonal stem cell disorder that is characterized by marked thrombocytosis and megakaryocytic hyperplasia[11,553,558,559,563,569,573,576,577,580–582,585,615,619–621]. The diagnosis of ET requires a sustained platelet count of ≥ 600 k/µl and exclusion of PV, CML, CIMF, MDS and reactive thrombocytosis. Patients may be asymptomatic or present with abnormal bleeding or symptoms related to vascular complications (thrombosis).

The peripheral blood (Figure 5.17A) shows an increase in number of platelets, which may display atypia and anisocytosis. Leukocytosis, if present, is mild. The bone marrow aspirate (Figure 5.17B) is hypercellular with numerous large, atypical megakaryocytes, which often cluster within spicules. The biopsy (Figure 5.17C and D) is hypercellular with panmyelosis and marked megakaryocytic hyperplasia with atypia. Megakaryocytes are often seen abnormally close to the bony trabeculae; usually, they are located in the deep interstitium. Reticulin fibers may be focally increased, but fibrosis generally occupies less than 25% of the marrow area (Figure 5.17E).

DIFFERENTIAL DIAGNOSIS OF CMPD

Figures 5.1 and 5.18 and Table 5.2 present general diagnostic criteria of CMPD. The subclassification is based on clinical, cytogenetic and morphologic data[11,558,563,565,566,569,572,573,576,577,584,622]. Morphologically, all

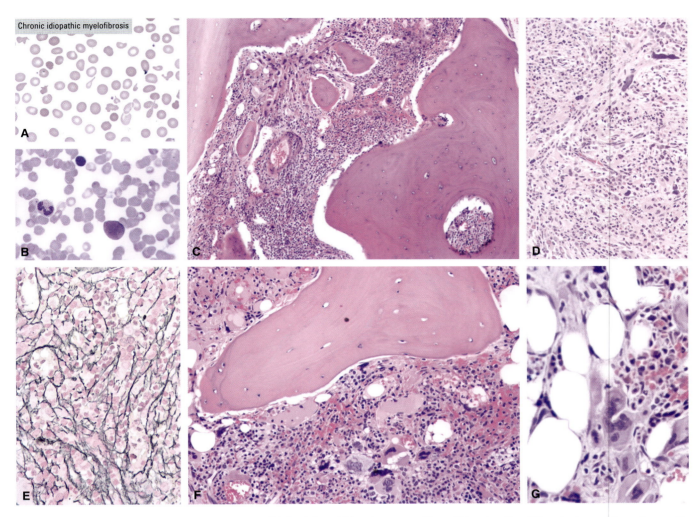

Figure 5.14 Chronic idiopathic myelofibrosis. (**A**) Peripheral blood smear with red blood cell poikilocytosis and tear drop cells. (**B**) Hypocellular, aspicular bone marrow aspirate (**C**) Hypercellular marrow with osteosclerosis and megakaryocytosis. (**D**) The cells appear to 'stream', an effect caused by fibrosis. (**E**) Increased reticulin fibers (silver staining). (**F** and **G**) Clusters of atypical megakaryocytes

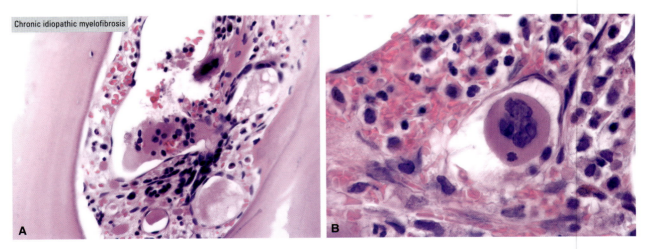

Figure 5.15 Chronic idiopathic myelofibrosis (CIMF). Dilated sinuses with intrasinusoidal hematopoiesis are characteristic for CIMF (**A**, intermediate magnification; **B**, high magnification)

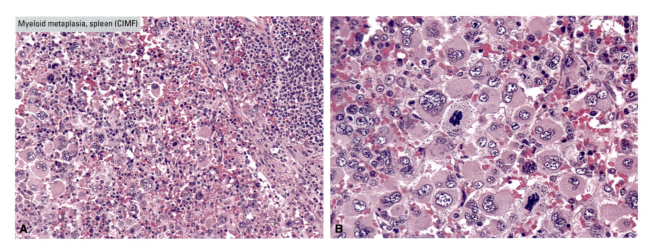

Figure 5.16   Chronic idiopathic myelofibrosis (CIMF) with extramedullary hematopoiesis in the spleen (**A**, intermediate magnification; **B**, high magnification)

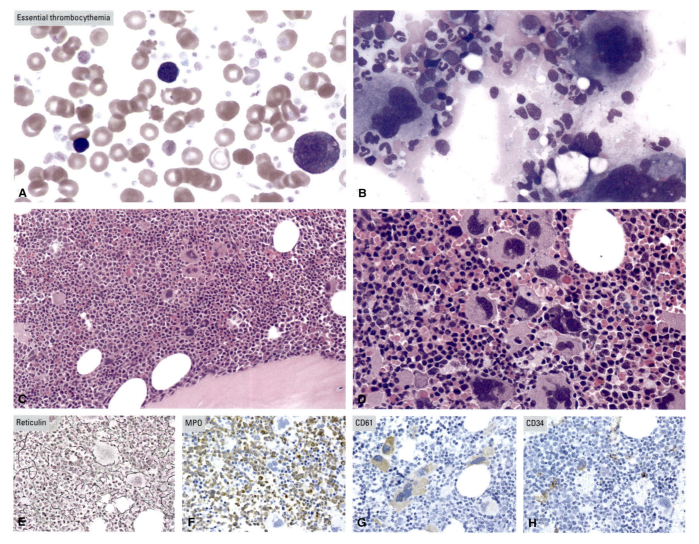

Figure 5.17   Essential thrombocythemia (ET). (**A**) Peripheral blood film with thrombocytosis and leukoerythroblastosis. (**B**) Hypercellular bone marrow aspirate with prominent megakaryocytic atypia. (**C** and **D**) Bone marrow core biopsy showing markedly hypercellular marrow with myeloid hyperplasia and megakaryocytic atypia with clustering. (**E**) Silver staining depicts mild diffuse increase in reticulin fibers. (**F–H**) Immunohistochemistry shows predominance of myeloid cells (**F**), atypical megakaryocytes (CD61 staining, **G**) and rare blasts (CD34 staining, **H**)

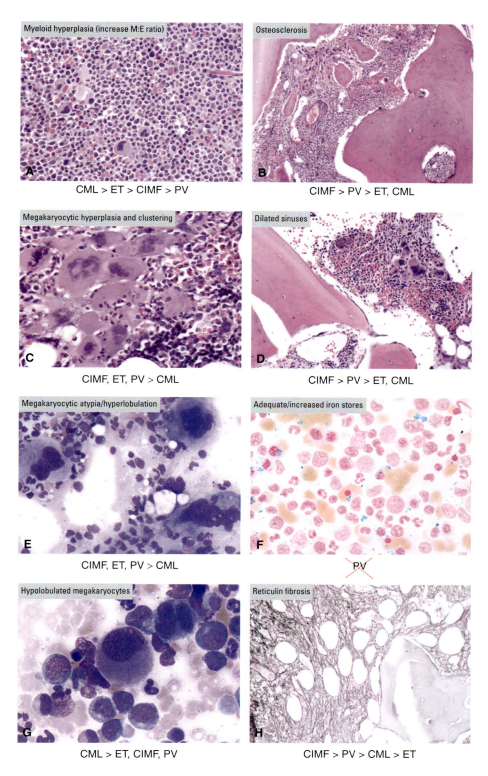

Myeloid hyperplasia (increase M:E ratio)

A

CML > ET > CIMF > PV

Osteosclerosis

B

CIMF > PV > ET, CML

Megakaryocytic hyperplasia and clustering

C

CIMF, ET, PV > CML

Dilated sinuses

D

CIMF > PV > ET, CML

Megakaryocytic atypia/hyperlobulation

E

CIMF, ET, PV > CML

Adequate/increased iron stores

F

PV

Hypolobulated megakaryocytes

G

CML > ET, CIMF, PV

Reticulin fibrosis

H

CIMF > PV > CML > ET

Figure 5.18   Comparison of morphologic features in chronic myeloproliferative disorders (CMPD). (**A**) Myeloid hyperplasia is present in all CMPD, but is most pronounced in CML. PV may show increased, normal or decreased M:E ratio. (**B**) Osteosclerosis is most typical for chronic idiopathic myelofibrosis (CIMF). (**C**) Marked megakaryocytic atypia with clustering and bizarre forms is usually seen in CIMF, ET, and PV. CML shows increased megakaryocytes, but they are usually hypolobated. (**D**) Dilated sinuses are associated with fibrosis and are typical for CIMF, especially when accompanied by intrasinusoidal hematopoiesis. (**E**) Aspirate smear with marked megakaryocytic atypia is seen in all three non-CML chronic myeloproliferative disorders. (**F**) The presence of adequate stainable iron does not favor PV. (**G**) Hypolobated megakaryocytes are characteristic of CML. (**H**) Diffuse reticulin fibrosis is most pronounced in CIMF but may occur in the later (fibrotic) stage of all CMPD

Table 5.2   Comparison of morphologic features of chronic myeloproliferative disorders

Feature	Disorder			
	CML	PV	CIMF	ET
M:E ratio	↑↑↑	Variable	Variable	Variable
Myeloid hyperplasia	+++	+	++	++
Erythroid hyperplasia	−	Variable	Variable	Variable
Megakaryocytosis	+	++	++	+++
Megakaryocytic atypia/pleomorphism	+	++	+++	++
Megakaryocytic clustering	+	++	+++	+++
Hyperlobulated and/or giant megakaryocytes	+	++	++	+++
Hypolobulated/small megakaryocytes	+++	+/−	+	+/−
Dilated sinuses	−/+	+	+++	+
Fibrosis	+	+/−	+++	+
Iron stores	Variable (generally ↓)	↓/Absent	Variable (generally ↓)	Variable (generally ↓)
Osteosclerosis	−	−	+	−
Marrow hypercellularity	+++	+	++	+

other conditions (reactive and neoplastic) which contain normally maturing hypercellular marrow with fibrosis, megakaryocytosis and/or panmyelosis need to be differentiated from the chronic myeloproliferative process. They include reactive megakaryocytosis in the marrow involved by malignant lymphoma (Figure 5.19A), myelodysplastic syndrome (Figure 5.19B), acute megakaryoblastic leukemia (Figure. 5.19C), mixed myelodysplastic/myeloproliferative disorder (e.g., CMML; Figure 5.19D), Hodgkin lymphoma with fibrosis and reactive myeloid hyperplasia due to endogenous cytokine production by Reed–Sternberg cells (Figure 5.19E), reactive myeloid hyperplasia (Figure 5.19F), metastatic tumor with fibrosis, severe anemia with reactive erythroid hyperplasia, treatment with colony-stimulating factors (G-CSF and rHUG-CSF) and acute myelofibrosis.

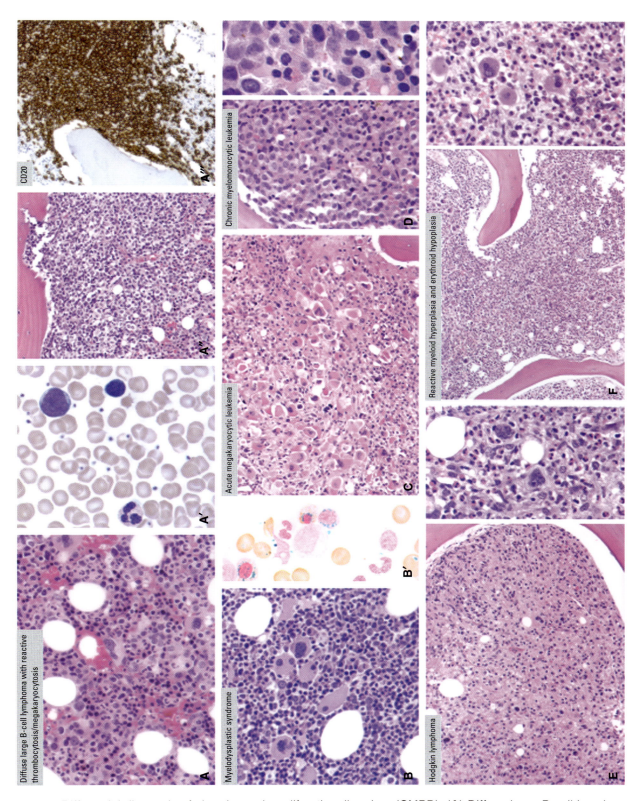

Figure 5.19   Differential diagnosis of chronic myeloproliferative disorders (CMPD). (**A**) Diffuse large B-cell lymphoma with reactive megakaryocytosis (A) and thrombocytosis (**A′**). Atypical paratrabecular large cell lymphoid infiltrate (**A″**) with strong expression of CD20 (**A‴**) is present. (**B**) Myelodysplastic syndrome (in this case RARS, **B′** shows ringed sideroblasts) displays atypical megakaryocytes. (**C**) Acute megakaryoblastic leukemia (AML-M7) shows prominent megakaryocytosis. (**D**) Chronic myelomonocytic leukemia may show similar histologic features to CMPD. Correlation with CBC data (number of monocytes), the presence of dysplasia in the marrow aspirate, and cytogenetic studies are needed for definite diagnosis. (**E**) Hodgkin lymphoma. Diffuse lymphohistiocytic infiltrate with atypical large cells which mimic megakaryocytes may be mistaken for CMPD. (**F**) Reactive processes or myeloid hyperplasia due to exogenous cytokine (G-CSF; Eo-CSF) stimulation may display morphologic features suggesting CMPD

CHAPTER 6

Myelodysplastic/ myeloproliferative diseases

The myelodysplastic/myeloproliferative diseases are clonal stem cell neoplasms with features of both cytopenia(s) and cytosis(es) giving rise to overlapping clinical, laboratory and morphologic features of myelodysplastic syndrome and chronic myeloproliferative disorders[78,574,623–630]. Table 6.1 presents the WHO classification of mixed myelodysplastic/myeloproliferative diseases.

CHRONIC MYELOMONOCYTIC LEUKEMIA

Chronic myelomonocytic leukemia is a mixed myelodysplastic/myeloproliferative disorder defined by persistent monocytosis ($>1 \times 10^9/l$) in the peripheral blood, fewer than 20% blasts and dysplastic features in one or more myeloid lineages[78,624–626,628,631–634]. Molecular/cytogenetic studies are negative for *bcr-abl* (Philadelphia chromosome). The monocytes are usually mature with focal nuclear and/or cytoplasmic atypia. Based on the number of blasts, CMML is divided into two categories: CMML-1 (< 5% blasts in blood, < 10% blasts in bone marrow) and CMML-2 (5–19% blasts in blood and 10–19% blasts in bone marrow). The bone marrow in CMML is hypercellular with prominent monocytosis, myeloid hyperplasia, megakaryocytic atypia and dysgranulopoiesis and/or dyserythropoiesis (Figures 6.1 and 6.2). Staining with NSE and MPO helps to differentiate between promonocytes, monocytes and dyspoietic granulocytic precursors. NSE (alpha naphthyl butyrate esterase) stains the cytoplasm of mature monocytes, and can help differentiate promonocytes from monocytes. The sum (promonocytes + monocytes) can be counted as 'monocytic' cells for purposes of classification. The ratio of monocytes, granulocytes and erythroid precursors varies. The neoplastic monocytes have the phenotype of mature monocytes with bright expression

Table 6.1 Classification of myelodysplastic/myeloproliferative disorders

Chronic myelomonocytic leukemia (CMML)
Atypical chronic myeloid leukemia
Juvenile myelomonocytic leukemia
Myelodysplastic/myeloproliferative diseases, unclassifiable

of CD11b, CD11c, CD14, CD33, CD45 and CD64 (Figure 6.3). A majority of cases express CD13, HLA-DR, and CD4. Lack of HLA-DR and CD13, and aberrant expression of CD16, CD23, CD56 and CD117, as well as the presence of abnormal granulocytes (with aberrant expression of CD10, CD11b, CD15, CD16, CD56 and HLA-DR) and increased numbers of blasts (< 20%), distinguishes CMML from reactive monocytosis. Table 6.2 presents phenotype of CMML based on flow cytometry evaluation.

Table 6.2 Immunophenotypic profile of chronic myelomonocytic leukemia (CMML)

Marker	% positive
CD2	34
CD4	76
CD7	9
CD10	28
CD11b	100
CD11c	100
CD13	95
CD14	100
CD16	29
CD23	9
CD33	100
CD34	0
CD45	100 (bright)
CD56	53
CD64	100
CD117	5
HLA-DR	71

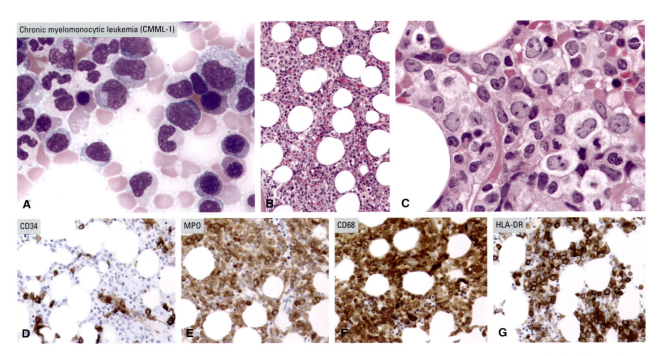

Figure 6.1   Chronic myelomonocytic leukemia (CMML). (**A**) Bone marrow aspirate with maturing myeloid cells and increased monocytes. (**B** and **C**) Bone marrow core biopsy is hypercellular with prominent monocytosis. Immunohistochemical staining (**D–G**) demonstrates slightly increased blasts (**D**; CD34 staining), and predominance of cells positive for MPO (**E**), CD68 (**F**) and HLA-DR (**G**)

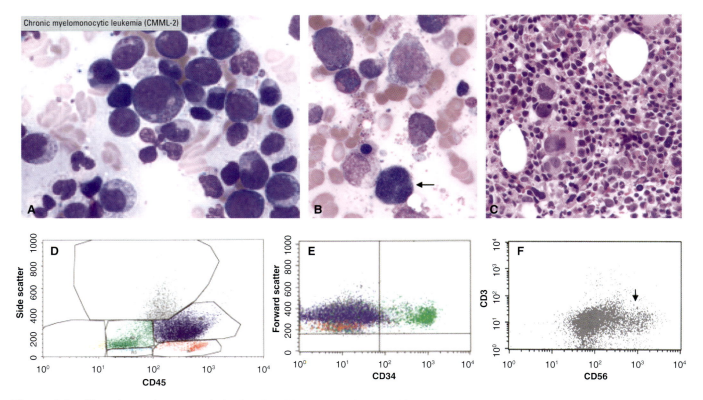

Figure 6.2   Chronic myelomonocytic leukemia with increased blasts (CMML-2). (**A**) Aspirate smear with maturing myeloid precursors and monocytes. (**B**) Red cell precursors show overt dyserythropoiesis (arrow). (**C**) Bone marrow core biopsy is hypercellular with megakaryocytic atypia and increased numbers of immature cells. Flow cytometry (**D–F**) shows a predominance of monocytes (blue; **D**), an increased number of myeloblasts (green, **E**) and dysmaturation of granulocytes (gray) with decreased side scatter (**D**) and upregulation of CD56 (**F**, arrow). In CMML-1 blasts do not exceed 10%. CMML-2 contains 11–19% blasts. Lesions with atypical monocytes and blasts of ≥ 20% are classified as acute myelomonocytic leukemia (AML-M4)

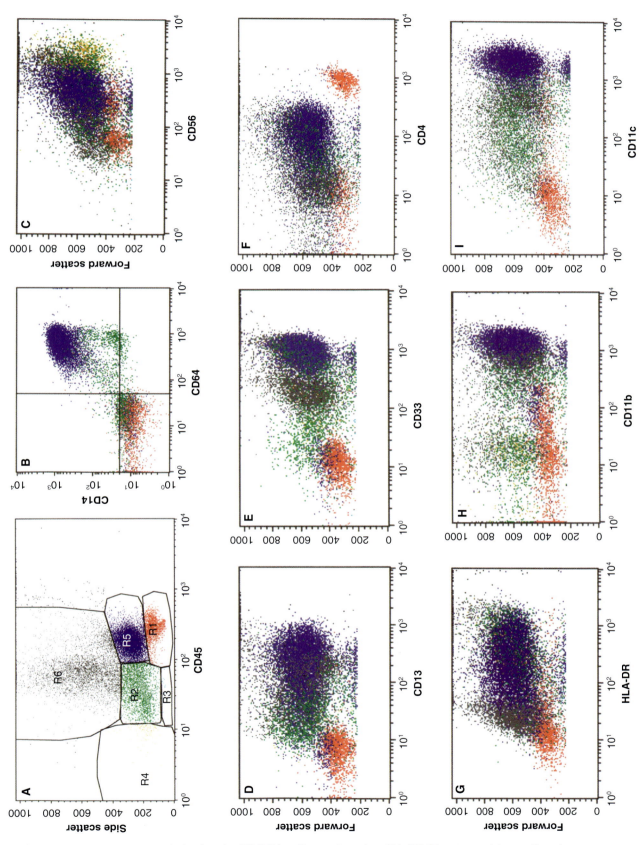

Figure 6.3 Chronic myelomonocytic leukemia (CMML) – flow cytometry. (**A**) CD45 versus side scatter shows numerous monocytes (blue), increased blasts (green), decreased granulocytes (gray) and a normal number of lymphocytes (red). Monocytes (blue) have a mature phenotype (CD14⁺/CD64⁺, **B**), show aberrant expression of CD56 (**C**), and are positive for CD13 (**D**), CD33 (**E**), CD4 (**F**), HLA-DR (**G**), CD11b (**H**) and CD11c (**I**)

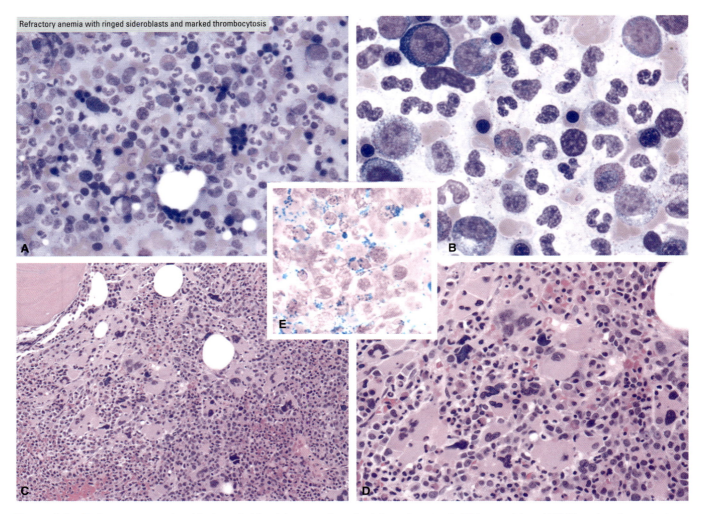

Refractory anemia with ringed sideroblasts and marked thrombocytosis

Figure 6.4   Refractory anemia with ringed sideroblasts and marked thrombocytosis. This provisional WHO entity shows features of myelodysplastic syndrome (such as RARS) overlapping with a chronic myeloproliferative disorder (such as ET). Bone marrow aspirate (**A** and **B**) and core biopsy (**C** and **D**) show hypercellular marrow with trilineage dyspoiesis. There is marked megakaryocytosis with atypia and clustering. An iron stain on a fresh aspirate (**E**) shows >15% ringed sideroblasts. Thrombocythemia is usually present (> 600 k/μl)

MYELODYSPLASTIC/MYELOPROLIFERATIVE DISEASE, UNCLASSIFIABLE

Myelodysplastic/myeloproliferative disease, unclassifiable, is a diagnosis of exclusion and is restricted to cases of mixed myelodysplastic/myeloproliferative disorders which do not fulfill the criteria for the diagnosis of CMML, atypical chronic myeloid leukemia and juvenile myelomonocytic leukemia, without prior history of any specific myeloid disorder. One or more of the myeloid lineages proliferates (as seen in chronic myeloproliferative disease), whereas the other lineages show dyspoiesis with ineffective hematopoiesis (as seen in myelodysplastic syndromes). Occasional cases of mixed myeloproliferative/myelodysplastic diseases (Figure 6.4) show features of refractory anemia with ringed sideroblasts with a markedly elevated platelet count (> 600k/μl)[635,636].

CHAPTER 7

Myelodysplastic syndromes

INTRODUCTION

Myelodysplastic syndrome (MDS) represents a heterogeneous group of malignant hematologic stem cell disorders characterized by cytopenia(s) with a variably cellular bone marrow which exhibits ineffective hematopoiesis[600,623,632,633,637–649]. MDS is a discrete entity that is different from AML and is characterized primarily by increased apoptosis in early and mature hematopoietic cells[56,601,637,650,651]. The reticulocyte count is correspondingly low for the patient's anemia. MDS can arise *de novo* or can be related to therapy (chemotherapy, radiotherapy, or of combined modality therapy for another tumor)[638,639,652–659]. The dysplastic process may involve one or more of the major myeloid lineages (granulocytes, erythroid cells and megakaryocytes). The dysmaturation in erythroid cells (dyserythropoiesis), granulocytes (dysgranulopoiesis) and/or megakaryocytes (dysmegakaryopoiesis) may be associated with an increased number of myeloblasts (the current threshold to differentiate MDS from acute myelogenous leukemia is 20%)[78]. The diagnosis and classification of MDS is based on morphologic evaluation of a peripheral blood smear, bone marrow aspirate (Wright–Giemsa and iron stains) and trephine core biopsy, immunophenotyping, cytogenetic studies and pertinent laboratory data[30,63,632,640,648,660–671]. Based on the number of myeloblasts, the degree of dysgranulopoiesis, dyserythropoiesis and the morphology of megakaryocytes, and the presence of ringed sideroblasts, WHO classification[78] (Table 7.1) recognizes the following categories of MDS: refractory anemia (RA), refractory anemia with ringed sideroblasts (RARS), refractory cytopenia with multilineage dysplasia (RCMD), refractory anemia with excess blasts (RAEB, types 1 and 2), del(5q) syndrome (MDS associated with isolated del5(q)) and MDS, unclassifiable[78,632,637,639–641,671,672]. Rare forms of MDS include the hypocellular variant of MDS and MDS with bone marrow fibrosis[673–675].

Table 7.1 Classification of myelodysplastic syndromes

Refractory anemia (RA)
Refractory anemia with ringed sideroblasts (RARS)
Refractory cytopenia with multilineage dysplasia (RCMD)
Refractory anemia with excess blasts (RAEB)
Myelodysplastic syndrome associated with isolated del (5q)
Myelodysplastic syndrome, unclassifiable

MORPHOLOGIC FEATURES

Dysplastic normoblasts (dyserythropoiesis) are characterized by nuclear and cytoplasmic abnormalities (Figure 7.1). Dysplastic nuclear features include asymmetric budding, multinucleation, hyperchromasia, internuclear bridging, and karyorrhexis. Cytoplasmic abnormalities include dyssynchronous maturation (nuclear–cytoplasmic dyssynchrony) and ringed sideroblastosis. Findings which may be seen in MDS but are more non-specific include irregular (shaggy) cytoplasmic borders and vacuolization. Although there is usually erythroid hyperplasia, occasional cases of MDS display erythroid hypoplasia (they respond well to cyclosporine A therapy). This variant shares features with aplastic anemia; in fact, aplastic anemia and hypocellular MDS likely represent a spectrum of the same disease process. Dysgranulopoiesis is characterized by hypogranular cytoplasm, pseudo-Pelger–Huet cells (nuclear hypolobation) and hypersegmentation (Figure 7.2). Dysplastic features of megakaryocytes include micromegakaryocytes, hypolobated or non-lobated nuclei, hyperchromasia and numerous, widely separated nuclei (Figure 7.3). The recommended percentage of cells with dysplasia is 10%[632,640]. Increased numbers of blasts, the presence of ringed sideroblasts, micromegakaryocytes and pseudo-Pelger–Huet cells correlates most strongly with the presence of clonal cytogenetic abnormalities in MDS.

The cytomorphologic findings are complemented by histologic features (Figure 7.4), which include increased number of megakaryocytes, megakaryocytic

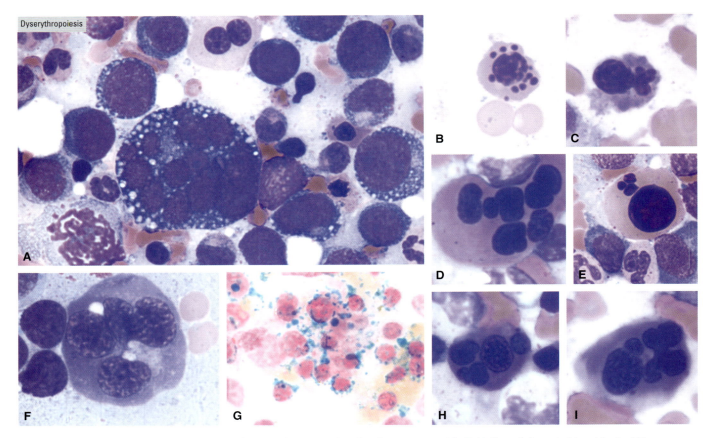

Figure 7.1   Dyserythropoiesis. Bizarre, often multinucleated red cell precursors (**A–F, H, I**) and ringed sideroblasts (**G**)

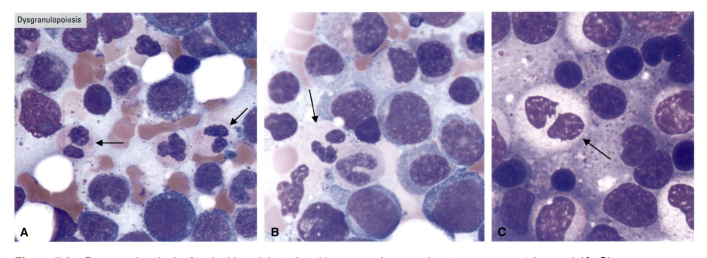

Figure 7.2   Dysgranulopoiesis. Atypical hypolobated and hypogranular granulocytes are present (arrows) (**A–C**)

atypia, abnormal localization of immature precursors (ALIP) and/or increased reticulin fibrosis.

Phenotypic features (flow cytometry)

Ancillary techniques, including flow cytometry, have been utilized in the diagnosis of patients with MDS[34,640,662,670]

to determine features of dysmaturation and to exclude other disorders, which share clinical features with MDS. Flow cytometry does not evaluate red cell precursors for features of dyserythropoiesis, since they are lysed together with red blood cells during sample preparation. Therefore, flow cytometric analysis in MDS concentrates on granulocytes (megakaryocytes are too scanty to be harvested for analysis). Flow cytometric features suggesting

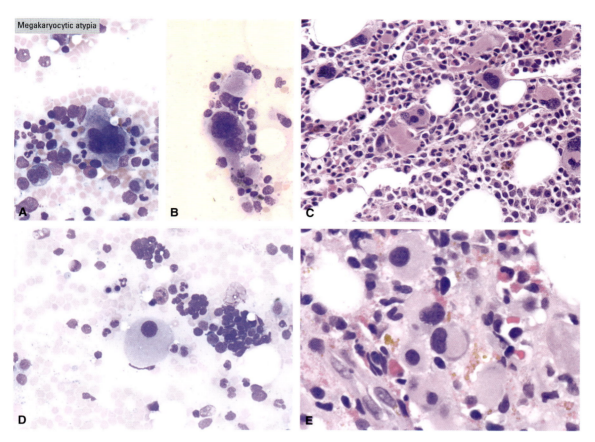

Figure 7.3   Megakaryocytic atypia. (**A**–**C**) Atypical megakaryocytes with hyperlobulated nuclei. (**D** and **E**) Atypical hypolobulated megakaryocytes, characteristic for 5q-syndrome

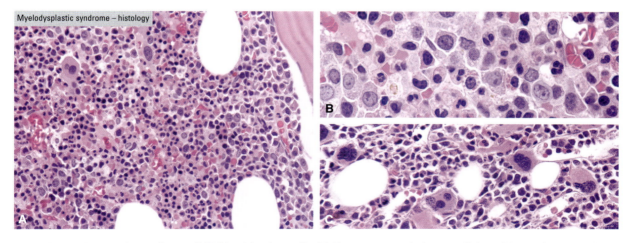

Figure 7.4   Myelodysplastic syndrome (MDS) – histology. (**A**–**C**) Bone marrow is hypercellular with atypical megakaryocytes. Immature cells (**B**) often show an abnormal interstitial localization (away from bony trabeculae)

dysmaturation include decreased side scatter and aberrant expression of CD10, CD11b, CD15, CD16, CD56 and HLA-DR. The first four markers may be downregulated, while the latter two may be upregulated in MDS. All flow cytometric features may be present on a subset of cells or involve the entire population. The intensity (degree) of aberrant expression is also variable, but often correlates with the degree of myelodysplasia. Low-grade MDS tends to have less obvious changes, whereas high-grade MDS (e.g., RAEB) shows pronounced changes, often involving more than one antigen. Decreased side scatter (Figure 7.5) reflects hypogranularity. Figures 7.6–7.8 present examples of aberrant expression of CD10, CD11b/HLA-DR and CD56 in MDS, respectively.

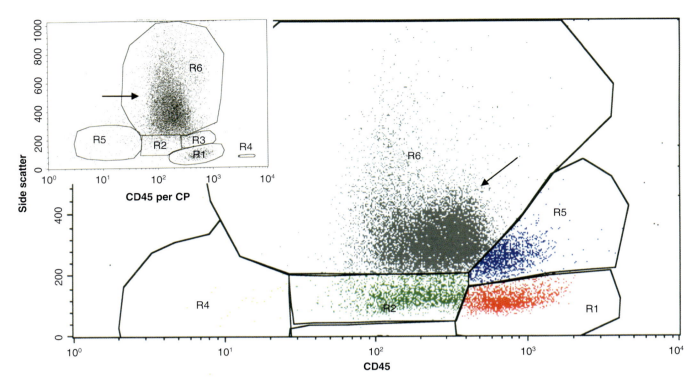

Figure 7.5   Myelodysplastic syndrome (MDS) – flow cytometry (dysgranulopoiesis). Granulocytes display markedly decreased orthogonal side scatter (arrow), indicating decreased granularity. Compare with normal bone marrow (inset)

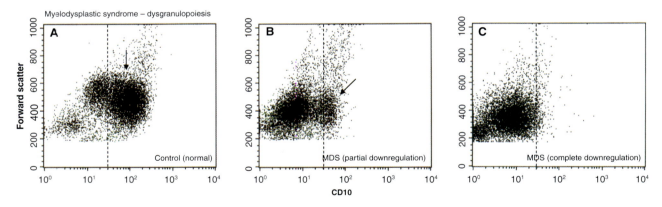

Figure 7.6   Myelodysplastic syndrome (MDS) – flow cytometry (dysgranulopoiesis). Granulocytes show decreased expression of CD10. (**A**) Normal (control) sample. Note positive CD10 expression (arrow). (**B**) MDS with partial loss of CD10 expression. Only a minute subset of granulocytes (arrow) is CD10⁺. (**C**) MDS with complete lack of CD10 expression by granulocytes

Cytogenetics

Cytogenetic analysis should be performed in all patients with a clinical impression of MDS. Chromosomal studies play an important role not only by confirming clonal myeloid disorder, but also by helping in subclassification of MDS and serving as an independent prognostic marker[676–679]. Complex chromosomal abnormalities are associated with unfavorable clinical course. The

de novo 5q(-) syndrome (isolated del(5q)), is associated with good prognosis and low risk of progression into acute leukemia.

REFRACTORY ANEMIA (RA)

RA is characterized by ineffective hematopoiesis leading to anemia. Bone marrow (Figure 7.9) shows unilineage dysplasia of erythroid series (dyserythropoiesis), less than

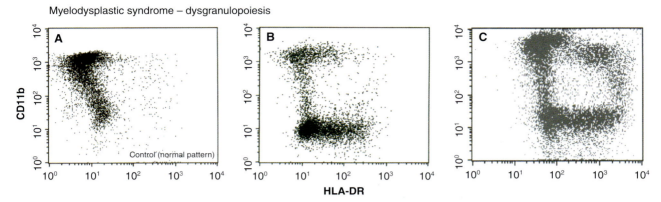

Myelodysplastic syndrome – dysgranulopoiesis

Figure 7.7 Myelodysplastic syndrome (MDS) – flow cytometry (dysgranulopoiesis). (**A**) Normal (control) sample. (**B** and **C**) Granulocytes in MDS show decreased CD11b expression and increased HLA-DR expression. In pronounced cases a typical 'window' pattern (**C**) is evident (compare with **A**)

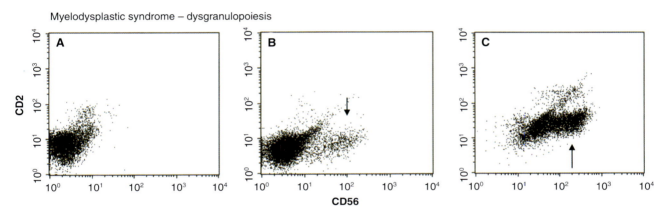

Myelodysplastic syndrome – dysgranulopoiesis

Figure 7.8 Myelodysplastic syndrome (MDS) – flow cytometry (dysgranulopoiesis). Upregulation of CD56 expression in MDS. (**A**) Normal (control) sample. (**B**) MDS with upregulation of CD56 on a minute subset of granulocytes (arrow). (**C**) MDS with marked upregulation of CD56 (arrow)

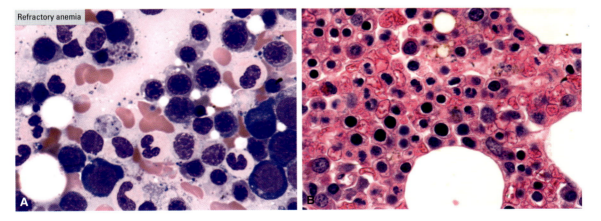

Figure 7.9 Refractory anemia (RA). (**A**) Bone marrow aspirate with erythroid hyperplasia and dyserythropoiesis. (**B**) Hypercellular marrow (core biopsy) with prominent erythroid hyperplasia. In many cases of RA, the morphologic changes are subtle and not diagnostic. To some degree, it remains a diagnosis of exclusion

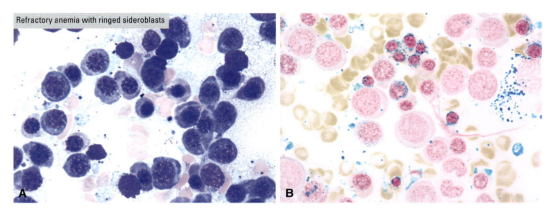

Figure 7.10 Refractory anemia with ringed sideroblasts (RARS). (**A**) Bone marrow aspirate shows erythroid hyperplasia with dyserythropoiesis and megaloblastoid changes. (**B**) Ringed sideroblasts exceed 15% of all red cell precursors

5% blasts (< 1% in peripheral blood) and less than 15% ringed sideroblasts. There are no Auer rods, and dysgranulopoiesis or megakaryocytic atypia is either minimal or not present. It is often a diagnosis of exclusion.

REFRACTORY ANEMIA WITH RINGED SIDEROBLASTS (RARS)

RARS is characterized by 15% or more ringed sideroblasts (among erythroid precursors) in the bone marrow (Figure 7.10). Other findings in the bone marrow and peripheral blood are similar to refractory anemia: bone marrow shows unilineage dysplasia of erythroid series and less than 5% blasts, and peripheral blood shows less than 1% blasts. There are no Auer rods, and dysgranulopoiesis or megakaryocytic atypia is either minimal or not present.

The differential diagnosis includes mixed myeloproliferative/myelodysplastic diseases (e.g., refractory anemia with ringed sideroblasts and marked thrombocytosis) and other myelodysplastic disorders with ringed sideroblasts (e.g., RAEB, del(5q) syndrome, and refractory cytopenia with multilineage dysplasia and ringed sideroblasts). Secondary causes of ringed sideroblasts (ethanolism, heavy metal exposure, pyridoxine deficiency) should also be excluded.

REFRACTORY CYTOPENIA WITH MULTILINEAGE DYSPLASIA (RCMD)

RCMD is characterized by bicytopenia or pancytopenia with less than 1% blasts in peripheral blood and less than 5% blasts in the bone marrow. Dysplastic features are present in 10% or more of the cells in two or more myeloid lineages and are usually more obvious (Figure 7.11) than in RA or RARS[78,661,664,680]. Clonal chromosomal changes

are seen more often than in RA or RARS – they can be found in up to 50% of patients. More common abnormalities include monosomy 5, monosomy 7, trisomy 8, del(5q) and del(20q), as well as complex abnormalities. A subset of cases may present with increased (15% or more) ringed sideroblasts (RCMD-ringed sideroblasts) (Figure 7.12).

REFRACTORY ANEMIA WITH EXCESS BLASTS (RAEB)

RAEB is characterized by at least 5% bone marrow blasts[78,651,672]. Based on the number of blasts in the bone marrow and peripheral blood, RAEB is divided into two categories: RAEB-1 and RAEB-2. RAEB-1 has 5–9% blasts in bone marrow and < 5% blasts in the peripheral blood. RAEB-2 has 10–19% blasts in the bone marrow. Cases of RAEB with Auer rods are classified as RAEB-2, regardless of the blast count. Peripheral blood smear and bone marrow aspirate show overt dysmaturation in one to three lineages (Figure 7.13). Bone marrow biopsy (Figure 7.13B) is variably cellular and most often hypercellular marrow with increased number of immature cells, which are found in aggregates in the interstitium, away from the vicinity of the bone trabeculae or vessels (abnormal localization of immature precursors; ALIP).

5q(-) SYNDROME (del(5q) SYNDROME)

MDS with isolated del(5q) chromosome occurs most often in elderly women who present with RA and a preserved or elevated platelet count[71,574,661,665,679,681–683]. The most characteristic morphologic feature on bone marrow examination is hypolobated micromegakaryocytes (Figure 7.14). The erythroid series may show subtle dyserythropoiesis. The

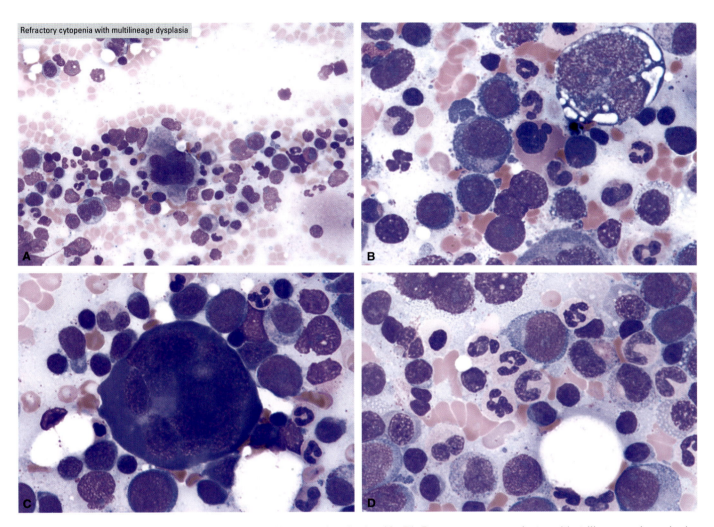

Figure 7.11   Refractory cytopenia with multilineage dysplasia. (**A–D**) Bone marrow aspirate with trilineage dyspoiesis. (**A**) Atypical megakaryocyte. (**B** and **C**) Marked dyserythropoiesis. (**D**) Dysgranulopoiesis in the form of hypogranular granulocytes

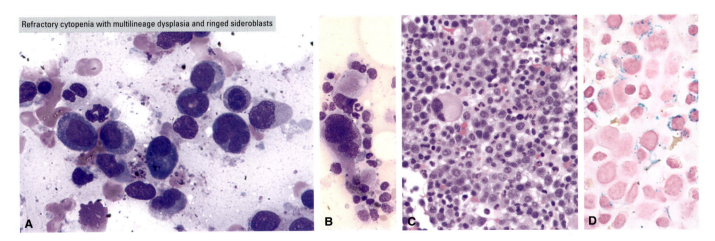

Figure 7.12   Refractory cytopenia with multilineage dysplasia and ringed sideroblasts. (**A**) Bone marrow aspirate with dysplastic normoblasts. (**B**) Atypical megakaryocyte. (**C**) Core biopsy: hypercellular marrow with atypical megakaryocytes. (**D**) Aspirate (iron stain) with ringed sideroblasts

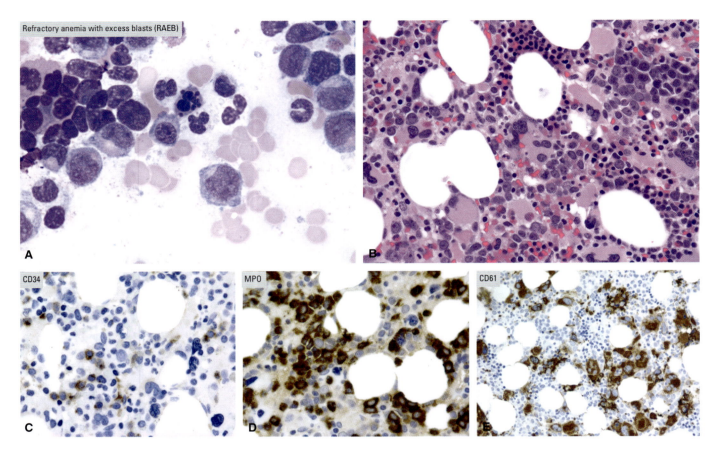

Figure 7.13 Refractory anemia with excess blasts (RAEB). (**A**) Bone marrow aspirate with dyserythropoiesis. (**B**) Core biopsy: hypercellular marrow with atypical megakaryocytosis and increased number of blasts. (**C–E**) Immunohistochemical staining shows increased number of CD34+ blasts (**C**), myeloid cells with leftward shift (**D**, MPO staining) and megakaryocytic hyperplasia (**E**, CD61 staining)

sole cytogenetic abnormality involves a deletion between bands q31 and 33 on chromosome 5 (Figure 7.14).

DIFFERENTIAL DIAGNOSIS OF MDS

The diagnosis of MDS is complex and requires correlation between multiple technologies, including morphology, cytogenetics, immunophenotyping, molecular tests and routine laboratory tests. Although the diagnosis is straightforward in cases with profound dyspoiesis in one or more of the myeloid lineages, it is often challenging. There are no strictly defined minimal diagnostic criteria for MDS. In patients with early stages of MDS, a single isolated cytopenia or isolated macrocytosis (where histomorphologic changes are very subtle), it may be difficult to make a definite diagnosis. This is a group of patients in which cytogenetic studies are often negative (the chance of positive cytogenetics studies rises in advanced stages of MDS). Generally, karyotypic abnormalities are present

in only 20–60% of MDS cases[63]. If there is no definite morphologic evidence of dyspoiesis and cytogenetics studies are negative, patients should be followed up with peripheral blood tests and/or repeated bone marrow evaluation at appropriate clinical intervals, providing other causes of the associated cytopenias have been eliminated. Figure 1.30 (Chapter 1) presents an approach (algorithm) to patients with anemia.

The presence of dysplastic features (morphology and/or flow cytometry immunophenotyping) does not, per se, make a diagnosis of MDS. Dysmaturation may be seen in healthy individuals and in conditions other than MDS, such as B$_{12}$/folate deficiency, treatment with granulocyte colony-stimulating factors, exposure to heavy metals (especially arsenic), drugs and toxins, paroxysmal nocturnal hemoglobinuria, viral infections including parvovirus and immunologic disorders.

Figure 7.15 presents the entities which clinically and/or morphologically require differentiation from MDS.

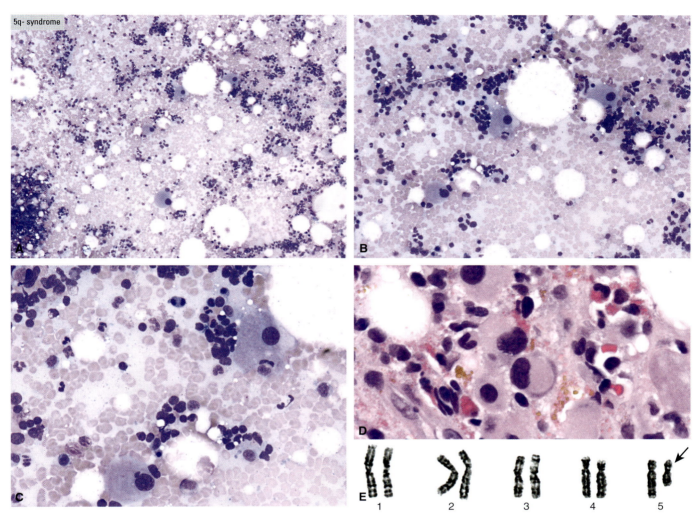

Figure 7.14 5q(-) syndrome. (**A–C**) Bone marrow aspirate (**A**, low; **B**, intermediate; **C**, high magnification) showing maturing trilineage hematopoiesis and hypolobated megakaryocytes. (**D**) Core biopsy with typical megakaryocytic morphology. (**E**) Cytogenetic karyotype with deletion of '*q*' portion of chromosome 5 (arrow)

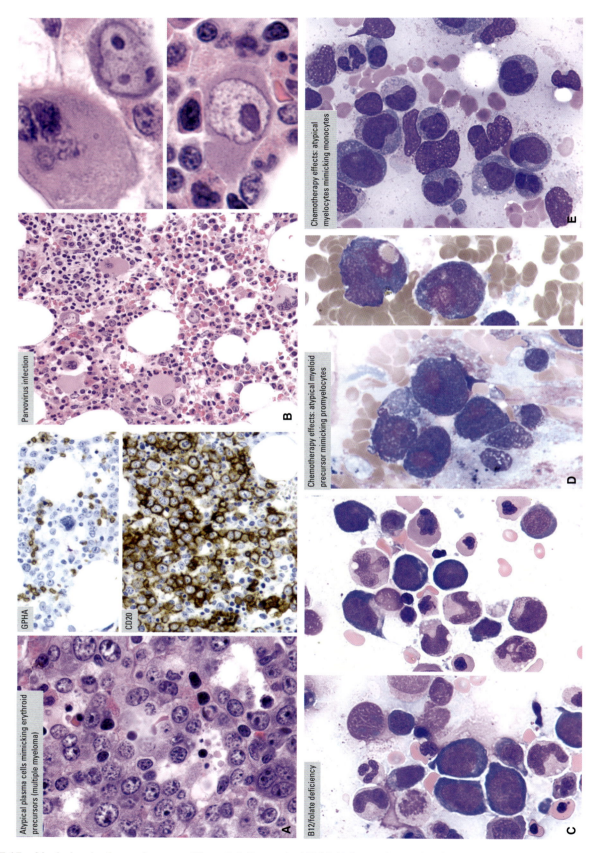

Figure 7.15   Myelodysplastic syndrome – differential diagnosis. (**A**) Multiple myeloma. Atypical plasma cells mimic dysplastic red cell precursors. GPHA staining is negative and CD20 staining is positive. (**B**) Parvovirus infection. (**C**) B$_{12}$/folate deficiency. (**D** and **E**) Post-treatment dyspoiesis. (**F**) Chronic myelomonocytic leukemia. (**G**) Chronic myeloproliferative disorders (PV, left; ET, right). (**H**) Reactive erythroid hyperplasia associated with hemolysis. (**I**) Acute erythroid leukemia (AML-M6)

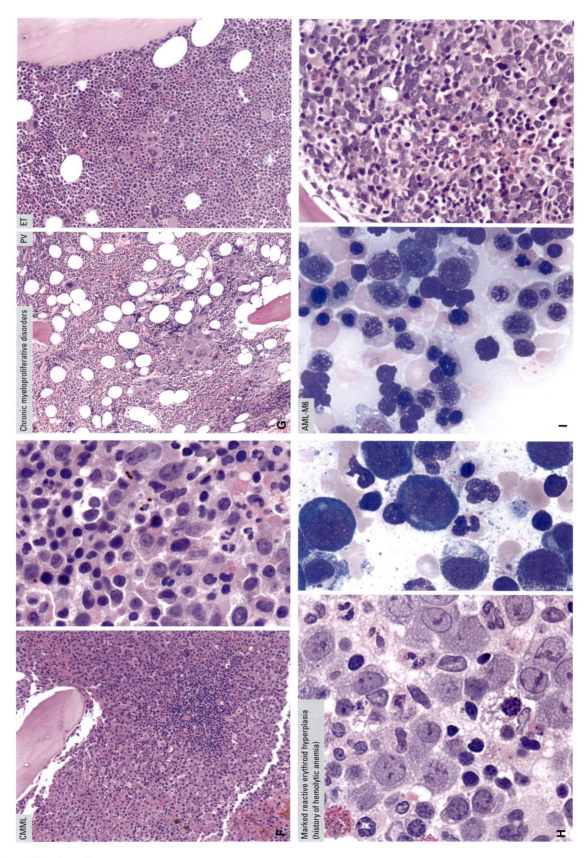

Figure 7.15 *(Continued)*

CHAPTER 8

Acute myeloid leukemia

INTRODUCTION

Acute myeloid leukemia (AML) is a clonal proliferation of immature hematopoietic precursor cells involving primarily the bone marrow and peripheral blood. The classification of acute leukemia is based on morphologic, immunophenotypic, cytogenetic, molecular and clinical data[45,48,50,64,65,160,684–690]. Generally, acute leukemias are divided into acute lymphoblastic leukemia (ALL) and AML, with a subset of leukemias displaying features of both (acute biphenotypic leukemia). Precursor B- and T-lymphoblastic leukemias are discussed in Chapter 9.

The WHO classification divides AML into four major categories: (i) AML with recurrent genetic abnormalities, (ii) AML with multilineage dysplasia, (iii) AML and myelodysplastic syndrome, therapy related, and (iv) AML not otherwise categorized (Table 8.1). The prognosis of AML with recurrent genetic abnormalities [t(15;17), inv(16) and t(8;21)] is relatively favorable, unlike all other categories of AML[64,65,685,688,691–693].

The requisite minimum of blasts for a diagnosis of acute leukemia is 20% in the bone marrow or peripheral blood, as recommended in the WHO classification. Acute myeloid leukemia associated with certain recurrent translocations, such as t(15;17)(q22;q12), t(8;21)(q22;q22) and inv16(p13q22), is diagnosed even with < 20% blasts/immature precursors. For the purposes of diagnosing acute leukemia, abnormal promyelocytes (acute promyelocytic leukemia), monoblasts/promonocytes (acute monoblastic leukemia) and megakaryoblasts (acute megakaryoblastic leukemia) are considered blast equivalents.

General morphologic features

Three major types of myeloblasts are recognized by nuclear and cytoplasmic characteristics. Type 1 myeloblasts (Figure 8.1A) have scanty, agranular cytoplasm, round or

Table 8.1 Classification of acute myeloid leukemia (AML)

AML with t(8;21) (AML1/ETO)
AML with inv(16)(p13q22) or t(16;16)(p13;q22) (acute myelomonocytic leukemia with eosinophilia; AML-M4Eo)
Acute promyelocytic leukemia [AML with t(15;17)(q22;q12)], APL (AML-M3)
Acute myeloid leukemia with multilineage dysplasia with prior myelodysplastic syndrome without prior myelodysplastic syndrome
Acute myeloid leukemia and myelodysplastic syndrome, therapy-related
Acute myeloid leukemia, minimally differentiated (AML-M0)
Acute myeloid leukemia without maturation (AML-M1)
Acute myeloid leukemia with maturation (AML-M2)
Acute myelomonocytic leukemia (AML-M4)
Acute monoblastic leukemia (AML-M5)
Acute erythroid leukemia (AML-M6)
Acute megakaryoblastic leukemia (AML-M7)
Acute basophilic leukemia
Acute panmyelosis with myelofibrosis
Myeloid sarcoma

slightly irregular nuclei, fine chromatin and a prominent nucleolus (usually more than one). A few granules in the cytoplasm may be occasionally seen. Type 2 myeloblasts (Figure 8.1B) are similar to type 1 except for the pauci-granular cytoplasm (< 15 primary azurophilic granules). Type 3 myeloblasts (Figure 8.1C) are characterized by numerous cytoplasmic granules (> 20 granules). Abnormal promyelocytes from acute promyelocytic leukemia (hypergranular variant) are characterized by the presence of numerous small azurophilic cytoplasmic granules and Auer rods (Figure 8.1D and E). In the microgranular variant of APL, the atypical promyelocytes have a characteristic bilobed or dumbbell-shaped nuclei with delicate chromatin, bearing some resemblance to monoblasts (Figure 8.1F). Monoblasts (Figure 8.1G) have large nuclei which are often folded or convoluted, finely dispersed chromatin and abundant pale cytoplasm. Occasional blasts may display erythrophagocytosis (Figure 8.1H). This phenomenon is most commonly associated with monoblastic differentiation. Promonocytes

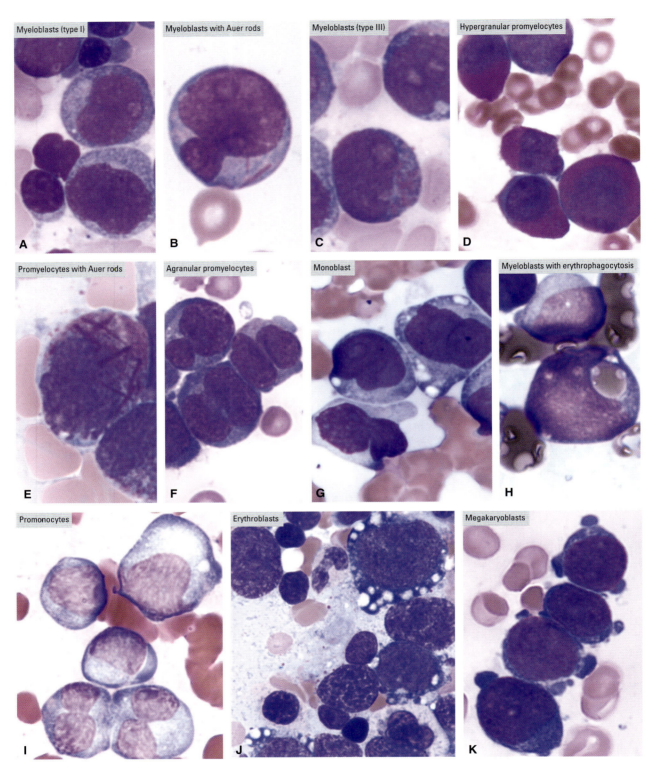

Figure 8.1   Acute myeloid leukemia – cytology. (**A**) Agranular myeloblasts. (**B**) Myeloblast with Auer rods. (**C**) Granulated myeloblasts. (**D**) Hypergranular promyelocytes. (**E**) Promyelocytes with numerous Auer rods. (**F**) Agranular promyelocytes. (**G**) Monoblasts. (**H**) Myeloblasts with erythrophagocytosis. (**I**) Promonocytes. (**J**) Erythroblasts. (**K**) Megakaryoblasts

(Figure 8.1I) are intermediate cells in maturation between monocytes and monoblasts; they are large with abundant, pale cytoplasm, which may contain azurophilic granules. The nuclei are round or folded with finely dispersed chromatin and contain several inconspicuous nucleoli. Immature erythroid precursors (Figure 8.1J) have markedly basophilic cytoplasm with focally prominent vacuolation. Nuclei are large with coarse chromatin, irregular contours and multinucleation. Dyserythropoietic features are prominent. Megakaryoblasts vary in morphologic appearance depending on the degree of differentiation. The most immature forms resemble myeloblasts, whereas cells with intermediate differentiation (promegakaryocytes) have more abundant cytoplasm with pseudopod formation (Figure 8.1K).

Evaluation of bone marrow core biopsy reveals a hypercellular marrow with sheets of immature cells. Occasional acute leukemia presents with a hypocellular marrow or prominent fibrosis. Immunohistochemical staining of the core biopsy for CD34, TdT and CD117 is very useful in establishing the diagnosis of AML in these situations.

Phenotypic features of acute leukemias

Immunophenotyping (by flow cytometry and/or immunohistochemistry) plays an important role in the diagnosis and subclassification of acute leukemias[14,15,23,26,28,31,48,684,691,694–706]. Side scatter and phenotypic characteristics of blasts differentiate between major types of acute leukemia (e.g., minimally differentiated AML versus ALL, acute monoblastic leukemia versus NK-cell lymphoma/leukemia, or B-ALL versus T-ALL) and allows to make specific diagnoses, such as acute promyelocytic leukemia, acute megakaryoblastic leukemia or acute monoblastic leukemia. The major markers used for the diagnosis and subclassification of AML are presented in Table 1.2 (Chapter 1). The panel should be broad since there is an overlap in the expression of some of the markers throughout acute leukemias of different lineages; thus, CD33 may be positive in precursor B- or T-lymphoblastic leukemia, CD19 may be positive in a subset of AML-M2, and some of the pan-T antigens (CD2 and CD7) are often expressed in AML.

AML (FAB M0, M1 and M2) is positive for CD4 (dim), CD11c (dim to moderate), CD13 (moderate), CD33 (moderate), CD34, CD117 and HLA-DR.

Acute promyelocytic leukemia (hypergranular variant; APL) is positive for CD4, CD13 (dim), CD33 (bright), and CD117; it displays increased side scatter and is negative for HLA-DR and CD34. Hypogranular APL is positive for CD2, CD4, CD13, CD33, CD34, CD64 and CD117.

Acute myelomonocytic leukemia (AML-M4) shows two populations: blasts with the phenotype similar to AML-M2, and monocytic cells, which are positive for CD11b, CD11c, CD14 and CD64.

Acute monocytic leukemia (AML-M5) is positive for CD4, CD11b, CD11c, CD13 (dim), CD33 (bright), CD56 and HLA-DR. Lack of CD14 favors acute monocytic leukemia over CMML.

Acute erythroid leukemia is positive for GPHA and hemoglobin A and acute megakaryoblastic leukemia is positive for CD41 and CD61.

AML WITH t(8;21)(q22;q22) (AML1/ETO)

AML with t(8;21)(q22;q22) most often displays the morphology of AML with maturation (AML-M2)[707–710]. Blasts are large with a variable number of azurophilic cytoplasmic granules and Auer rods. Phenotypically, they are positive for pan-myeloid antigens (CD13, CD33), blastic markers (CD34, CD117) and characteristically for CD19 and CD56 (Figure 8.2). Occasional cases may show lack of surface pan-myeloid antigens[691]. The translocation t(8;21)(q22;q22) (Figure 8.3) involves the *AML1* gene and *ETO* gene.

AML WITH inv(16)(p13q22) OR t(16;16)(p13;q22)

AML with inv(16)(p13q22) or t(16;16)(p13;q22) is a variant of acute myelomonocytic leukemia (AML-M4) characterized by increased eosinophils in the bone marrow (Figures 8.4 and 8.5). The eosinophils are atypical with large basophilic granules. Inv(16)(p13q22) and t(16;16)(p13;q22) results in the fusion of the *CBFβ* gene and the smooth muscle *myosin heavy-chain* gene[692].

ACUTE PROMYELOCYTIC LEUKEMIA (APL, AML-M3; AML WITH t(15;17)(q22;q12))

Acute leukemia with t(15;17)(q22;q12) is characterized by a proliferation of abnormal promyelocytes (Figure 8.6). It is often accompanied by disseminated intravascular coagulation and particular response to treatment with all-*trans*-retinoic acid, which induces maturation[60,688,711–713].

APL is divided into hypergranular and hypogranular variants. The hypergranular variant of APL contains abnormal promyelocytes (Figure 8.6) characterized by numerous azurophilic granules. A subset of promyelocytes may contain one or more delicate Auer rods ('faggot cells'). The bone marrow biopsy (Figure 8.7) is hypercellular and completely replaced by promyelocytes with

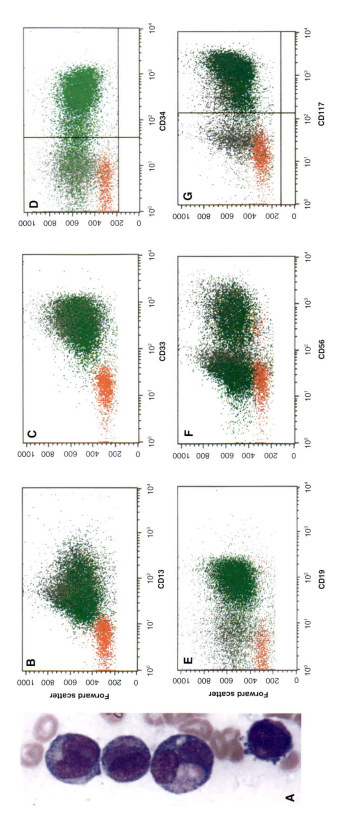

Figure 8.2 Acute myeloid leukemia with t(8;21) – flow cytometry. Myeloblasts have granular cytoplasm (**A**). They are positive for CD13 (**B**), CD33 (**C**), CD34 (**D**), CD19 (**E**), CD56 (**F**) and CD117 (**G**)

Acute myeloid leukemia with t(8;21)

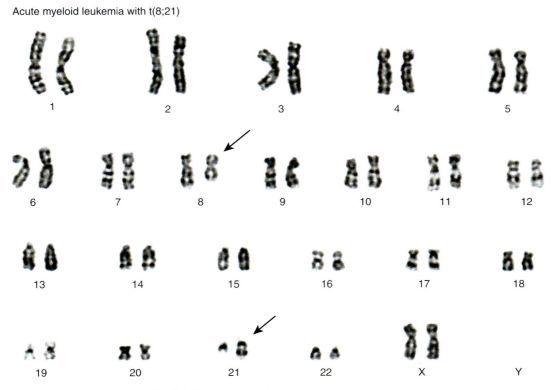

Figure 8.3 Acute myeloid leukemia with t(8;21) – cytogenetics

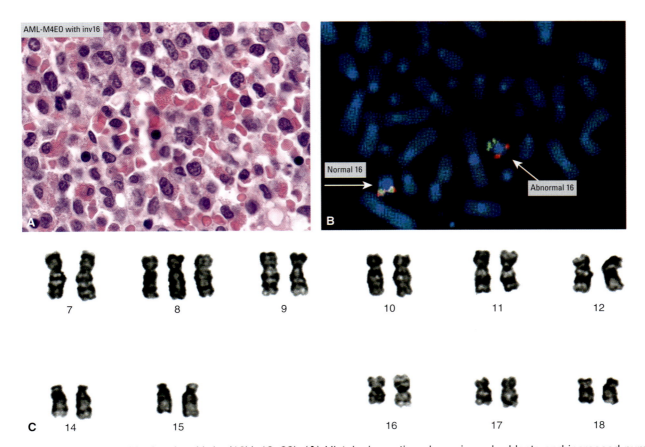

Figure 8.4 Acute myeloid leukemia with inv(16)(p13q22). (**A**) Histologic section shows irregular blasts and increased number of eosinophils. (**B** and **C**) FISH and cytogenetic studies show abnormal chromosome 16

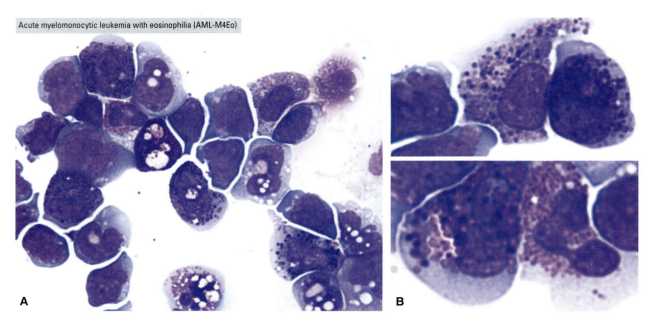

Figure 8.5   Acute myeloid leukemia with inv(16)(p13q22) – cytology. Abnormal eosinophils with large basophilic colored granules (**A** and **B**)

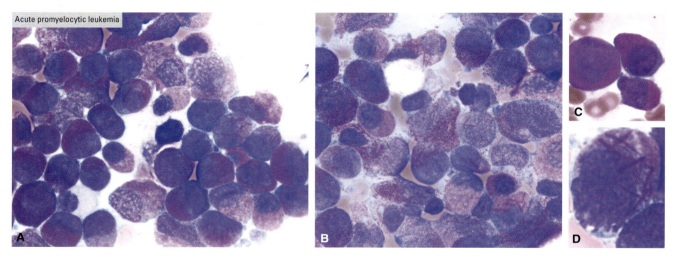

Figure 8.6   Acute promyelocytic leukemia – cytology. (**A–D**) Aspirate smear with hypergranular promyelocytes and promyelocytes with numerous Auer rods ('faggot cells')

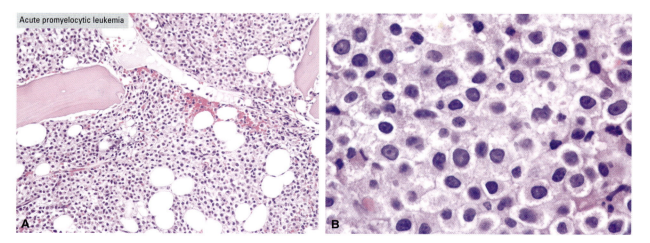

Figure 8.7   Acute promyelocytic leukemia (APL) – histology. Low (**A**) and high (**B**) magnification of APL. Bone marrow is replaced by abnormal promyelocytes with abundant cytoplasm and conspicuous borders, mimicking fried eggs or plant cells

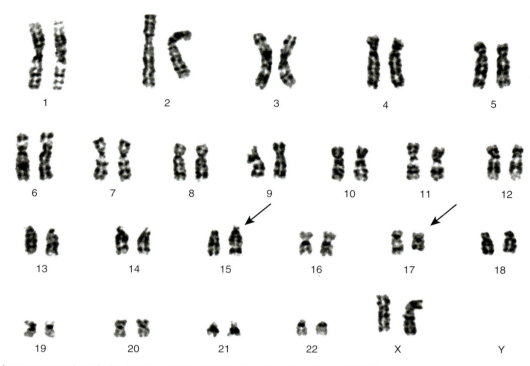

Figure 8.8 Acute promyelocytic leukemia – cytogenetics. The translocation t(15;17)

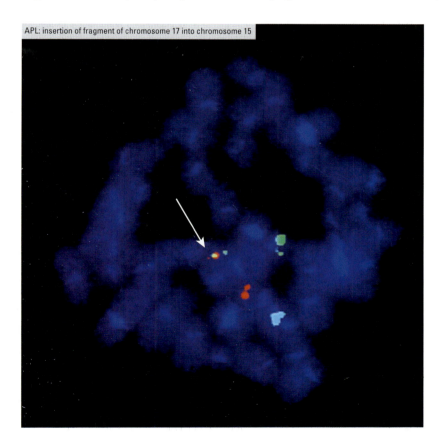

Figure 8.9 Acute promyelocytic leukemia (APL) – FISH study showing t(15;17) (arrow)

abundant pale or eosinophilic cytoplasm with distinct borders mimicking fried eggs or plant cells.

T(15;17)(q22;q12) results in fusion of the retinoic acid receptor-alpha (*RARα*) gene on chromosome 17 with a nuclear regulatory factor (*PML* gene) on chromosome 15

(Figures 8.8 and 8.9). A minority of APL cases lack the classic t(15;17)(q22;q12). In the majority of these cases, the *PML/RARα* rearrangements are due to insertions or more complex mechanisms, including three-way and simple variant translocations[64,65,688,700,714].

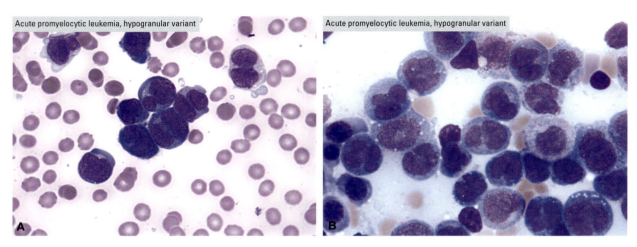

Figure 8.10   Acute promyelocytic leukemia – two examples of hypogranular variant (**A** and **B**, cytology). The hypogranular (microgranular) variant of APL is characterized by agranular cytoplasm and a bilobed nucleus

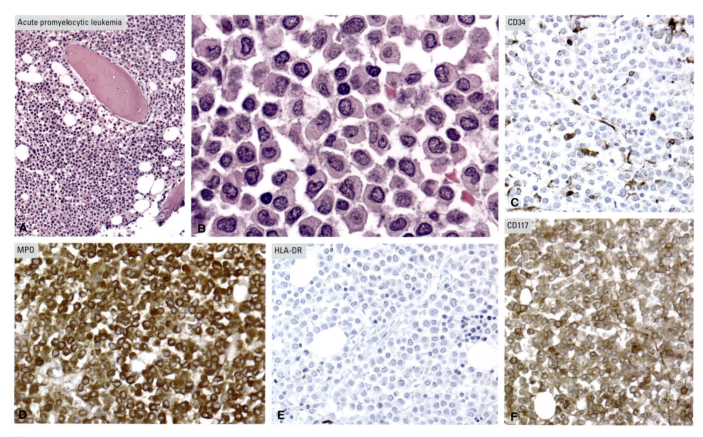

Figure 8.11   Acute promyelocytic leukemia – immunohistochemistry. (**A** and **B**) Histologic section shows hypercellular marrow with atypical promyelocytes. Neoplastic cells are negative for CD34 (**C**) and HLA-DR (**E**) and are positive for MPO (**D**) and CD117 (**F**)

The hypogranular (microgranular) variant of APL (APLv; Figure 8.10) is characterized by atypical promyelocytes with marked nuclear irregularities, mostly in the form of bilobation, folding or convolution. The cytoplasm is either agranular or hypogranular with finer azurophilic granulation when compared to typical APL.

APL has specific immunophenotypic features. Immunohistochemical analysis of hypergranular APL reveals lack of HLA-DR and CD34 and strong expression of MPO and CD117 (Figure 8.11). APL analyzed by flow cytometry (Figure 8.12) reveals increased side scatter, expression of CD13, CD33 and CD117, and lack of

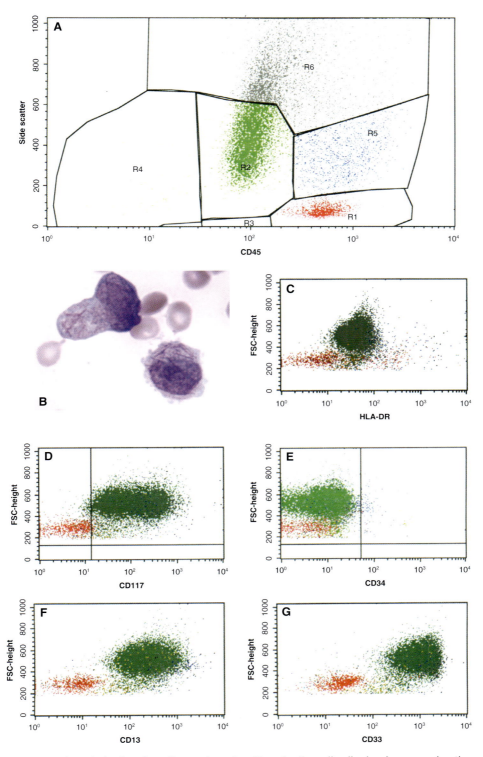

Figure 8.12   Acute promyelocytic leukemia – flow cytometry. Neoplastic cells display increased orthogonal side scatter (**A**) corresponding to hypergranular cytoplasm (**B**). Tumor cells are HLA-DR negative (**C**), CD117⁺ (**D**), CD34⁻ (**E**), CD13⁺ (**F**) and CD33⁺ (**G**)

HLA-DR and CD34. Hypogranular (microgranular) APL, apart from pan-myeloid antigens, is often positive for CD2, CD34 and CD117. Tables 8.2 and 8.3 summarize the phenotypic characteristics of hypergranular and hypogranular APL, respectively.

The differential diagnosis of APL includes atypical myeloid precursors associated with chemotherapy and/or recombinant granulocyte growth factor, acute monocytic leukemia and HLA-DR negative AML[48,696,705,714–716]. Myeloid precursors, following toxic insult to bone

Table 8.2   Immunophenotypic profile of acute promyelocytic leukemia (hypergranular variant)

Marker	% positive (intensity)
Side scatter	Markedly increased
CD2	10% (dim)
CD4	35% (dim)
CD11b	0
CD11c	0
CD13	100% (dim, 45%; moderate, 55%)
CD14	0
CD16	0
CD19	0
CD33	100% (moderate, 30%; bright, 70%)
CD34	0 (16% of cases shows minute subset of CD34+ cells)
CD38	84% (dim)
CD45	100% (moderate)
CD56	25%
CD64	90% (dim)
CD117	100% (moderate)
HLA-DR	0

Table 8.3   Immunophenotypic profile of acute promyelocytic leukemia (microgranular variant)

Marker	% positive (intensity)
Side scatter	Decreased (blast region)
CD2	87% (dim to moderate)
CD4	62% (dim)
CD11b	0
CD11c	0
CD13	100% (dim, 75%; moderate, 25%)
CD14	0
CD16	0
CD19	0
CD33	100% (bright)
CD34	75% + (all cells positive); 13% +/− (subset cells +), 12% − (all cells negative)
CD38	88% (dim)
CD45	100% (moderate)
CD56	12.5%
CD64	100% (dim)
CD117	100% (moderate)
HLA-DR	0

marrow, show a predominance of late promyelocyte/early myelocyte forms with a prominent Golgi area, and may suggest APL (Figure 8.13). Recent history of the treatment and absence of Auer rods are distinguishing features. In abundant agranular basophilic cytoplasm and lobulated nuclei of APLv, they resemble immature monocytes; therefore, the differentiation between acute monocytic leukemia and microgranular APL is often difficult solely on cytomorphologic grounds. Lack of occasional cells with hypergranular cytoplasm, lack of Auer rods and positive cytochemical staining with non-specific esterase (NSE), and lack of staining with myeloperoxidase (MPO) are diagnostic for acute monocytic leukemia (Figure 8.14). Phenotypically, immature monocytes are usually positive for HLA-DR and are negative for both CD34 and CD117 (compare Tables 8.3 and 8.4). Positive MPO distinguishes APL from megakaryoblastic leukemia. Also included in the differential diagnosis is AML-M2, which rarely may be HLA-DR⁻ and CD34⁻ (Figure 8.15).

Based on the CD45 expression and side scatter characteristics, hypergranular APL resembles normally maturing myeloid cells (compare A and E, Figure 8.16): atypical hypergranular promyelocytes are located in the same area as normal granulocytes (gray). Analysis of CD11b versus HLA-DR (Figure 8.17) and CD10, CD16 and CD117 (Figure 8.18) distinguishes benign process from APL. The pattern of expression of CD117 and CD11b is helpful in differentiating APL from recovering benign myeloid proliferation[705].

ACUTE MYELOID LEUKEMIA (AML-M0, M1 AND M2)

AML, minimally differentiated (AML-M0), is acute leukemia with no cytomorphologic evidence of myeloid differentiation (< 3% blasts react for myeloperoxidase). Flow cytometry immunophenotyping reveals expression of one or more pan-myeloid antigens (CD13, CD33), CD34, CD117 and HLA-DR. TdT may be positive, but B- and pan-T markers are negative, which excludes precursor lymphoblastic leukemia. Moderate expression of CD117 is one of the most important markers, since both precursor B- and T-lymphoblastic leukemias may be occasionally positive for some of the pan-myeloid antigens, and cases of AML may be CD19+ or CD7+.

AML without maturation (AML-M1) is defined by ≥ 90% blasts of non-erythroid lineage (less than 10% of the marrow cells manifest evidence of maturation to promyelocytes or more mature granulocytes). At least 3% of blasts are positive for MPO. AML with maturation is defined by ≥ 20% blasts and evidence of myeloid maturation (promyelocytes and subsequent stages) in ≥ 10% of the bone marrow cells.

The myeloblasts vary from medium-sized to large. The cytoplasm may be agranular to paucigranular (myeloblasts types 1 and 2). Single Auer rods are occasionally seen. AML with maturation usually reveals prominent dyspoiesis of maturing elements. Nuclei are large and often irregular (Figure 8.19). Phenotyping by immunohistochemistry

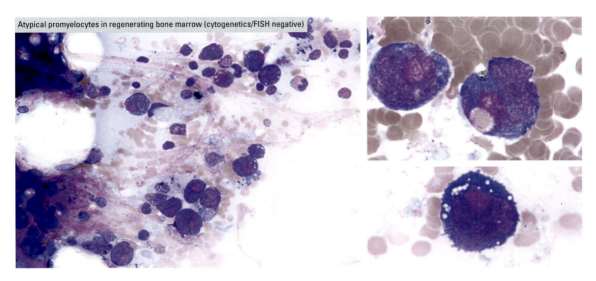

Figure 8.13 Differential diagnosis of APL: atypical myeloid precursors in regenerating bone marrow after chemotherapy

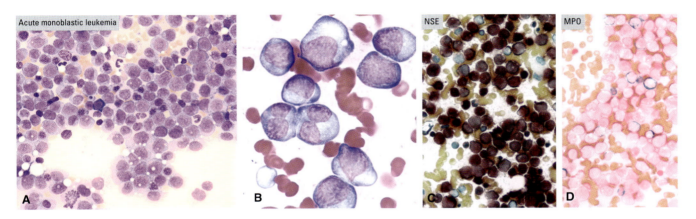

Figure 8.14 Differential diagnosis of APL: acute monoblastic leukemia. Monoblasts (**A** and **B**) have irregular nuclei, which look similar to hypogranular promyelocytes. In contrast to APL, neoplastic cells are NSE$^+$ (**C**) and MPO$^-$ (**D**)

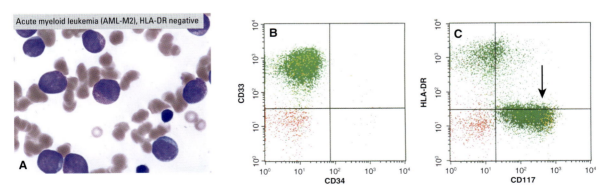

Figure 8.15 Differential diagnosis of APL: HLA-DR negative acute myeloid leukemia (AML-M2). Subset of acute myeloid leukemias (non-M3) shows similar phenotype to APL: lack of CD34 and HLA-DR. Correlation with cytomorphology and cytogenetic/FISH studies helps to distinguish between APL and HLA-DR$^-$ AML

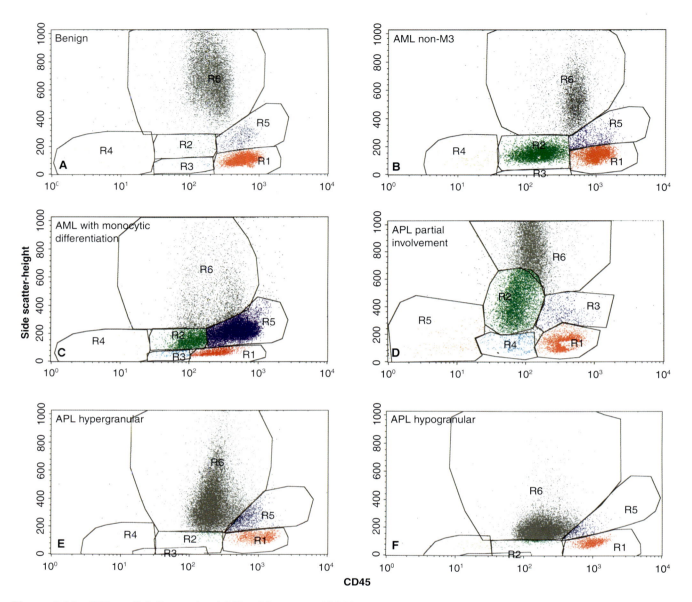

Figure 8.16 Differential diagnosis of APL: side scatter (SSC) characteristics of different types of acute myeloid leukemias. (**A**) Normal (control) sample. (**B**) AML (non-M3). Granulocytes (gray) have high SSC and blasts (green) have low SSC. (**C**) Neoplastic monocytes (blue) have low SSC and bright CD45 expression. (**D**) APL, partial bone marrow involvement. Promyelocytes have high SSC (green). (**E**) Hypergranular APL. Promyelocytes (gray) have increased SSC. (**F**) Hypogranular APL. Promyelocytes (gray) have low SSC, similar to regular myeloblasts (compare with **B**)

(Figure 8.19) or flow cytometry (Figure 8.20) reveals expression of myeloid markers (CD13, CD33, MPO), CD34, CD117, and HLA-DR in most cases. Most cases show blasts with low side scatter (Figure 8.20A), but rare cases have hypergranular blasts, which are located in granulocytic gate.

ACUTE MYELOMONOCYTIC LEUKEMIA (AML-M4)

This is acute leukemia characterized by the proliferation of both neutrophil and monocyte precursors with 20%

or more myeloblasts in the bone marrow. Monocytic and granulocytic lineages each comprise at least 20% of marrow cells. The number of monocytic cells and their precursors in peripheral blood is usually greater than $5 \times 10^9/l$. The bone marrow is hypercellular (Figure 8.21) and contains a mixed population of monocytes and their precursors and granulocytes and their precursors. The monoblasts are slightly larger than myeloblasts, have abundant cytoplasm and one prominent nucleolus or several nucleoli. The myeloblasts and maturing granulocytes show morphologic features similar to AML with maturation. At least 3% of blasts are MPO+.

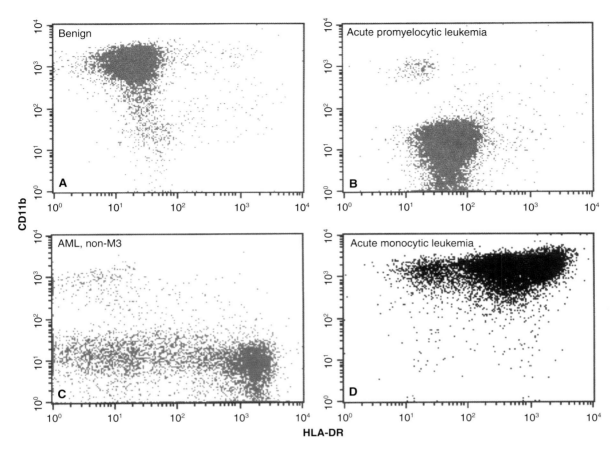

Figure 8.17   Differential diagnosis of APL: comparison of the expression of CD11b and HLA-DR in APL, non-M3 AML and acute monocytic leukemia. (**A**) Normal (control) sample. Granulocytes are brightly positive for CD11b and negative for HLA-DR. (**B**) APL. Promyelocytes lack the expression of CD11b and HLA-DR. (**C**) AML non-M3. Blasts are strongly positive for HLA-DR and negative for CD11b. (**D**) Monoblasts are positive for both CD11b and HLA-DR

Flow cytometry (Figure 8.22) reveals two distinct populations: blasts (moderate CD45 and low side scatter) and monocytic cells (bright CD45 and slightly increased side scatter). The monocytic component is positive for CD11b, CD11c, CD13, CD14, CD33, CD64 and HLA-DR, and myeloblasts are positive for CD13, CD33, CD34, CD117 and HLA-DR. A subset of AML-M4 shows expression of CD2, CD7, CD34 and CD56 by atypical monocytes.

ACUTE MONOCYTIC LEUKEMIA (AML-M5)

Acute monocytic (monoblastic) leukemia is defined as acute myeloid leukemia in which 80% or more of the leukemic cells are of monocytic lineage (monoblasts, promonocytes and monocytes)[78,717,718]. Leukemic monocytes have abundant cytoplasm, which may show irregular borders with pseudopods and cytoplasmic vacuoles

(Figure 8.23). The monoblasts have large and usually round nuclei with one prominent nucleolus or several nucleoli. Promonocytes tend to have irregular, folded nuclei and pale, slightly basophilic cytoplasm with occasional azurophilic granules. NSE is positive (Figure 8.24) in a majority of cases, although it may be weak. MPO is characteristically negative.

The bone marrow core biopsy is hypercellular and usually completely replaced by monoblasts, which are large and have prominent nucleoli (Figure 8.25). Immunohistochemistry reveals expression of HLA-DR, CD68 and CD56 (in most cases) and lack of MPO and CD34 (Figure 8.25B–F).

Flow cytometry (Figure 8.26) in AML-M5 usually reveals expression of CD4, CD11b, CD11c (bright), CD13 (dim), CD33 (bright), CD11c (moderate or bright), CD45 (moderate or bright), CD56, CD64 and HLA-DR. A subset of cases shows expression of

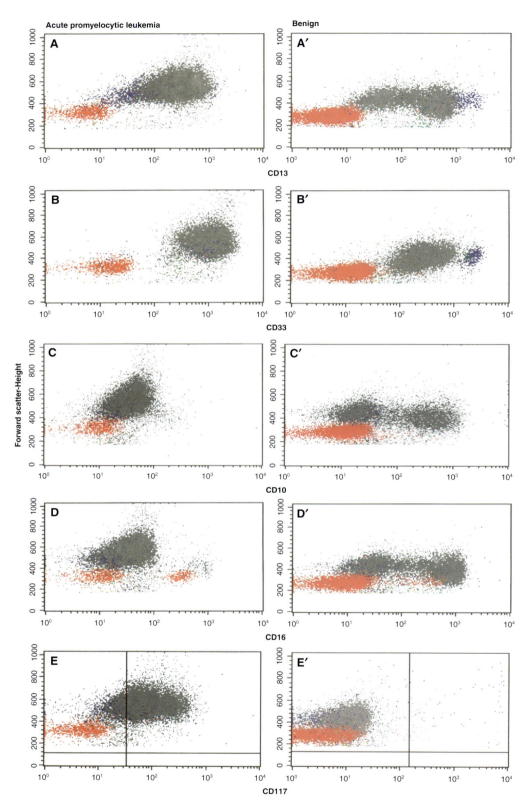

Figure 8.18 Differential diagnosis of APL: flow cytometric differences between promyelocytes (left column) and granulocytes (right column). Promyelocytes and granulocytes are positive for CD13 and CD33 (**A** and **B**). In contrast to granulocytes, promyelocytes do not express CD10 (**C**, compare with **C'**) and CD16 (**D**, compare with **D'**), and are positive for CD117 (**E**, compare with **E'**)

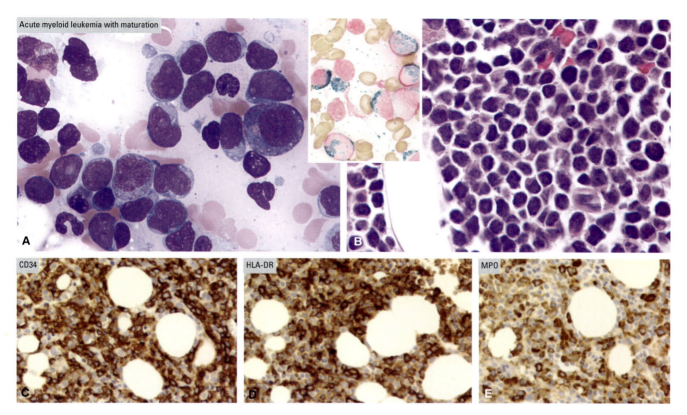

Figure 8.19 Acute myeloid leukemia with maturation (AML-M2). (**A**) Bone marrow aspirate shows large blasts with abundant granular cytoplasm, irregular nuclei and several nucleoli (inset: positive staining with MPO). (**B**) Histology section shows replacement of the marrow by immature mononuclear cells. Blasts are positive for CD34 (**C**), HLA-DR (**D**), and MPO (**E**) by immunohistochemistry

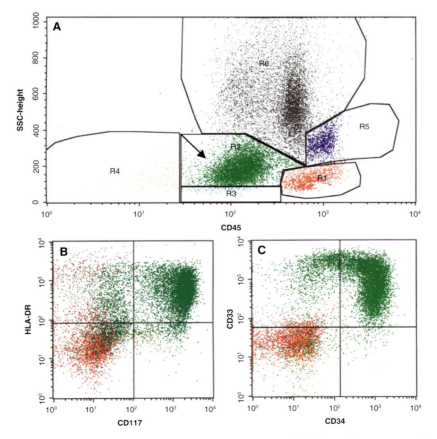

Figure 8.20 Acute myeloid leukemia with maturation – flow cytometry. (**A**) Blasts (green, arrow) have low side scatter and moderate expression of CD45. They are positive for CD117, HLA-DR, CD34 and CD33 (**B** and **C**)

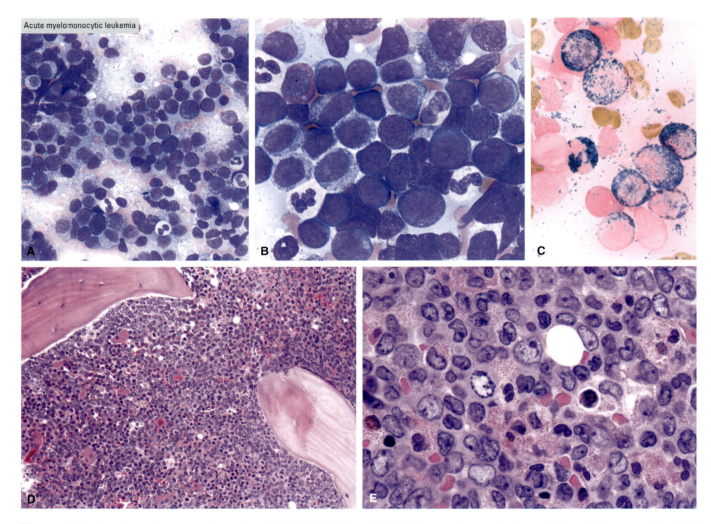

Acute myelomonocytic leukemia

Figure 8.21 Acute myelomonocytic leukemia (AML-M4). (**A** and **B**) Cytology shows mixed population of blasts and atypical monocytes. Blasts are expressing MPO (**C**). (**D** and **E**) Histology section shows hypercellular marrow with predominance of blasts and monocytes

CD2, CD7, CD10, CD23, and CD117 (see Table 8.4 for details).

The differential diagnosis of acute monocytic leukemia includes acute promyelocytic leukemia (microgranular variant), AML without maturation (AML-M0), minimally differentiated AML (AML-M1), chronic myelomonocytic leukemia (CMML), acute megakaryoblastic leukemia and acute myelomonocytic leukemia (AML-M4). Extramedullary myeloid tumors with monocytic differentiation (monoblastic sarcoma) may be confused with large cell lymphoma, carcinoma or sarcoma. Myeloblasts and abnormal promyelocytes are strongly MPO⁺, whereas monocytes are either weakly positive or negative. Monoblasts and promonocytes usually are positive with NSE staining, but a significant subset of acute monocytic leukemia is NSE⁻. Therefore, definite diagnosis often requires correlation of CBC data, cytologic features and cytochemistry with additional techniques such as immunophenotyping by flow cytometry, cytogenetics/ FISH and molecular tests.

ACUTE ERYTHROID LEUKEMIA (AML-M6)

Acute erythroid leukemia is characterized by a predominance of abnormal erythroid cells. The WHO recognizes two subtypes of AML-M6: erythroleukemia (erythroid/ myeloid leukemia) and pure erythroid leukemia[78,79,719]. Erythroleukemia is defined by ≥ 50% erythroid precursors (among all nucleated cells) and ≥ 20% myeloblasts of non-erythroid cells. Pure erythroid leukemia is defined by > 80% erythroid precursors among all nucleated marrow cells. Myelodysplastic

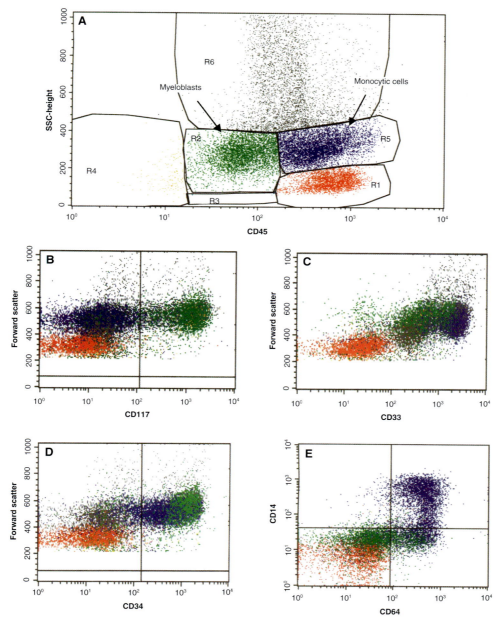

Figure 8.22   Acute myelomonocytic leukemia – flow cytometry. Flow cytometry shows predominance of two populations: blasts with low side scatter and moderate CD45 expression (**A**, green) and monocytes with low side scatter and bright CD45 expression (**A**, blue). Myeloblasts are positive for CD117 (**B**), CD33 (**C**) and CD34 (**D**). Monocytic population is negative for CD117 (**B**), and has bright expression of CD33 (**C**) and dim expression of CD34 (**D**). The majority of monocytes coexpress CD14 and CD64 (**E**)

syndrome differs from erythroleukemia by < 20% myeloblasts of non-erythroid cells (proerythroblasts are not included in the blast percentage).

The blood and bone marrow findings in erythroid leukemias are variable, depending on the degree of erythroid proliferation, maturation, dyserythropoiesis and proportion of myeloblasts. The erythroid precursors (Figure 8.27) are large with abundant basophilic cytoplasm with vacuoles. Cytoplasmic pseudopods similar to

those of acute megakaryoblastic leukemia may be present. Nuclei are round or irregular with lobulation and multinucleation and prominent megaloblastoid chromatin. Ringed sideroblasts are often present on iron preparations. The bone marrow core biopsy (Figure 8.28) is hypercellular with a predominance of erythroid precursors. Erythroblasts are positive for glycophorin A (GPHA) by flow cytometry or immunohistochemistry (Figure 8.28D and G) and hemoglobin A. They lack

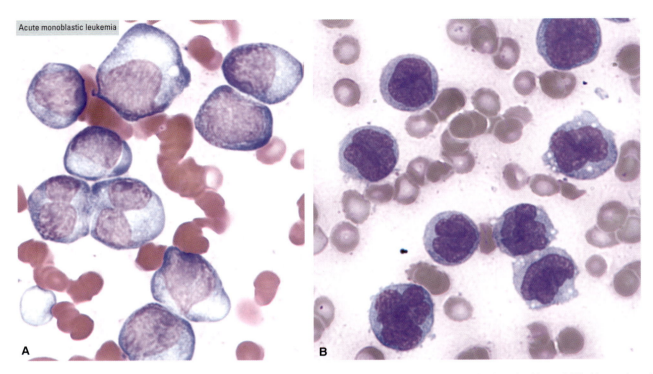

Figure 8.23   Acute monoblastic leukemia – cytology. Two examples of acute monoblastic leukemia (**A** and **B**). Note abundant cytoplasm, occasional cytoplasmic vacuoles and prominent nuclear irregularities

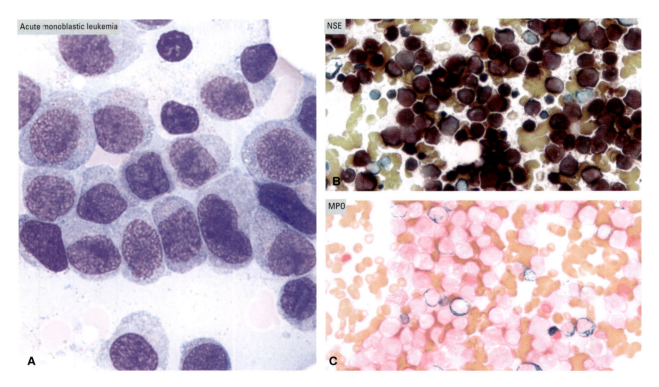

Figure 8.24   Acute monoblastic leukemia – cytochemistry. Neoplastic monocytes (**A**) are strongly positive for NSE (**B**) and do not stain for MPO (**C**)

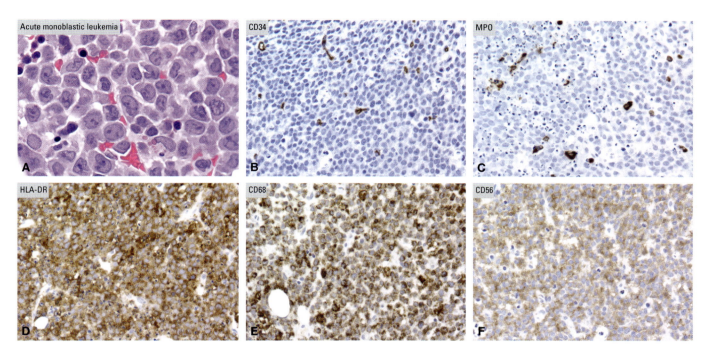

Figure 8.25 Acute monoblastic leukemia – immunohistochemistry. Monoblasts (**A**, histology section) are negative for CD34 (**B**) and MPO (**C**), and are positive for HLA-DR (**D**), CD68 (**E**) and CD56 (**F**)

MPO, CD34, CD45 and pan-myeloid antigens. CD117, CD43 and epithelial membrane antigen (EMA) are often positive (Figure 8.28J–L). Often, the early erythroblasts show coarse granular positivity for PAS (periodic acid-Schiff).

The differential diagnosis of acute erythroid leukemia includes high-grade myelodysplastic syndrome (refractory anemia with excess blasts), AML with multilineage dysplasia, erythroid hyperplasia with prominent megaloblastic changes due to B_{12}/folate deficiency, acute megakaryoblastic leukemia and other types of AML (AML-M0, M1, M2 and acute myelomonocytic leukemia).

ACUTE MEGAKARYOBLASTIC LEUKEMIA (AML-M7)

Acute megakaryoblastic leukemia is AML with ≥ 20% blasts, of which 50% or more are of megakaryocyte lineage. Cytomorphologic features vary, depending on the degree of maturation of megakaryoblasts. In the more differentiated cases, megakaryoblasts (Figure 8.29) are medium-sized to large with round or slightly irregular nucleus and basophilic, agranular cytoplasm with distinct blebs (pseudopods). In poorly differentiated cases, megakaryoblasts resemble myeloblasts or lymphoblasts, and their lineage can be revealed by immunophenotyping. The spectrum of morphologic features of acute

megakaryoblastic leukemia in bone marrow core biopsy (Figure 8.30) varies from predominance of poorly differentiated blasts (Figure 8.30A) to sheets of atypical megakaryocytes with predominance of micromegakaryocytes (Figure 8.30D).

Flow cytometry analysis (Figure 8.31) is characteristic and shows blasts with moderate CD34, dim CD117, negative to dim HLA-DR, negative CD13, bright CD33 and dim CD64. CD41 and CD61 are expressed (expression of CD41 and CD61 has to be interpreted with caution due to potential non-specific adsorption of platelets on other cells).

ACUTE BASOPHILIC LEUKEMIA

Acute basophilic leukemia (Figure 8.32) is a variant of acute myeloid leukemia with prominent basophilic differentiation[720]. Blood and bone marrow shows immature basophils with numerous, coarse, basophilic cytoplasmic granules.

DIFFERENTIAL DIAGNOSIS OF AML

Prominent bone marrow involvement by large mononuclear cells in various hematopoietic and non-hematopoietic lesions may imitate AML in trephine core biopsy (Figure 8.33).

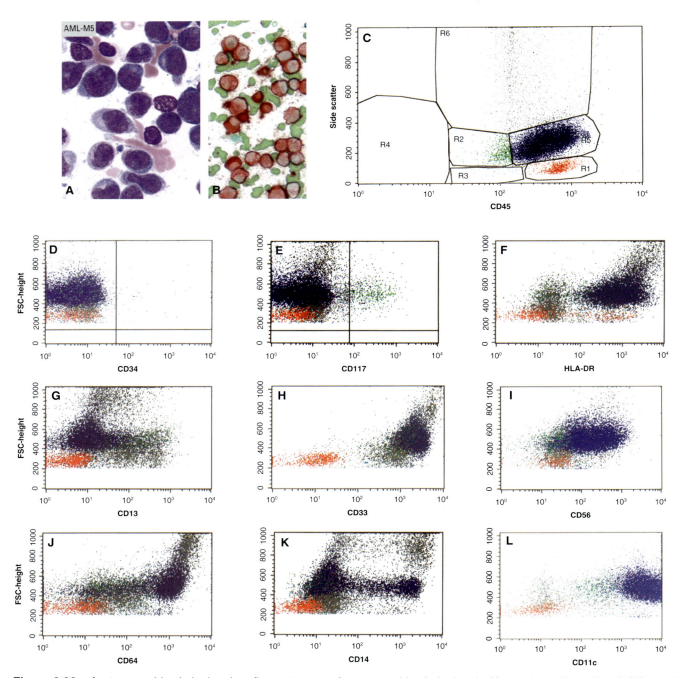

Figure 8.26 Acute monoblastic leukemia – flow cytometry. Acute monoblastic leukemia (**A**, cytology; **B**, positive NSE staining) shows bright expression of CD45 (**C**), negative CD34 (**D**), negative CD117 (**E**), bright HLA-DR (**F**), negative to dim CD13 (**G**), bright CD33 (**H**), positive CD56 (**I**), bright CD64 (**J**), variable expression of CD14 (**K**) and bright expression of CD11c (**L**)

Plasma cell myeloma (Figure 8.33A) with coarse chromatin and basophilic cytoplasm may occasionally mimic erythroleukemia. Both lesions may be positive for CD138, EMA, CD56 and CD117, but plasma cells express light- and heavy-chain immunoglobulins and are negative for GPHA. Poorly differentiated metastatic tumors, including breast carcinoma (Figure 8.33B), small cell carcinoma (Figure 8.33C), neuroblastoma (Figure 8.33D) and alveolar rhabdomyosarcoma (Figure 8.33E), are distinguished from AML by their

specific immunophenotypic profile. Blastic NK-cell lymphoma/leukemia (Figure 8.33F) is positive for CD4 and CD56 and does not coexpress CD13, CD33 and CD117 (rare cases of blastic NK-cell lymphoma/ leukemia may be positive for either CD33 or CD117). Regenerating marrow after chemotherapy (Figure 8.33G) or treatment with recombinant granulocyte growth factors, myelodysplastic syndrome (Figure 8.33H and I) and reactive erythroid hyperplasia (Figure 8.33J) due to hemolytic anemia is differentiated by the enumeration of blasts. Diffuse large B-cell lymphoma (Figure 8.33K and L), Burkitt lymphoma (Figure 8.33M), and hairy cell leukemia (Figure 8.33N) are distinguished by expression of B-cell markers and lack of both CD34 and CD117. Precursor T- and B-lymphoblastic leukemias (Figure 8.33O and P) are distinguished by cytochemical staining (lack of MPO or NSE) and immunophenotyping (see Chapter 9). Large T-cell lymphomas (Figure 8.33R and S) lack CD34, TdT, myeloid antigens and MPO. A subset of CD8+ T-cell lymphoproliferations, especially T-PLL, may be CD117+. Langerhans cell histiocytosis (Figure 8.33T) expresses S100 and CD1a.

Table 8.4 Immunophenotypic profile of acute monocytic leukemia

Marker	% positive
CD2	14
CD4	93
CD7	21
CD10	7
CD11b	75
CD11c	100
CD13	78
CD14	18
	(additional 36% shows positive expression on small subset)
CD16	4
CD23	32
CD33	100
CD34	3
CD45	100
CD56	86
CD64	89
CD117	25
HLA-DR	96

EXTRAMEDULLARY MYELOID TUMOR (EMT)

EMT (granulocytic sarcoma, myeloid sarcoma) is a tumor mass composed of immature myeloid cells (myeloblasts or monoblasts), which occurs outside the bone marrow. EMT may precede or occur concurrently with AML or a chronic myeloproliferative disorder. It involves bone, paranasal sinuses, lymph nodes and skin[721,722]. The most common type of EMT is the granulocytic sarcoma (Figure 8.34), which has a phenotype similar to AML, with or without maturation. EMT with the phenotype similar to acute monocytic leukemia may be termed 'monoblastic sarcoma' (Figure 8.35). EMT may occasionally display features of biphenotypic acute leukemia (Figure 8.36).

BIPHENOTYPIC ACUTE LEUKEMIA

Biphenotypic acute leukemia is a form of acute leukemia which has morphologic and immunophenotypic features of both myeloid and lymphoid lineages[723–727]. Table 8.5 presents the scoring system for the diagnosis of acute biphenotypic leukemia proposed by the European Group for the Immunologic Classification for Leukemia[78]. Two or more points in two categories are needed for the diagnosis of biphenotypic leukemia.

Figures 8.36 and 8.37 depict biphenotypic acute leukemia with blasts coexpressing myeloid and T-cell markers. Occasional cases are composed of two populations of blasts, each representing different lineage (Figure 8.38). This form of acute leukemia is termed 'bilineal acute leukemia'.

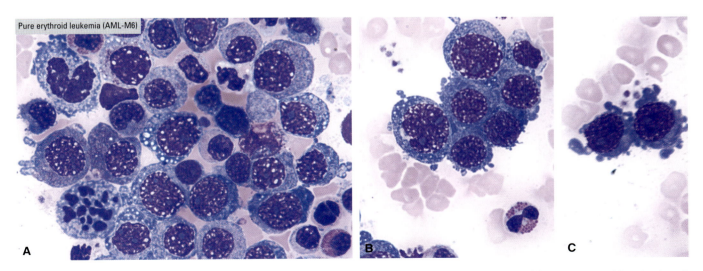

Figure 8.27 Acute erythroid leukemia (AML-M6) – cytology. (**A–C**) Numerous immature erythroid precursors with cytoplasmic vacuoles and occasionally irregular cytoplasmic borders are present

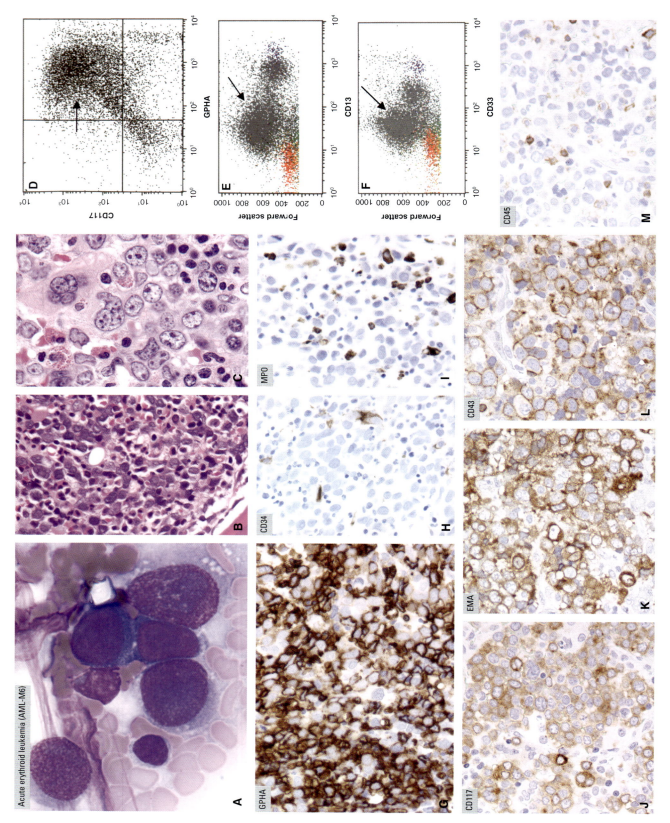

Figure 8.28   Acute erythroid leukemia (AML-M6) – immunophenotypic analysis. (**A**) Cytology shows immature erythroblasts with cytoplasmic vacuoles. (**B** and **C**) Histology shows replacement of the bone marrow by sheets of atypical erythroid precursors. Flow cytometry (**D**–**F**) shows expression of CD117 and glycophorin (**D**) and lack of CD13 and CD33 (**E** and **F**). Immunohistochemistry shows the following phenotype: GPHA⁺ (**G**), CD34⁻ (**H**), MPO⁻ (**I**), CD117⁺ (**J**), EMA⁺ (**K**), CD43⁺ (**L**) and CD45⁻ (**M**)

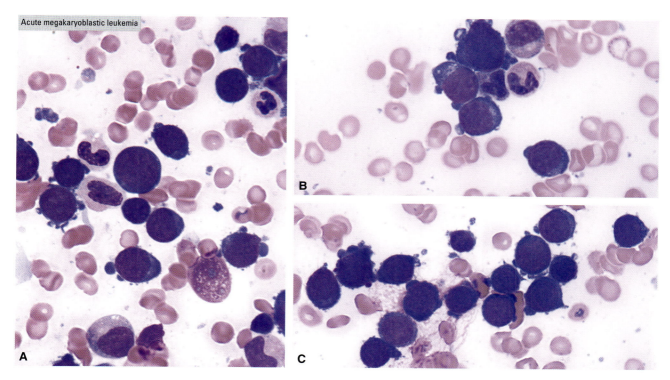

Figure 8.29 Acute megakaryoblastic leukemia (AML-M7) – cytology. (**A–C**) Aspirate smear with numerous blasts with basophilic cytoplasm, which shows distinct blebs or pseudopod formation

Table 8.5 Criteria for diagnosis of acute biphenotypic leukemia

B-lymphoid	T-lymphoid	Myeloid	Score
Cytoplasmic CD79a Cytoplasmic IgM Cytoplasmic CD22	CD3 Anti-TCR	MPO	2
CD19 CD20 CD10	CD2 CD5 CD8 CD10	CD117 CD13 CD33 CD65	1
TdT CD24	TdT CD7 CD1a	CD14 CD15 CD64	0.5

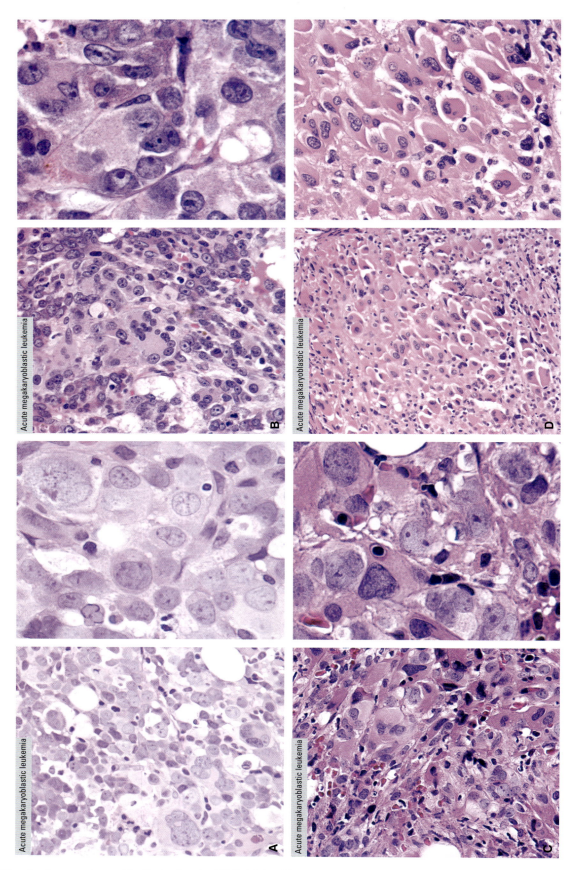

Figure 8.30   Acute megakaryoblastic leukemia (AML-M7) – histologic features of four different cases. Histologic features in acute megakaryoblastic leukemia vary from case to case. In some cases, poorly differentiated blasts predominate (**A**). In some cases, there is mixed population of highly atypical megakaryocytes, megakaryoblasts and blasts (**B** and **C**). In other cases, highly dysplastic megakaryocytes predominate (**D**)

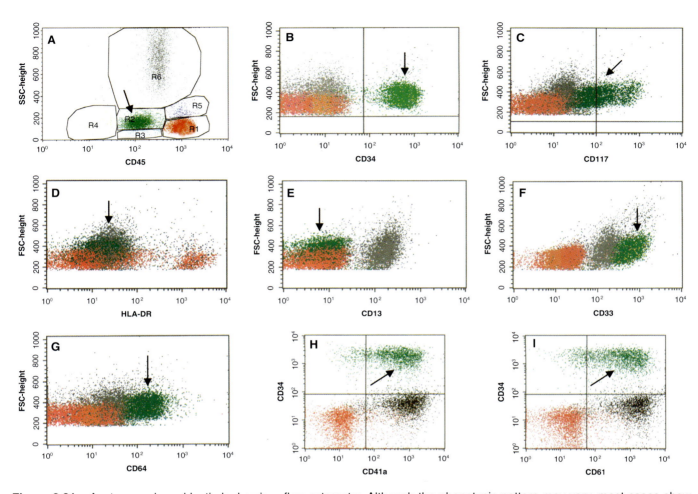

Figure 8.31   Acute megakaryoblastic leukemia – flow cytometry. Although the phenotypic pattern may vary, most cases show the following phenotype: low side scatter (**A**, arrow), CD34$^+$ (moderate expression; **B**), negative to dim expression of CD117 (**C**), negative HLA-DR (**D**), negative CD13 (**E**), bright expression of CD33 (**F**), dim expression of CD64 (**G**), and co-expression of CD41a and CD61 (**H** and **I**)

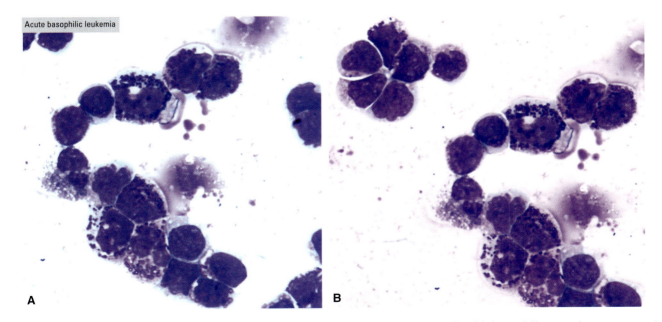

Figure 8.32   Acute basophilic leukemia – cytology. (**A** and **B**) Numerous immature cells with basophilic granules are present

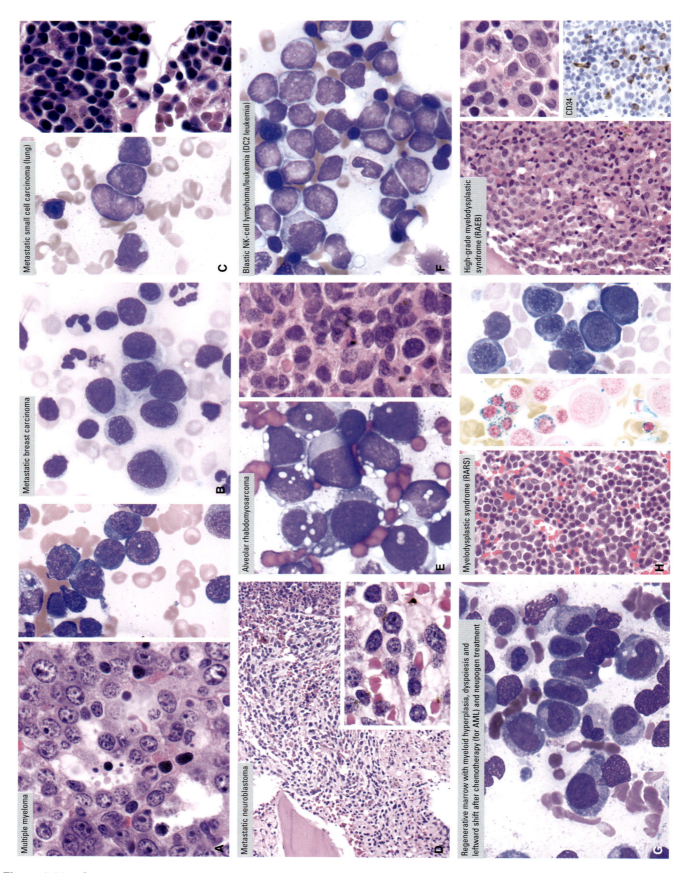

Figure 8.33   *See page 234 for legend*

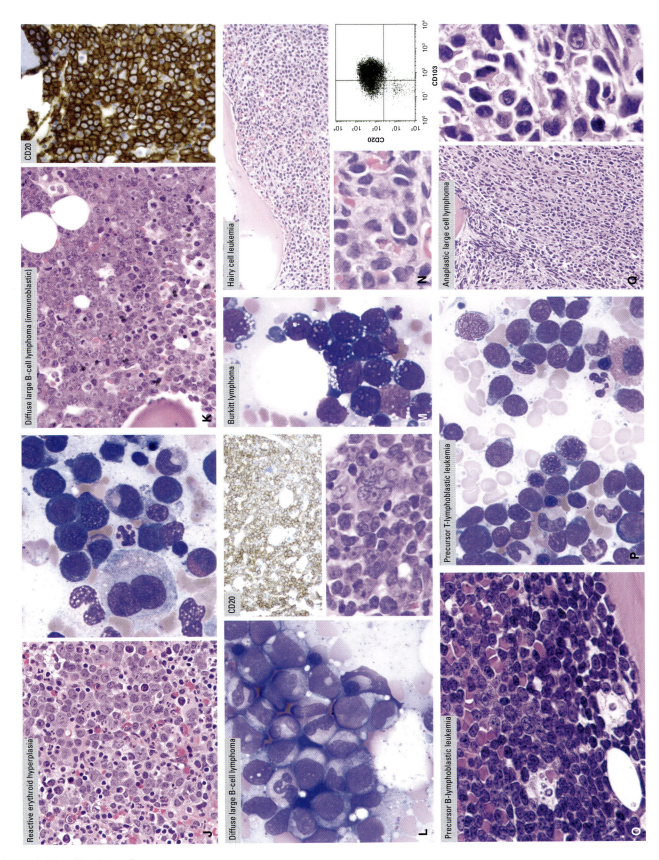

Figure 8.33   *(Continued)*

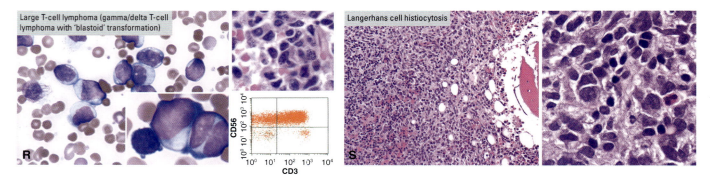

Figure 8.33   Acute myeloid leukemia – differential diagnosis (bone marrow). (**A**) Multiple myeloma. (**B**) Metastatic breast carcinoma. (**C**) Metastatic small cell carcinoma (lung primary). (**D**) Metastatic neuroblastoma. (**E**) Alveolar rhabdomyosarcoma. (**F**) Blastic NK-cell lymphoma/leukemia. (**G**) Regenerative marrow with myeloid hyperplasia, dyspoiesis and leftward shift following chemotherapy. (**H**) Myelodysplastic syndrome (refractory anemia with ringed sideroblasts). (**I**) Myelodysplastic syndrome, high grade (refractory anemia with excess blasts). (**J**) Diffuse large B-cell lymphoma. (**K**) Burkitt lymphoma. (**L**) Hairy cell leukemia. (**M**) Precursor B-lymphoblastic lymphoma/leukemia. (**N**) Precursor T-lymphoblastic lymphoma/leukemia. (**O**) Anaplastic large cell lymphoma. (**P**) Peripheral T-cell lymphoma, large cell type. (**Q**) Langerhans cell histiocytosis. (**R**) Immunoblastic lymphoma. (**S**) Reactive erythroid hyperplasia

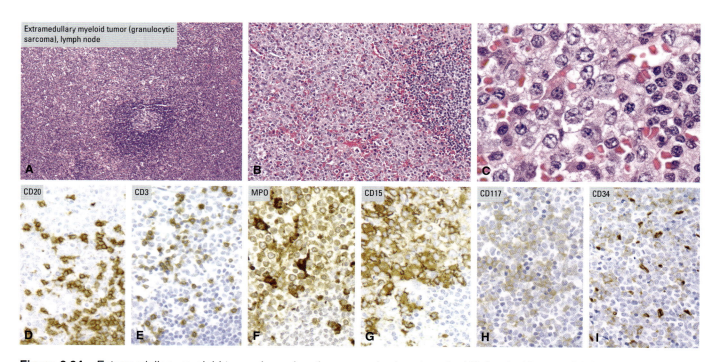

Figure 8.34   Extramedullary myeloid tumor (granulocytic sarcoma) – lymph node. (**A**) Atypical large cell infiltrate in the interfollicular area. (**B** and **C**) Higher magnification shows mononuclear cells with blastoid appearance. Neoplastic cells have the following phenotype: CD20⁻ (**D**), CD3⁻ (**E**), MPO⁺ (**F**), CD15⁺ (**G**), CD117⁺ (dim, **H**), CD34⁺ (**I**)

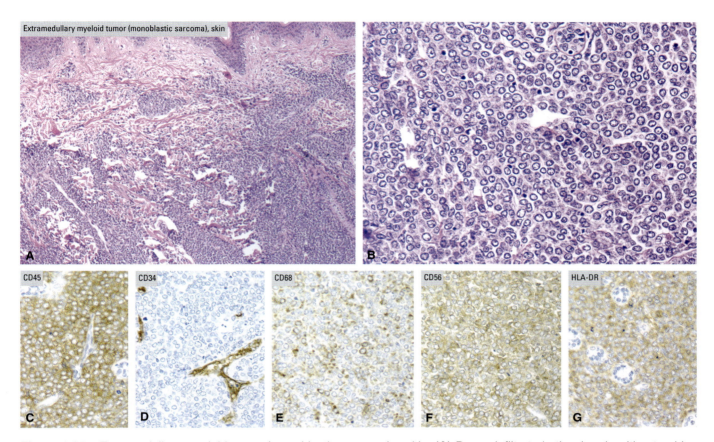

Figure 8.35   Extramedullary myeloid tumor (monoblastic sarcoma) – skin. (**A**) Dense infiltrate in the dermis without epidermotropism. (**B**) High magnification shows mononuclear cells with irregular nuclei. Tumor cells are positive for CD45 (**C**), CD68 (**E**), CD56 (**F**) and HLA-DR (**G**). CD34 is not expressed (**D**)

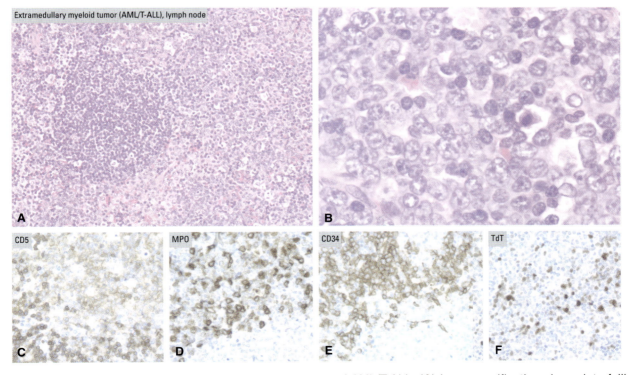

Figure 8.36   Extramedullary myeloid tumor with the phenotype of AML/T-ALL. (**A**) Low magnification shows interfollicular/paracortical infiltrate. (**B**) Large magnification shows blastic appearance of neoplastic cells. The phenotype of blasts fulfilled the criteria proposed by European Group for the Immunologic Classification of Leukemia for acute biphenotypic leukemia. Immunohistochemistry (**C–F**) shows positive expression of CD5 (**C**), MPO (**D**), CD34 (**E**) and TdT (**F**)

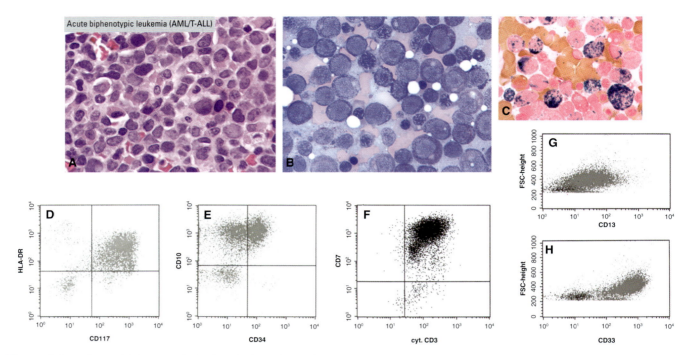

Figure 8.37   Acute biphenotypic leukemia (AML/T-ALL) – bone marrow. (**A**) Hypercellular bone marrow showing complete replacement by large blasts. (**B**) Aspirate smear showing blasts and rare erythroid precursors. (**C**) Blasts are positive for MPO. (**D–H**) Flow cytometry analysis shows the following phenotype of blasts: HLA-DR⁺ (**D**), CD117⁺ (**D**), CD34⁺ (**E**), CD10⁺ (**E**), CD7⁺ (**F**), cytoplasmic CD3⁺ (**F**), CD13⁺ (dim, **G**) and CD33⁺ (**H**)

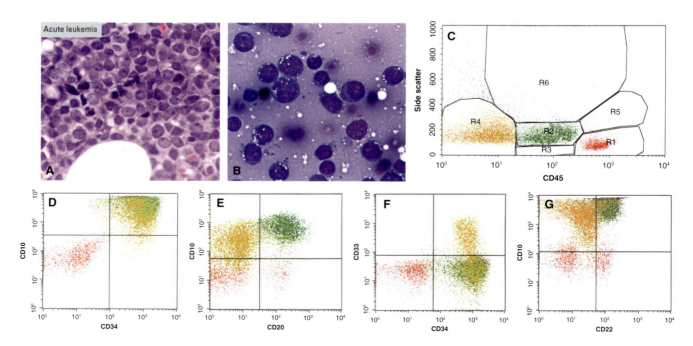

Figure 8.38   Bilineal acute leukemia (AML/B-ALL) – bone marrow. (**A**) Hypercellular bone marrow showing replacement by blasts. (**B**) Aspirate smear showing blasts with vacuolated cytoplasm. (**C–G**) Flow cytometry. Side scatter versus CD45 (**C**) shows two populations of blasts: CD45⁺ blasts (green) and CD45⁻ blasts (orange). CD45 blasts (green) have a phenotype compatible with B-ALL: CD34⁺ (**D**), bright CD10⁺ (**D**), CD20⁺ (**E**), CD33⁻ (**F**) and CD22⁺ (**G**). The other population of blasts (CD45⁻ orange) is CD34⁺ (**D**), CD33⁺ (**F**) and negative for B-cell markers (**E** and **G**). Alternatively, this leukemia can be classified as B-ALL with a distinct subset of blasts negative for CD45 and positive for CD33

CHAPTER 9

Precursor neoplasms

PRECURSOR B-LYMPHOBLASTIC LEUKEMIA/LYMPHOMA (B-ALL/LBL)

Precursor B-lymphoblastic leukemia/lymphoma (B-ALL/LBL) is a neoplasm of B-lymphoblasts. B-ALL involves bone marrow and blood, and B-LBL involves mediastinum, testes, central nervous system, skin, lymph nodes, bone, breast and soft tissue[27,327–329,696,728–734]. The chromosomal abnormalities in B-ALL include t(9;22)(q34;q11.2), t(8;14)(q24;q32), t(12;21)(p13;q22) and t(1;19)(q23;p13.3)[45,604,728,731,733,735].

Lymphoblasts are medium-sized with increased nuclear:cytoplasmic ratio and dispersed nuclear chromatin, and they may have vacuolated cytoplasm (Figure 9.1A). The bone marrow shows a diffuse and monotonous infiltrate of cells with immature vesicular chromatin, inconspicuous nucleoli and scanty cytoplasm (Figure 9.1B). Immunohistochemical staining of marrow core biopsy reveals expression of CD10, CD22, CD79a, Fli-1, Pax-5, TdT and CD45. The proliferation fraction (Ki-67 labeling) is moderate.

Flow cytometry (FC) immunophenotyping plays an important role in the diagnosis, subclassification, differential diagnosis and detection of minimal residual disease in B-ALL[14,18,29,31,32,696,728,731,733,734,736]. FC shows variable expression of CD45 (Figure 9.2). Many cases of B-ALL/LBL are CD45− or display dim expression of CD45. Most cases are positive for CD19 and cCD79a, CD10, HLA-DR and TdT (Figure 9.3). Characteristically, the expression of CD10 is bright (Figure 9.3A). A subset of cases is positive for CD20, CD22, CD34 and cIgM. Table 9.2 summarizes the B-ALL/LBL phenotype. Occasional cases have CD13 expression, which is often associated with Philadelphia chromosome[733].

Table 9.1 Classification of precursor neoplasms

Precursor B-cell neoplasms
Precursor B-lymphoblastic leukemia/lymphoma (B-ALL/LBL)
Precursor T-neoplasms
Precursor T-lymphoblastic leukemia/lymphoma (T-ALL/LBL)
Blastic NK-cell leukemia/lymphoma (DC2 acute leukemia)

Involvement of the lymph nodes by B-LBL is either diffuse or paracortical with preservation of germinal centers (Figure 9.4).

The differential diagnosis of B-ALL/LBL (Figure 9.5) includes malignant lymphomas, acute myeloid leukemia, precursor T-lymphoblastic lymphoma/leukemia, hematogones and metastatic small, blue-cell tumors[232,260,286,304,605,737]. B-cell lymphomas, including the leukemic phase of follicular lymphoma (Figure 9.5A), diffuse large B-cell lymphoma (Figure 9.5B), Burkitt lymphoma (Figure 9.5C) and immunoblastic lymphoma (Figure 9.5D), are differentiated from B-ALL/LBL by expression of surface light-chain immunoglobulins and lack of blastic markers (TdT and CD34). Blastic mantle cell leukemia is positive for B-cell markers and CD5. Plasma cell myeloma (Figure 9.5E) lacks TdT and CD34 expression and is positive for CD138. Pax-5 is negative in the majority of cases. Precursor T-lymphoblastic leukemia/lymphoma (Figure 9.5F) is positive for pan-T antigens (most often CD7) and lacks B-cell antigens. Acute myeloid leukemia (M0 and M1) is differentiated by expression of CD117 and lack of B-cell antigens (a subset of B-ALL/LBL will express CD13 or CD33, and a minute subset of AML may express CD19). Acute erythroid leukemia (Figure 9.5H) is strongly positive for glycophorin A and hemoglobin A. Prolymphocytic leukemias (both of

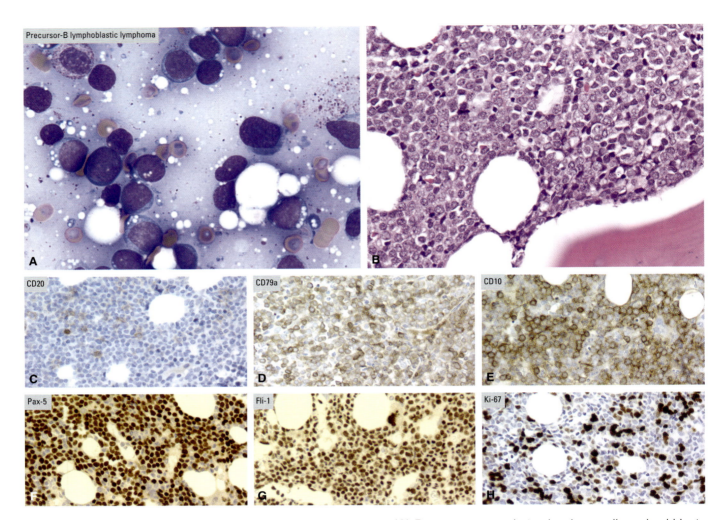

Figure 9.1 Precursor B-lymphoblastic leukemia – bone marrow. (**A**) Bone marrow aspirate showing medium-sized blasts with vacuolated cytoplasm. (**B**) Bone marrow core biopsy shows complete replacement of marrow by lymphoblasts. (**C–G**) Immunohistochemistry. Blasts are negative for CD20 (**C**), and positive for CD79a (**D**), CD10 (**E**), Pax-5 (**F**), Fli-1 (**G**) and focally Ki-67 (**H**)

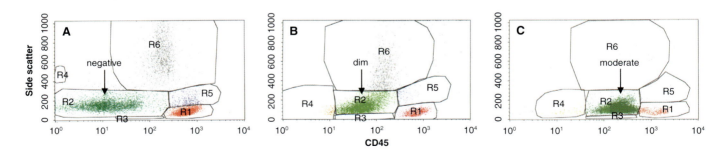

Figure 9.2 Precursor B-lymphoblastic lymphoma/leukemia – CD45 expression by flow cytometry. (**A**) Blasts (arrow) negative for CD45. (**B**) Dim expression of CD45. (**C**) Moderate expression of CD45. Lymphoblasts show low side scatter properties (**A–C**)

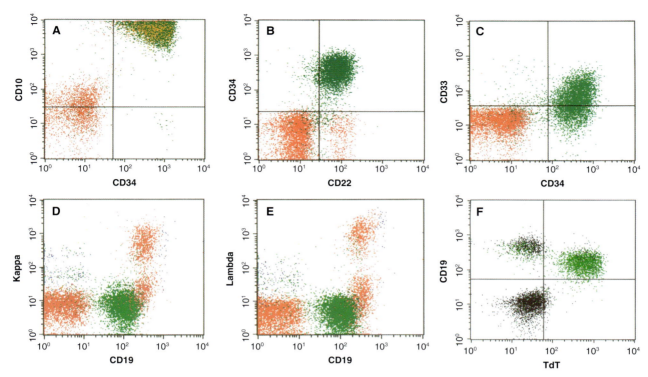

Figure 9.3 Precursor B-lymphoblastic lymphoma/leukemia – flow cytometry. B-lymphoblasts show bright expression of CD10 (**A**), positive expression of CD34 (**A** and **B**), CD22 (**B**), CD33 (**C**), CD19 (**D** and **E**) and TdT (**F**). Surface immunoglobulins are negative (**D** and **E**)

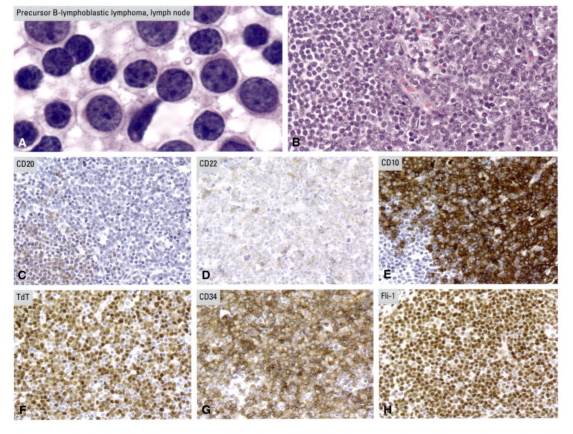

Figure 9.4 Precursor B-lymphoblastic lymphoma – lymph node. (**A**) Touch smear shows blasts with round regular nuclei and few inconspicuous nucleoli. (**B**) Histologic section of the lymph node shows sheets of lymphoblasts. Residual small lymphocytes are also noted (left side). (**C–H**) Immunohistochemistry. Blasts are negative for CD20 (**C**) and are positive for CD22 (**D**), CD10 (**E**), TdT (**F**), CD34 (**G**) and Fli-1 (**H**). Residual small lymphocytes are positive for CD20 (**C**) and negative for CD10 (**E**)

Table 9.2   Immunophenotypic profile of precursor B-lymphoblastic leukemia/lymphoma

Age	3–92 years old (average 51.4)
Female to male ratio	1.3:1
CD10+	89%
CD13+	7%
CD19+	100%
CD20+	25%
CD22+	68%
CD33+	35%
CD34+	64%
CD45+ (moderate)	46%
CD45+ (dim)	36%
CD45-	18%
CD56+	7%
CD117+	0
Cytoplasmic IgM+	21%
HLA-DR+	96%
TdT+	93%

Table 9.3   Immunophenotypic profile of precursor T-lymphoblastic leukemia/lymphoma

Age	6–78 years old (average 34.7)
Female to male ratio	0.2:1
CD2+	65% (including 6% dim expression)
CD3+	41% (including 18% dim expression)
CD5+	87% (including 30% dim expression)
CD7+	98% (including 4% dim expression)
CD1a+	30%
CD4+	11%
CD8+	9%
Dual CD4/CD8+	39%
Dual CD4/CD8-	41%
CD10+	24%
CD11b+	4%
CD11c+	0
CD13+	17%
CD33+	22%
CD34+	37%
CD45+ (moderate to bright)	69%
CD45+ (dim)	31%
CD56+	24%
CD117+	11%
HLA-DR+	9%
TCRαβ+	31%
TCRγδ+	17%
TCR-	52%
TdT+	87%

B- and T-cell origin) are distinguished by lack of TdT, CD10, and CD34 expression (Figure 9.5I and J). Metastatic tumors (Figure 9.5K and L) are distinguished by immunohistochemical analysis.

Hematogones (Figure 9.6) show very low side scatter by flow cytometry and variable (smeared) expression of CD20 and CD34. A subset of hematogones with dim CD45 is usually CD34+, and a subset of hematogones with moderate CD45 is CD34- (Figure 9.6A and B).

PRECURSOR T-LYMPHOBLASTIC LYMPHOMA/LEUKEMIA (T-ALL/LBL)

Precursor T-lymphoblastic leukemia/lymphoma (T-ALL/LBL) is a neoplasm of T-lymphoblasts. T-ALL involves bone marrow and blood, and T-LBL involves the mediastinum and, less commonly, lymph nodes, skin, gonads and central nervous system. Mediastinal involvement and adenopathy are more common in younger patients than in patients older than 60 years[78,330].

Morphologically, T-lymphoblasts are similar to B-lymphoblasts. They are medium-sized with scanty, often eccentric cytoplasm, which occasionally creates a 'hand-mirror' appearance (Figure 9.7). Chromatin is finely granular and evenly dispersed. Nucleoli are present but are inconspicuous. T-ALL/LBL, regardless of the site of involvement, shows replacement by normal elements by a diffuse monotonous infiltrate of medium-sized cells, often with a 'starry-sky' pattern (Figures 9.8 and 9.9).

T-lymphoblasts are positive for TdT, CD1a, pan-T antigens and CD45. CD45 expression is dim to moderate, which differs from bright expression of mature T-cells

(Figure 9.10). Almost all cases of T-ALL/LBL display aberrant expression of pan-T markers (loss or diminished expression; Figure 9.10). Among pan-T antigens, CD7 is most often expressed, and surface CD3 is least often positive. Most of the cases are dual CD4/CD8 negative or dual CD4/CD8 positive. Rare cases are either CD4+ or CD8+. T-ALL/LBL most often lacks TCR expression (Figure 9.10), about one-third of cases are TCRαβ+, and only rare cases are TCRγδ+ (Figure 9.11). A subset of T-ALL/LBL is positive for CD10, CD56 and pan-myeloid antigens (Figure 9.12). Table 9.3 presents a summary of the phenotypic features of T-ALL/LBL.

The differential diagnosis of T-ALL/LBL is similar to B-ALL (see above).

Thymocytes versus precursor T-lymphoblastic lymphoma

Dual positive expression of CD4/CD8 is rarely observed in peripheral (mature/post-thymic) T-cell lymphoproliferative disorders; therefore, when present, it suggests an immature T-cell population (precursor T-lymphoblastic lymphoma/leukemia shows coexpression of CD4 and CD8 in ~40% of cases). Thymocytes from either hyperplastic thymus or thymoma (Figures 9.13 and 9.14) are

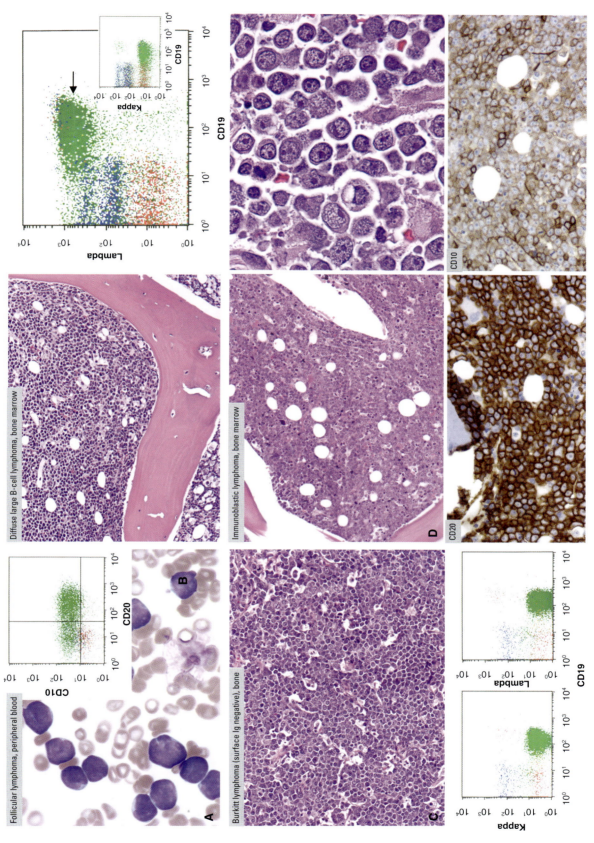

Figure 9.5 Precursor B-lymphoblastic lymphoma leukemia – differential diagnosis. (**A**) Follicular lymphoma (leukemic phase in the peripheral blood). (**B**) Diffuse large B-cell lymphoma involving the bone marrow. (**C**) Burkitt lymphoma. (**D**) Immunoblastic lymphoma. (**E**) Multiple myeloma. (**F**) T-lymphoblastic lymphoma/leukemia. (**G**) Acute myeloid leukemia. (**H**) Acute erythroid leukemia. (**I**) B-cell prolymphocytic leukemia. (**J**) T-cell prolymphocytic leukemia. (**K**) Metastatic small cell carcinoma. (**L**) Metastatic neuroblastoma

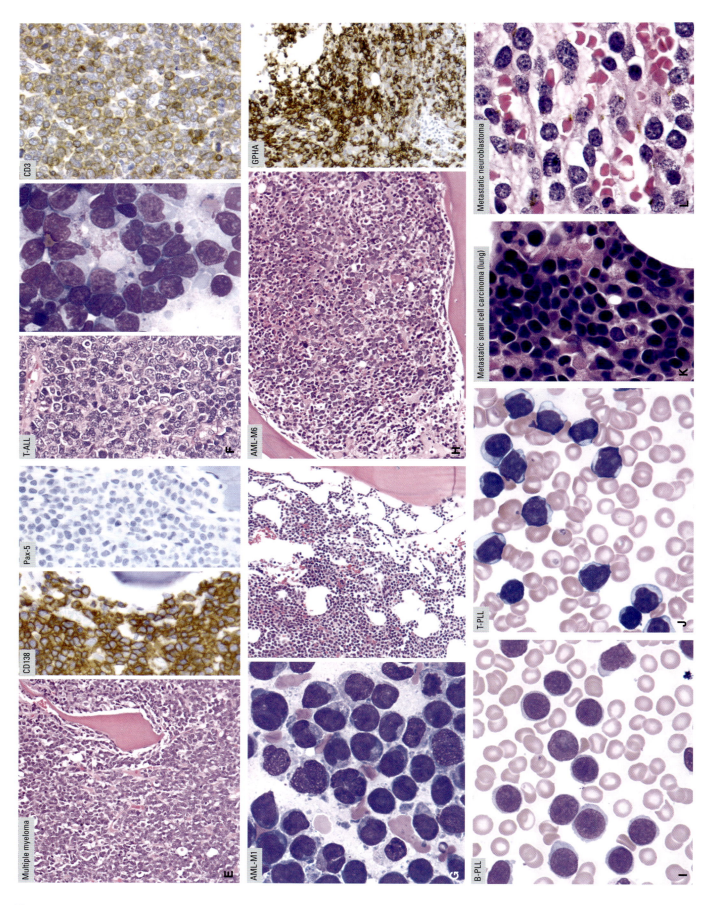

Figure 9.5 *(Continued)*

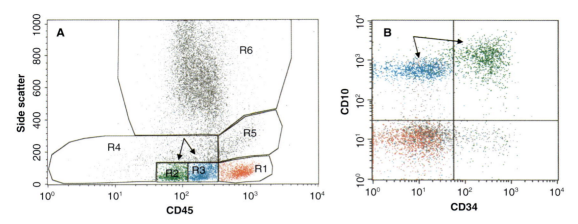

Figure 9.6   Hematogones. Flow cytometry shows two populations of B-cells with low side scatter (**A**, arrow). More mature cells with moderate CD45 expression (**A**, blue) are negative for CD34 (**B**). Less mature cells with dim CD45 expression (**A**, green) are coexpressing CD10 and CD34 (**B**)

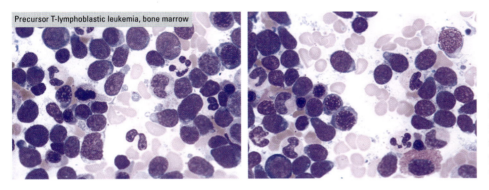

Figure 9.7   Precursor T-lymphoblastic lymphoma/leukemia – cytology. Bone marrow aspirate with numerous blasts with delicate chromatin, round eccentric nuclei with nucleoli and occasional 'hand-mirror' appearance

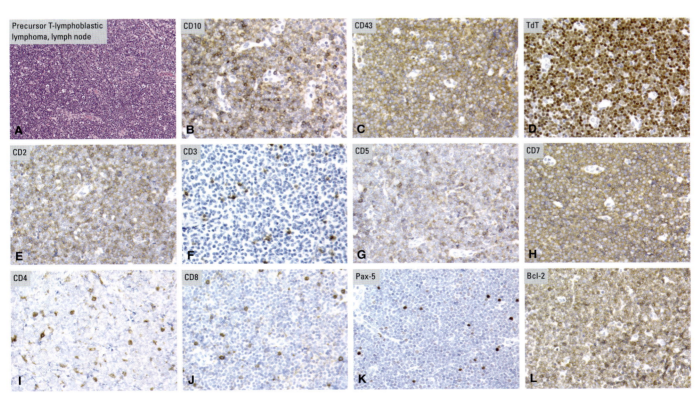

Figure 9.8   Precursor T-lymphoblastic lymphoma – immunohistochemistry (lymph node). (**A**) Histologic section shows monotonous lymphoid infiltrate with blastic appearance. (**B–L**) Immunohistochemistry. T-lymphoblasts are positive for CD10 (**B**), CD43 (**C**), TdT (**D**), CD2 (**E**), CD5 (**G**), CD7 (**H**) and bcl-2 (**L**). There is no immunoreactivity with CD3 (**F**), CD4 (**I**), CD8 (**J**) and Pax-5 (**K**)

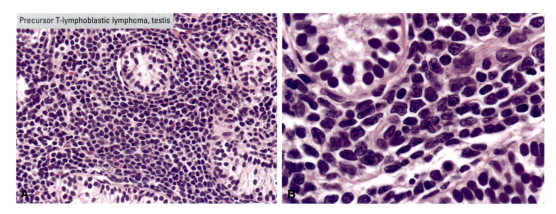

Figure 9.9 Precursor T-lymphoblastic lymphoma – testis. Dense infiltrate of the testicular parenchyma by lymphoblasts

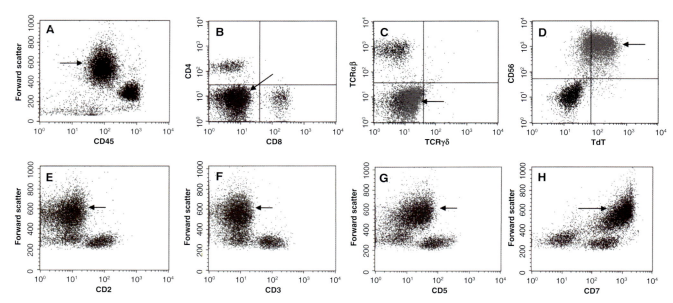

Figure 9.10 Precursor T-lymphoblastic lymphoma – flow cytometry (lymph node). Blasts show increased forward scatter (**A**, arrow), dual negative expression of CD4/CD8 (**B**), lack of TCR (**C**), and positive expression of TdT (**D**) and CD56 (**D**). Among pan-T antigens, three antigens are missing (**E–G**), and only CD7 is positive (**H**)

always CD4/CD8 positive; therefore, the diagnosis of mediastinal T-ALL/LBL cannot be based on the presence of CD4/CD8 coexpression. Regardless of whether from thymoma or benign thymic hyperplasia, benign immature T-cells (thymocytes) display characteristic variable expression of surface CD3 antigen (Figures 9.13D and 9.14A)[21]. The majority of cells (small T-cells) show positive but variable (smeared-like) CD3 expression, whereas larger T-cells are CD3 negative. This smeared pattern is never observed in surface CD3+ T-ALL/LBL. Small more mature T-cells from thymoma/ thymic hyperplasia are CD10−, and larger immature T-cells (surface CD3−) show positive expression of CD10 (Figure 9.14A and B).

BLASTIC NK-CELL LYMPHOMA (DC2 ACUTE LEUKEMIA)

Blastic NK-cell lymphoma, also known as DC2 acute leukemia or CD4+/CD56+ hematodermic neoplasm[447,497,738–744], is a distinct clinicopathologic entity characterized by skin tropism, bone marrow involvement (with or without a leukemic phase), poor prognosis and coexpression of CD4, CD56, CD43 and HLA-DR. It is

Table 9.4 Summary of the phenotypic characteristics of blastic NK-cell lymphoma / leukemia

Age (years)	68	88	81	80	85	78	79	67	79	85	88	76	83
Sex	M	M	M	F	F	M	M	F	M	F	M	M	M
Site	BM	skin	PB	LN	skin	BM	PB	BM	BM	BM	PB	BM + skin	LN
% cells	60	60	64	90	72	46	44	90	70	85	40	40	80
CD2	–	++	++	–	–	+	–	++	–	++	–	+	–
CD3	–	–	–	–	–	–	–	–	–	–	–	–	–
CD4	+/++	+	++	+/++	+	+++	+	++	++	++	+	+++	++
CD5	–	–	–	–	–	–	–	–	–	–	–	–	–
CD7	+	+	+	++	++	++	+/++	–	++	++	+	+	+
CD8	–	–	–	–	–	–	–	–	–	–	–	–	–
CD10	–	–	–	–	–	–	–	+	–	–	+	–	–
CD13	–	–	–	–	–	–	–	–	–	–	–	–	–
CD16	–	–	–	–	–	–	–	–	–	–	–	–	–
CD19/CD20	–	–	–	–	–	–	–	–	–	–	–	–	–
CD23	–	–	–	–	–	–	–	–	–	–	–	–	–
CD33	–	–	+	+	–	+	–	–	–	–	+	+	–
CD34	–	–	–	–	–	–	–	–	–	–	–	–	–
CD45	+	++	++	++	++	++	+	++	+	+/++	++	++	++
CD56	+++	+++	+++	++	+++	+++	++	+/+++	++	++	+++	++	+++
CD57	–	–	–	–	–	–	–	–	–	–	–	–	–
HLA-DR	++	+	+	+	+	+	+	+	+	+	+	+++	+
TdT	–	++	–	–	–	–	+	–	–	–	–	–	–
CD117	–	–	–	–	+	–	+	+	+	–	–	–	–
CD25	–	–	–	–	–	–	–	–	–	–	–	–	–
TCR	–	–	–	–	–	–	–	–	–	–	–	–	–
CD38	–	–	+++	–	+	s+	+	–	–	–	–	++	–
CD64	–	–	–	–	–	–	–	–	–	–	–	–	–
CD43	–	–	+	–	+	–	–	–	–	–	–	–	+
CD103	–	–	–	–	–	–	–	–	+	–	–	–	–
CD11b	–	–	–	–	–	–	–	–	–	–	–	–	–
CD11c	–	–	s+	–	–	s+	–	–	–	–	–	–	–

M, male; F, female; BM, bone marrow; PB, peripheral blood; LN, lymph node +, positive (+, dim; ++, moderate; +++, bright); –, negative; s, subset.

always positive   often positive   may be positive (**no** dual CD33/CD117 positive expression).

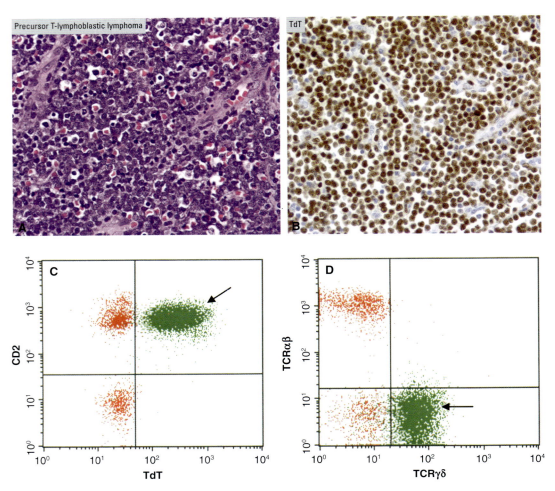

Figure 9.11   Precursor T-lymphoblastic lymphoma with TCRγδ phenotype. (**A**) Complete replacement of the lymph node by lymphoblasts. (**B**) Positive expression of TdT. (**C** and **D**) Flow cytometry. Lymphoblasts are positive for CD2 (**C**), TdT (**C**) and TCRγδ (**D**)

suggested that they arise due to oncogenic transformation of CD56[+] 'plasmacytoid' monocyte-like dendritic cells (DC-2)[740,742–744].

Blastic NK-cell lymphoma is composed of medium-sized cells resembling lymphoblasts (Figure 9.15). The clinical presentation is typically that of cutaneous nodule(s) associated with adenopathy and/or splenomegaly and cytopenia. Massive bone marrow involvement is seen in a majority of cases[740]. Blastic NK-cell lymphoma is defined by coexpression of CD4 and CD56, and lack of coexpression of pan-myeloid antigens and CD117, negative surface and cytoplasmic CD3, B-cell markers, plasma cell markers

and TCR (Figure 9.16). Figures 9.17 and 9.18 depict blastic NK-cell lymphoma involving skin and lymph node, respectively. Most cases have clonal and complex chromosomal aberrations[742]. Table 9.4 depicts detailed flow cytometric findings in blastic NK-cell lymphoma/leukemia.

The differential diagnosis includes acute monocytic leukemia, acute myeloid leukemia with NK-cell differentiation/CD56 expression, large B- and T-cell lymphoma, precursor T-lymphoblastic leukemia/lymphoma, histiocytic sarcoma, NK-cell lymphoma/leukemia and other small, 'blue-cell' tumors.

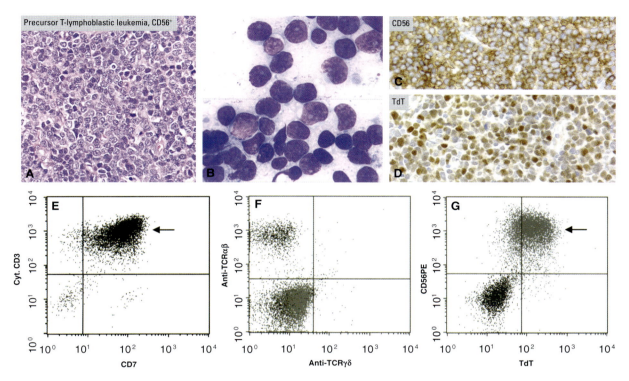

Figure 9.12 Precursor T-lymphoblastic leukemia with CD56 expression. (**A**) Histologic section shows diffuse infiltrate of the bone marrow by lymphoblasts. (**B**) Bone marrow aspirate shows blasts with high nuclear-cytoplasmic ratio and prominent nucleoli. (**C** and **D**) Immunohistochemical staining shows expression of CD56 (**C**) and TdT (**D**). (**E** and **G**) Flow cytometry: blasts are positive for cytoplasmic CD3 (**E**) and CD7 (**E**), negative for TCRαβ/TCRαγ (**F**) and positive for CD56 (**G**)

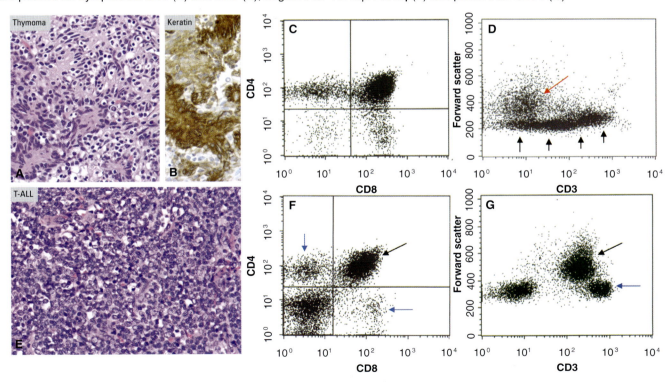

Figure 9.13 Flow cytometric comparison between thymocytes (**A–D**) and T-lymphoblasts (**E–G**). (**A** and **B**) Histologic section of thymoma. Tumor cells are positive for cytokeratin (AE1/AE3). Flow cytometric analysis reveals immature T-cells with dual expression of CD4/CD8 (**C**) and variable (smeared) expression of surface CD3 (**D**; black arrows). There is additional population of larger T-cells with negative expression of CD3 (red arrow). (**E**) T-lymphoblastic lymphoma (mediastinum). Lymphoblasts are dual positive for CD4/CD8 (**F**). There are distinct populations of benign T-cells expressing CD4 or CD8 (blue arrows). In contrast, thymocytes (**C**) show gradual transition from CD4+/CD8− cells to CD4−/CD8+ cells with a majority of cells positive for both antigens. T-lymphoblasts (black arrow) show moderate expression of surface CD3 (**G**) without variability, as seen in thymocytes (compare with **D**). Normal (benign) T-cells (blue arrow, **G**) show brighter CD3 expression and lower forward scatter than lymphoblasts

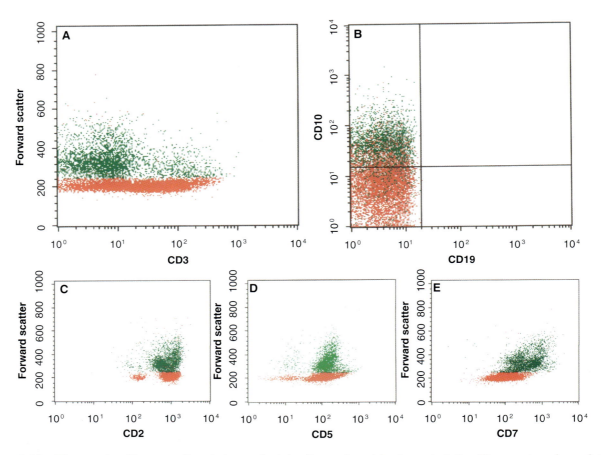

Figure 9.14 Thymocytes (thymoma/thymic hyperplasia) – flow cytometric characteristics. Thymocytes show characteristic smeared (variable) expression of surface CD3 on flow cytometric analysis (**A**). Small cells (red) have variable expression of CD3, whereas larger cells (green) with increased forward scatter are CD3 negative (**A**). Those larger cells coexpress CD10 (**B**). Both T-cell populations are positive for CD2 (**C**), CD5 (**D**) and CD7 (**E**)

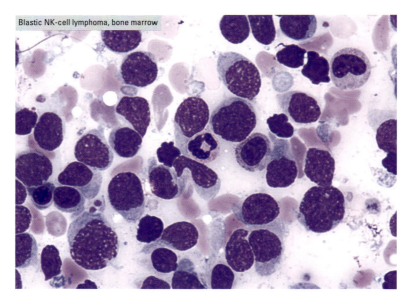

Figure 9.15 Blastic NK-cell lymphoma – cytology. Bone marrow aspirate with predominance of blasts. Tumor cells have irregular nuclei, inconspicuous nucleoli and pale basophilic cytoplasm

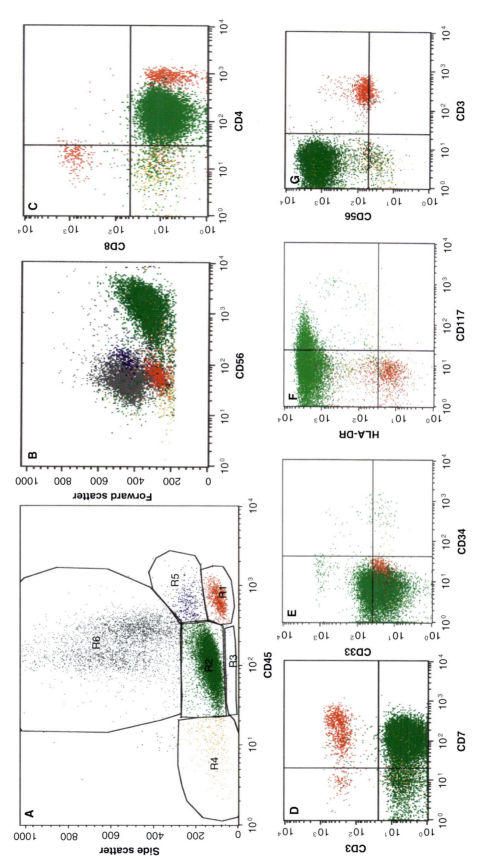

Figure 9.16   Blastic NK-cell lymphoma – flow cytometry. Blasts have low orthogonal side scatter (**A**, green) and are positive for CD45 (**A**), CD56 (**B**), CD4 (**C**), CD7 (**D**) and HLA-DR (**F**). CD34 (**E**) and CD3 (**G**) are negative

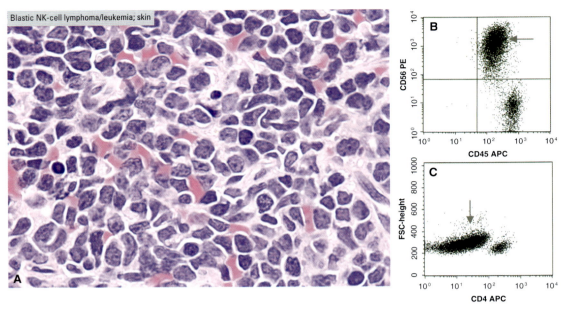

Figure 9.17   Blastic NK-cell lymphoma – skin. (**A**) Histologic section shows blasts with high nuclear/cytoplasmic ratio and irregular nuclei. Flow cytometry revealed expression of CD56 (**B**) and dim expression of CD4 (**C**)

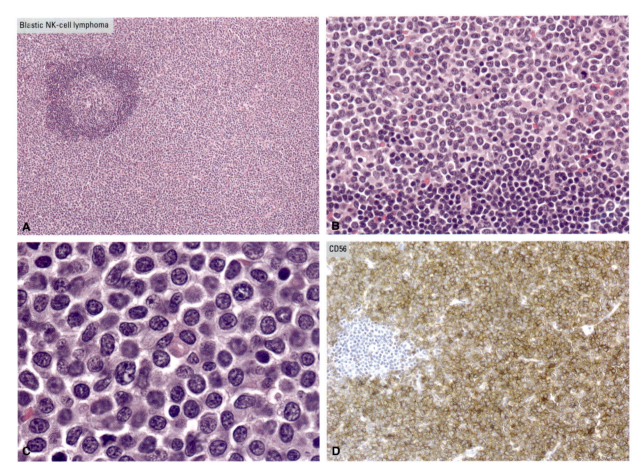

Figure 9.18   Blastic NK-cell lymphoma – lymph node. (**A**) Low magnification shows a dense interfollicular infiltrate. (**B** and **C**) Higher magnification shows predominance of blasts with round nuclei, prominent nucleoli and scanty to moderate cytoplasm. (**D**) Blasts are strongly positive for CD56

CHAPTER 10

Histiocytic and dendritic cell tumors

Table 10.1 depicts the WHO classification of histiocytic and dendritic cell neoplasms. Table 10.2 depicts the immunophenotypic profile of Langerhans cells, histiocytes/monocytes (macrophage cells), interdigitating dendritic cells and follicular dendritic cells.

HISTIOCYTIC SARCOMA

Histiocytic sarcoma is a malignant tumor of the macrophage lineage[745–753]. It occurs in lymph nodes and extranodal locations including skin, abdominal organs (intestinal tract), soft tissue and spleen. The cytomorphologic features are highly variable (compare Figures 10.1 and 10.2). The neoplastic cells are large and pleomorphic with abundant eosinophilic cytoplasm or foamy cytoplasm and bizarre nuclei. Nucleoli are prominent. Many cells are multinucleated. The overall morphologic features resemble anaplastic large cell lymphoma or malignant melanoma. Neoplastic cells lack immunoreactivity with B- and T-cell markers, epithelial markers (EMA, cytokeratin), blastic markers (CD34, TdT, CD117), HMB-45, CD21, CD30, ALK-1 and myeloperoxidase. Histiocytic sarcomas are positive for CD4, CD11c, CD14, CD43, CD45, CD68, HAM56 and HLA-DR. Staining with S100 may be positive but is usually focal and weak[745,749]. The diagnosis of histiocytic sarcoma is largely based on marked cytologic atypia, exclusion of diffuse large B-cell lymphoma, anaplastic large cell lymphoma, melanoma and carcinoma, and expression of CD45 and histiocytic markers.

Table 10.1 Classification of histiocytic and dendritic cell neoplasms

Histiocytic sarcoma
Langerhans cell histiocytosis/Langerhans cell sarcoma
Interdigiting dendritic cell sarcoma
Follicular dendritic cell sarcoma
Dendritic cell sarcoma, NOS

Table 10.2 Phenotypic features of histiocytic and dendritic cells/tumors

Marker	Langerhans cells	Interdigitating dendritic cells	Follicular dendritic sarcoma	Macrophages	Histiocytic sarcoma	Langerhans cell histiocytosis	Rosai–Dorfman disease
CD1a	+	−	−	−	−	+	+
CD2	−	−	−	−	−	−	−
CD4	+	−	−	+	+	+	−
CD20	−	−	−	−	−	−	−
CD21	−	−	++	+/−	−	−	−
CD23	−	−	+	−	−	−	−
CD30	−	−	−	−	−	−	−
CD45	+	−	−	+	+	+/−	+
CD68	−	−	−/+	+	+	+/−	−/+
S100	+	+	−/+	−/+	−	+	+
Lysozyme	−	−	−	+	+	+/−	−
Non-specific esterase	−	−	−	+	+	−	−
HMB-45	−	−	−	−	−	−	−
HLA-DR	+	−	+	+	+	+	+

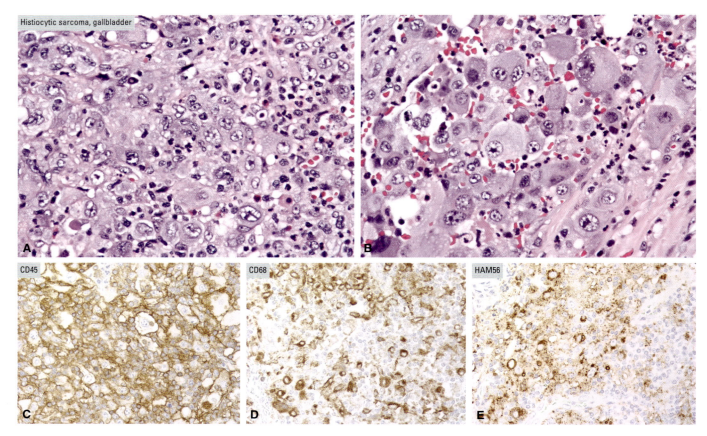

Figure 10.1   Histiocytic sarcoma – gallbladder. (**A** and **B**) Histologic sections show diffuse infiltrate of large pleomorphic cells with abundant cytoplasm and highly atypical nuclei. (**C–E**) Immunohistochemistry: tumor cells are positive for CD45 (**C**) and histiocytic/macrophage markers (CD68 and HAM56; **D** and **E**)

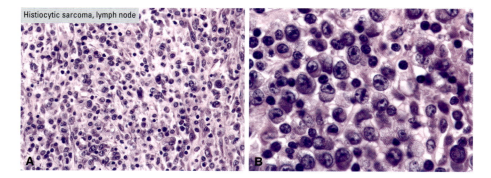

Figure 10.2   Histiocytic sarcoma – lymph node. (**A**) Diffuse infiltrate of the lymph node by atypical large cells. (**B**) High magnification shows large mononuclear cells. The distinction from large cell hematopoietic tumors, including large cell lymphomas, should be based on a broad panel of immunophenotypic markers

LANGERHANS CELL HISTIOCYTOSIS

Langerhans cell histiocytosis is a neoplastic proliferation of Langerhans cells, which invariably express CD1a and S100[754–758]. Unifocal tumors, termed 'eosinophilic granulomas', usually involve bone, skin, lymph nodes and lung.

Multifocal Langerhans cell histiocytosis of bone is also known as Hand–Schuller–Christian disease and frequently involves the skull. Disseminated disease, termed Letterer–Siwe disease, occurs predominantly in children and involves the bone, liver, spleen, skin and lymph nodes (Figure 10.3). Patients with isolated bone

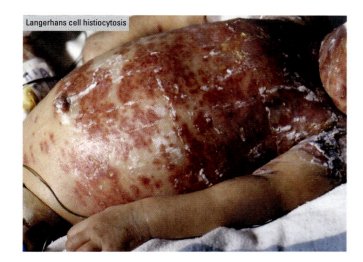

Langerhans cell histiocytosis

Figure 10.3   Langerhans cell histiocytosis – infant with skin involvement by multifocal, multisystem disease (Letterer–Siwe disease)

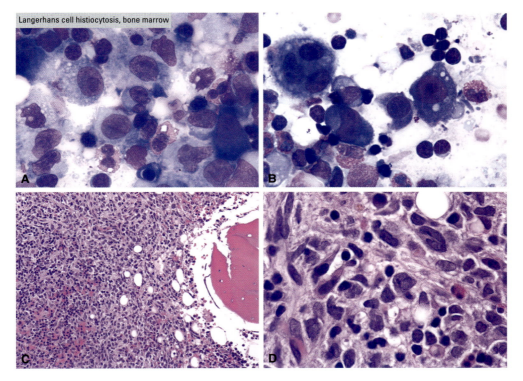

Langerhans cell histiocytosis, bone marrow

Figure 10.4   Langerhans cell histiocytosis – bone marrow. (**A** and **B**) Bone marrow aspirate with large cells with abundant cytoplasm, prominent nucleoli and occasional nuclear irregularities. (**C** and **D**) Bone marrow core biopsy. Diffuse large cell infiltrate replacing normal bone marrow elements (**C**). High magnification shows characteristic nuclear irregularities (**D**). Scattered eosinophils are present

Langerhans cell histiocytosis have a better prognosis than patients with multisystem involvement[756].

Morphologically, Langerhans cell histiocytosis is recognized by the presence of Langerhans cells (Figure 10.4), which are polygonal or elongated, bean-shaped cells with characteristic nuclear grooves (linear nuclear clefts and indentations), seen in an inflammatory background of eosinophils, histiocytes, neutrophils and small lymphocytes. Lymph nodes show either an intrasinusoidal distribution or prominent paracortical involvement (Figure 10.5). Langerhans cells express CD1a, S100, vimentin, HLA-DR and CD45. The expression of CD68 is weak and focal.

The differential diagnosis of Langerhans cell histiocytosis involving lymph nodes includes benign histiocytic lesions, such as Rosai–Dorfman disease[759] (Figure 10.6),

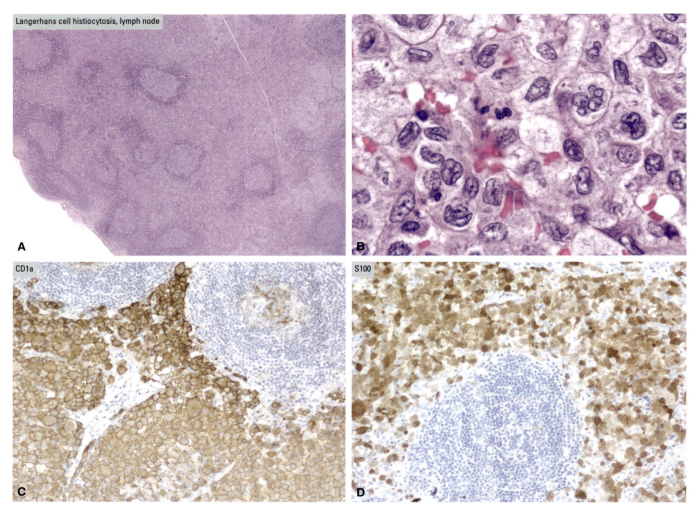

Figure 10.5   Langerhans cell histiocytosis – lymph node. (**A**) Low magnification shows prominent interfollicular/paracortical infiltrate. (**B**) High magnification displays typical nuclear grooves (folding). (**C** and **D**) Immunohistochemistry: tumor cells are positive for CD1a (**C**) and S100 (**D**)

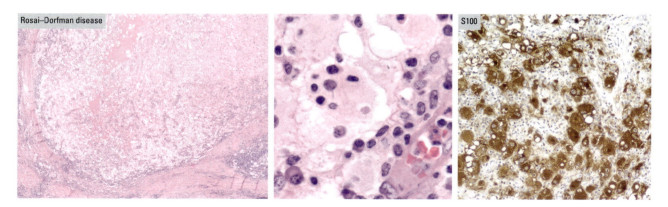

Figure 10.6   Rosai–Dorfman disease. Numerous histiocytes with abundant foamy cytoplasm demonstrating emperipolesis (center). S100 staining is strongly positive

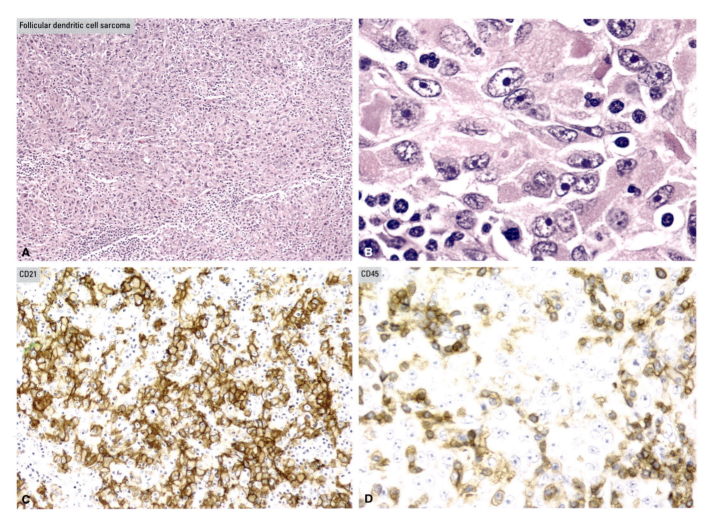

Follicular dendritic cell sarcoma

CD21

CD45

Figure 10.7 Follicular dendritic cell sarcoma. (**A**) Low magnification shows nests of atypical plump cells with abundant eosinophilic cytoplasm. (**B**) High magnification shows pleomorphic cells with abundant eosinophilic and somewhat granular cytoplasm. Nuclei have prominent nucleoli. (**C** and **D**) Immunohistochemistry: tumor cells are positive for CD21 (**C**) and negative for CD45 (**D**)

Erdheim–Chester disease, dermatopathic lymphadenopathy, metastatic tumors and malignant lymphoma, especially those with a sinusoidal distribution, such as ALCL or malignant lymphoma with erythrophagocytosis[760].

FOLLICULAR DENDRITIC CELL SARCOMA

Follicular dendritic cell sarcoma is a spindle-cell neoplasm with positive immunoreactivity for CD21 and CD23, which usually lacks CD45. It occurs primarily in lymph nodes, but extranodal sites have been reported[463,537,761–765]. Lymph nodes (Figures 10.7 and Figure 10.8) contain clusters or sheets of spindle cells with elongated nuclei,

eosinophilic cytoplasm and mild to moderate pleomorphism. Nucleoli are present and may be conspicuous. The tumor cells are mixed with small lymphocytes, with a prominent perivascular cuffing[463,765]. The uninvolved lymphoid tissue contains small lymphocytes with occasional germinal centers. Follicular dendritic cell sarcomas are positive for CD21, CD23, vimentin and occasionally S100 and CD68. They lack CD45, B- and T-cell markers, cytokeratin and CD30 expression. The behavior of follicular dendritic cell sarcoma is more reminiscent of a low-grade soft tissue sarcoma than a malignant lymphoma and is characterized by local recurrence and occasional metastases[463,763,765].

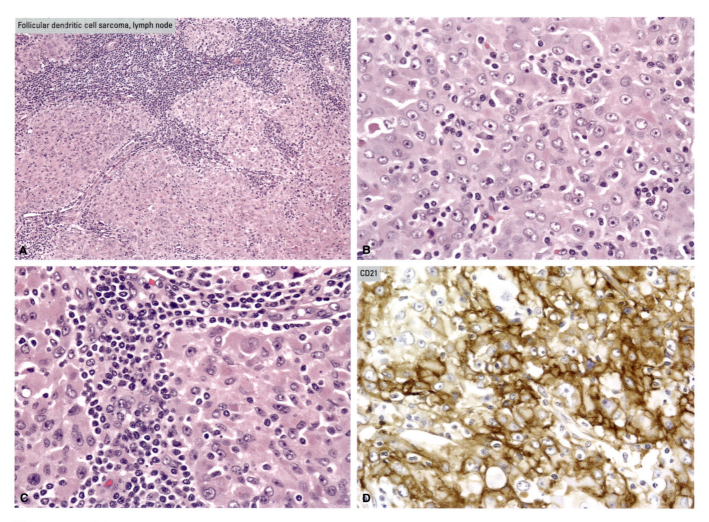

Figure 10.8   Follicular dendritic cell sarcoma. (**A–C**) Histology. (**D**) Immunohistochemistry: tumor cells are positive for CD21

CHAPTER 11

Mastocytosis

Mastocytosis is a heterogeneous group of disorders characterized by proliferation and abnormal accumulation of mast cells in one or more organ systems[78,721,766–786]. They range from urticaria pigmentosa to disseminated diseases with an aggressive clinical course. Table 11.1 presents the WHO classification of mast cell diseases.

Mast cells in the bone marrow aspirate have round to oval nuclei and dark cytoplasm, packed with small basophilic granules. The cytoplasmic granules are usually so abundant that they obscure the nucleus. Mast cells may range from round to polygonal, but atypical forms, including spindle cells, multilobated cells and metachromatically granulated blast-like cells, may be present. Systemic and more aggressive variants of mast cell disease more often display atypical cytomorphologic features. Figure 11.1 depicts spindle-cell variants of mast cells. A bone marrow core biopsy (Figure 11.2) shows multiple, well-demarcated foci of mast cells within a fibrohistiocytic matrix, with a tendency to perivascular and/or paratrabecular locations. Mast cells are accompanied by lymphocytes, histiocytes,

Table 11.1 Classification of mast cell proliferations

Mastocytosis
  Custaneous mastocytosis
  Indolent systemic mastocytosis
  Systemic mastocytosis with associated clonal hematological
    disease
  Aggressive systemic mastocytosis
  Mast cell leukemia
  Mast cell sarcoma

eosinophils and fibroblasts. In lymph nodes (Figure 11.3), mast cells may form inconspicuous clusters or a prominent infiltrate replacing the normal lymph node architecture. Systemic mastocytosis may be associated with other hematopoietic neoplasms, such as acute leukemia (Figure 11.4), myelodysplastic syndromes, malignant lymphoma or chronic myeloproliferative disorders.

Immunophenotypic studies of neoplastic mast cells reveal expression of CD2, CD25, CD43, CD45, CD68, CD117 and mast cell tryptase[776,777,781,782]. Normal (benign) mast cells lack expression of CD2 and CD25.

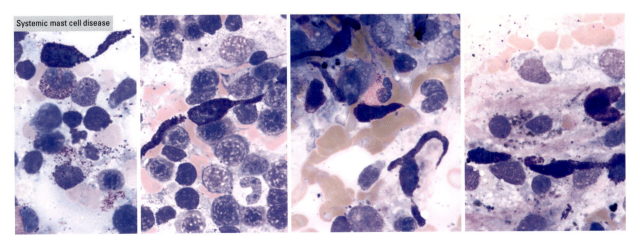

Figure 11.1   Mastocytosis – cytology (bone marrow aspirate). Aspirate smear from bone marrow with systemic mastocytosis. Numerous spindle mast cells with dark cytoplasmic granules are present

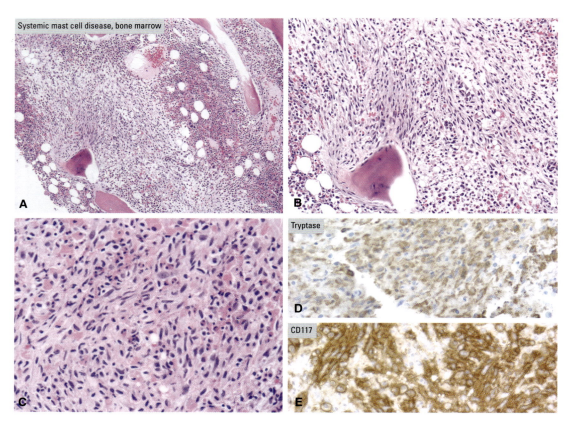

Figure 11.2   Mastocytosis – histology. (**A–C**) Bone marrow core biopsy with systemic mastocytosis. Large sheets of atypical, predominantly spindle cells with pale and clear cytoplasm are present. (**D** and **E**) Immunohistochemistry: mast cells are positive for tryptase (**D**) and CD117 (**E**)

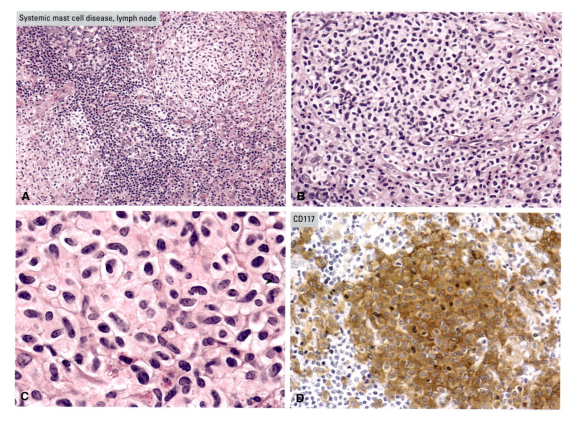

Figure 11.3   Mastocytosis – lymph node. (**A–C**) Histologic section from lymph node with systemic mastocytosis shows cohesive clusters of clear cells with elongated and often irregular nuclei. (**D**) Mast cells are strongly positive for CD117

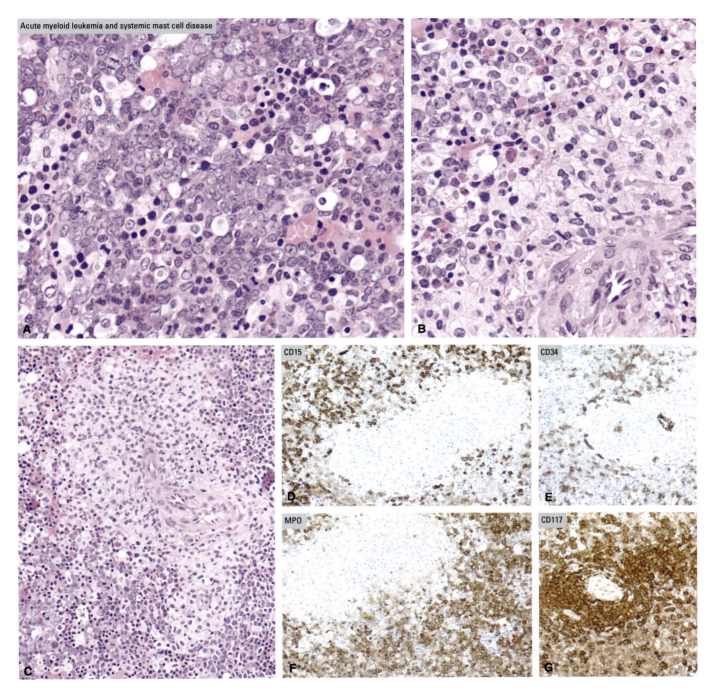

Figure 11.4 Acute myeloid leukemia and systemic mast cell disease – bone marrow. (**A**) Bone marrow area with predominance of blasts. (**B**) Another area with numerous mast cells. (**C**) Low magnification showing mast cells (perivascular aggregate) and blasts (compare with immunohistochemical staining, **D–G**). (**D–G**) Immunohistochemistry: myeloblasts are positive for CD15 (**D**), CD34 (**E**), MPO (**F**) and CD117 (dim expression, **G**). Mast cells are strongly positive for CD117 (**G**)

CHAPTER 12

Composite hematolymphoid tumors

Composite lymphoma is defined as more than one distinct lymphoma variant occurring in the same anatomic site irrespective of the clonal relationship between those components[61,130,787–790]. The most frequent type of composite lymphoma is a combination of two different types of B-cell lymphoma. The concurrence of Hodgkin lymphoma and B-cell lymphoma or composite lymphoma composed of T- and B-cell lymphoma occurs less often. Figures 12.1 to 12.9 depict examples of composite lymphomas, and Figure 12.10 presents concurrence of plasma cell myeloma and acute myeloid leukemia.

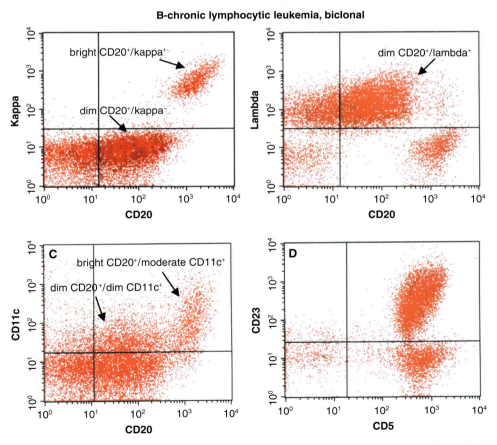

B-chronic lymphocytic leukemia, biclonal

Figure 12.1 'Biclonal' B-chronic lymphocytic leukemia. Flow cytometry analysis reveals two clonal B-cell populations. B-cells with bright CD20 expression are positive for kappa (**A**) and B-cells with dim CD20 expression are positive for lambda (**B**). Both populations express CD11c (**C**) and coexpress CD5 and CD23 (**D**)

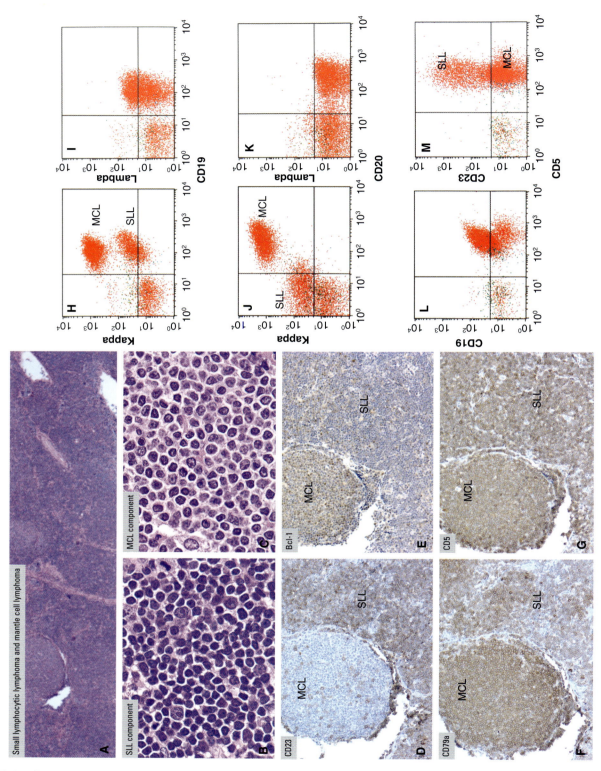

Figure 12.2   Small lymphocytic lymphoma (SLL) and mantle cell lymphoma (MCL) – lymph node. (**A–G**) Histology and immunohistochemistry. (**A**) Low magnification shows vaguely nodular lymphoid infiltrate. (**B** and **C**) High magnification shows small lymphocytes in the diffuse areas (small lymphocytic lymphoma component, **B**) and slightly larger lymphocytes with less compact chromatin in the nodular areas (mantle cell component, **C**). SLL is positive for CD23 (**D**), CD79a (dim expression, **F**) and CD5 (**G**). MCL is positive for bcl-1 (**E**), CD79a (strong expression, **F**) and CD5 (**G**). (**H–M**) Flow cytometry. Both SLL and MCL are kappa positive (**H**, compare with lambda – **I**). SLL shows dim expression of kappa and MCL shows moderate to bright expression of kappa. MCL shows moderate expression of CD20, whereas SLL shows dim expression (**J** and **K**). Both populations are CD5 positive (**L**). SLL is expressing CD23 and MCL, CD23⁻ (**M**)

Small lymphocytic lymphoma and follicular lymphoma

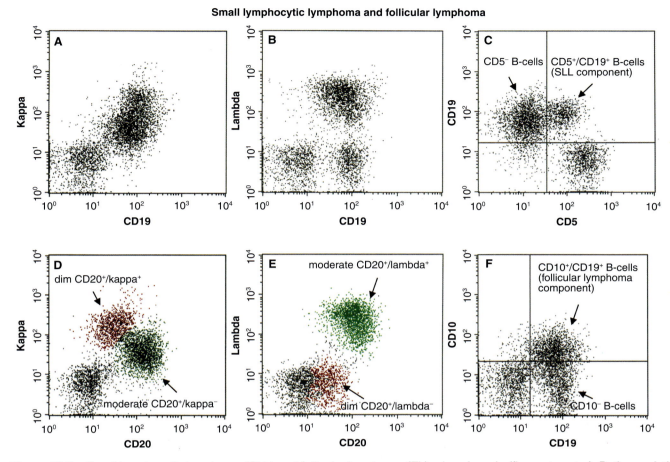

Figure 12.3   Small lymphocytic lymphoma (SLL) and follicular lymphoma (FL) – lymph node (flow cytometry). Both populations are positive for CD19 (**A–C**). FL (green) shows moderate expression of CD20 (**D** and **E**), lambda (**E**) and CD10 (**F**). Small lymphocytic lymphoma shows expression of kappa (**D**) and CD5 (**C**)

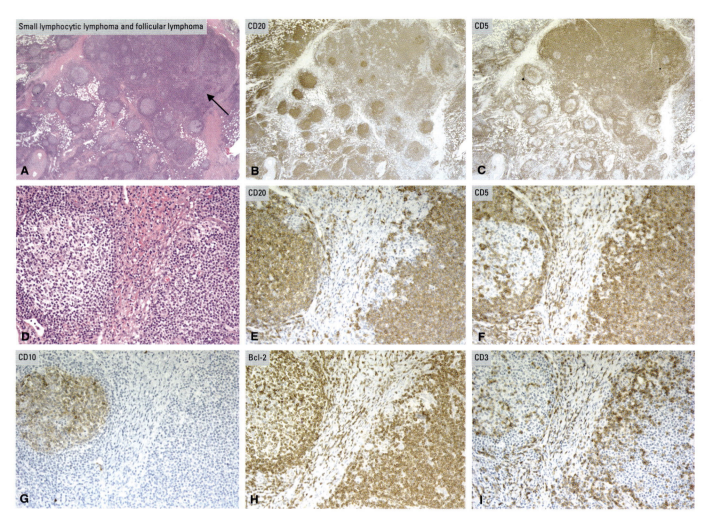

Figure 12.4   Small lymphocytic lymphoma (SLL) and follicular lymphoma (FL) – immunohistochemistry. Low magnification (**A**) shows distinct nodular architecture with focal diffuse infiltrate (arrow). Both components express CD20 (**B**), and SLL expresses CD5 (**C**). Follicular component (**D**) is positive for CD20 (**E**), CD10 (**G**) and bcl-2 (**H**). SLL component is positive for CD20 (**B** and **E**), CD5 (**C** and **F**; compare with CD3 staining, **I**) and bcl-2 (**H**)

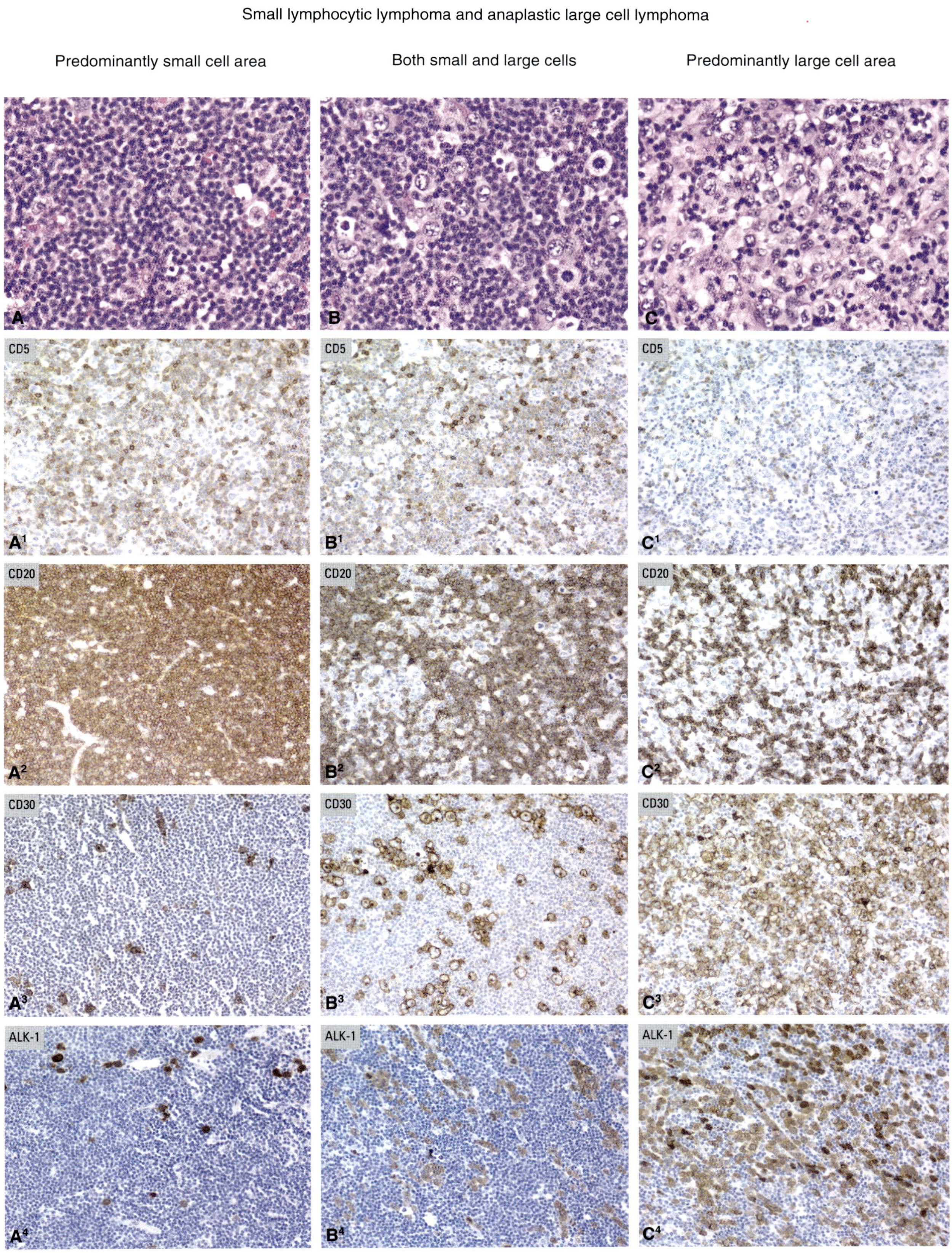

Small lymphocytic lymphoma and anaplastic large cell lymphoma

Predominantly small cell area | Both small and large cells | Predominantly large cell area

Figure 12.5 B-small lymphocytic lymphoma and anaplastic large lymphoma (ALCL; T-cell) – lymph node. Low magnification of the lymph node shows a diffuse small lymphocytic infiltrate intermixed with a variable proportion of large cells. Column **A** (left panels) shows histology and immunohistochemistry of area with predominance of small lymphocytes (B-SLL component). Column **B** (middle panels) shows mixed population of small and large lymphocytes (B-SLL and ALCL), and column **C** (right panels) shows predominance of large cells (ALCL component). B-SLL is positive for CD5 (**A¹**, **B¹**) and CD20 (**A²**, **B²**), whereas ALCL is positive for CD30 (**B³**, **C³**) and ALK-1 (**B⁴**, **C⁴**)

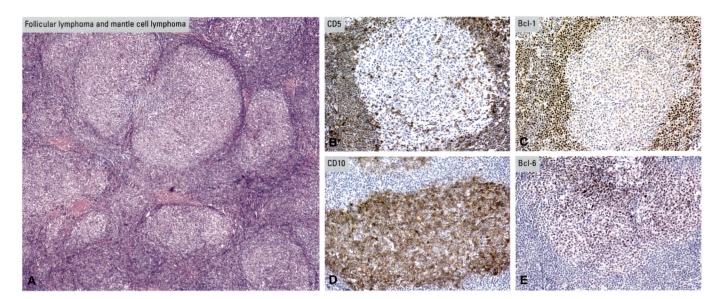

Figure 12.6 Follicular lymphoma (FL) and mantle cell lymphoma (MCL) – lymph node. (**A**) Low magnification shows distinct nodular architecture with inconspicuous mantle zone. MCL was not suspected by histologic examination and was revealed with immunohistochemical staining. (**B–E**) Immunohistochemistry. MCL component shows positive staining with CD5 (**B**) and bcl-1 (**C**), whereas FL component is positive for CD10 (**D**) and bcl-6 (**E**)

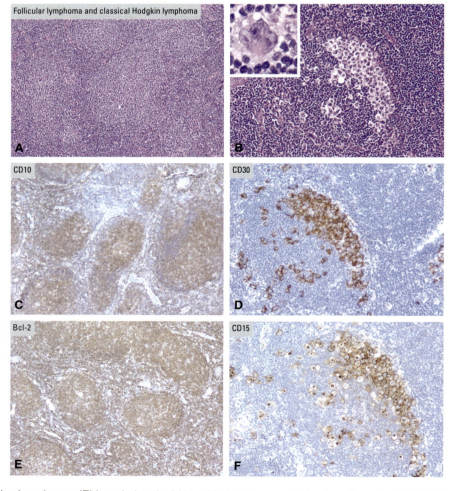

Figure 12.7 Follicular lymphoma (FL) and classical Hodgkin lymphoma (HL) – lymph node. (**A**) Histology of FL component. (**B**) Area of lymph node with cluster of Reed–Sternberg (R–S) and Hodgkin cells (inset: multilobated R–S cell). FL component is positive for CD10 (**C**) and bcl-2 (**E**), and HL component is positive for CD30 (**D**) and CD15 (**F**)

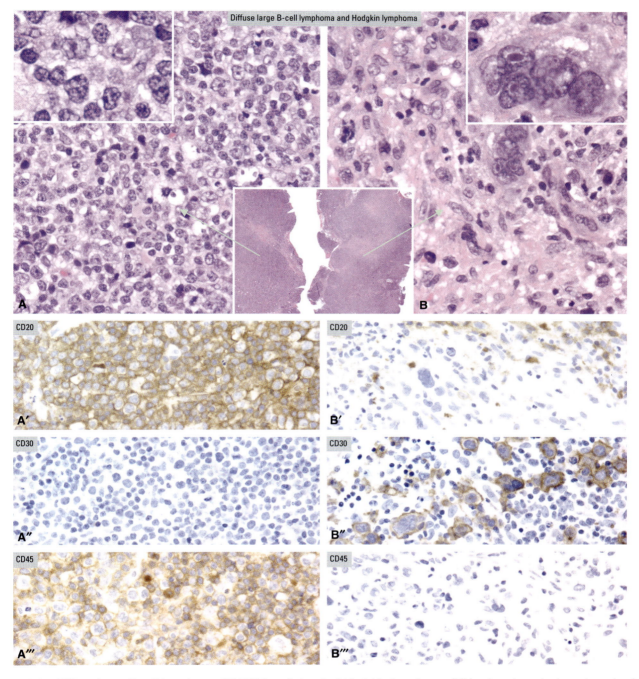

Figure 12.8   Diffuse large B-cell lymphoma (DLBCL) and classical Hodgkin lymphoma (HL) – lymph node. Lymph node shows diffuse area of large lymphoid infiltrate (**A**) and few 'pink' areas with scattered large multinucleated cells with macronucleoli (**B**). Inset shows high magnification of tumor cells in both areas. DLBCL is positive for CD20 (**A′**), negative for CD30 (**A″**) and positive for CD45 (**A‴**). HL shows reversed pattern of staining: large cells are negative for CD20 (**B′**), positive for C30 (**B″**) and negative for CD45 (**B‴**)

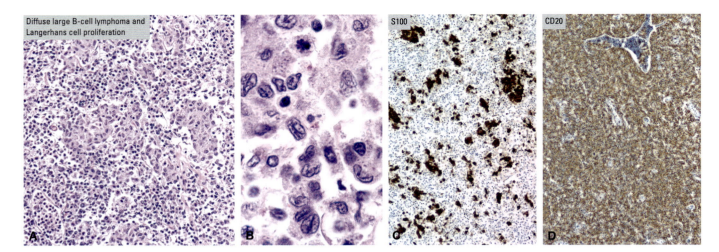

Figure 12.9   Diffuse large B-cell lymphoma (DLBCL) and Langerhans cell proliferation – lymph node. (**A**) Lymph node shows diffuse large cell lymphoid infiltrate with clusters of cells with abundant pale cytoplasm (Langerhans cells). (**B**) High magnification shows typical nuclear features of Langerhans cells. (**C** and **D**) Immunohistochemistry: Langerhans cells are strongly positive for S100 (**C**), and DLBCL is positive for CD20 (**D**)

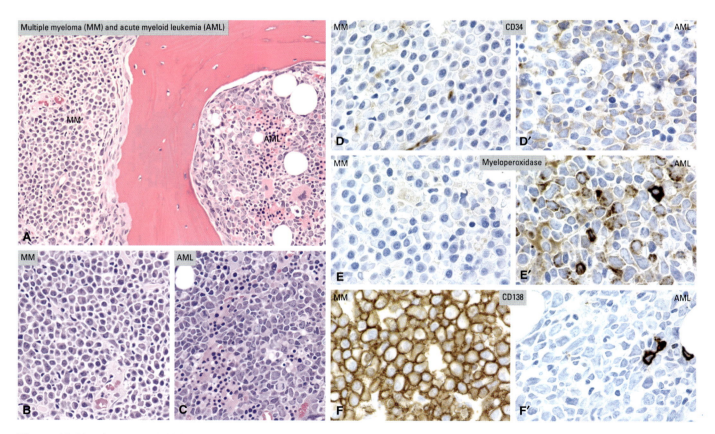

Figure 12.10   Acute myeloid leukemia (AML) and plasma cell myeloma (MM) – bone marrow. (**A**) Low magnification shows two components separated by bony trabeculae: plasma cell myeloma (MM, left) and AML (right). (**B**) High magnification of plasma cell myeloma. (**C**) High magnification of AML. (**D–F**) Immunohistochemistry. Neoplastic plasma cells are negative for CD34 (**D**) and MPO (**E**) and are positive for CD138 (**F**). AML shows reversed staining: blasts are positive for CD34 (**D′**) and MPO (**E′**) and are negative for CD138 (**F′**)

CHAPTER 13

Differential diagnosis – morphology

1. **Vacuolated cells (Figure 13.1):**
   A. Alveolar rhabdomyosarcoma
   B. Burkitt lymphoma
   C. Plasma cell myeloma (Mott cell)
   D. Monoblasts
   E. Erythroblasts (AML-M6)
   F. Pronormoblasts
   G. Langerhans cells
   H. Anaplastic large cell lymphoma.

2. **Lymph node with diffuse small lymphocytic infiltrate (Figure 13.2):**
   A. B-small lymphocytic lymphoma (B-SLL/CLL)
   B. Mantle cell lymphoma
   C. Marginal zone B-cell lymphoma
   D. Hairy cell leukemia
   E. Follicular lymphoma with fibrosis [not shown: diffuse follicle center cell lymphoma, grade 1 of 2 (see Figure 2.69 Chapter 2)]
   F. Lymphoplasmacytic lymphoma
   G. T-cell prolymphocytic leukemia
   H. Peripheral T-cell lymphoma (small cell type)
   I. Adult T-cell lymphoma/leukemia.

3. **Lymph node with diffuse, mixed small, medium-sized and large cell infiltrate (Figure 13.3):**
   A. B-small lymphocytic lymphoma with increased proliferation centers
   B. Marginal zone B-cell lymphoma with increased number of large cells
   C. Diffuse follicle center cell lymphoma, grade 2 of 2
   D. Mantle cell lymphoma, pleomorphic variant
   E. T-cell-rich large B-cell lymphoma
   F. Angioimmunoblastic T-cell lymphoma
   G. Reactive lymphoid hyperplasia
   H. Classical Hodgkin lymphoma, syncytial variant of nodular sclerosis

   I. Classical Hodgkin lymphoma, mixed cellularity type
   J. Peripheral T-cell lymphoma
   K. Lennert's lymphoma
   L. Langerhans cell histiocytosis.

4. **Lymph node with diffuse large cell infiltrate (Figure 13.4):**
   A. Diffuse large B-cell lymphoma
   B. Peripheral T-cell lymphoma (large cell type)
   C. Mantle cell lymphoma, blastoid variant
   D. Extramedullary myeloid tumor (granulocytic sarcoma)
   E. Anaplastic large cell lymphoma
   F. Dendritic cell sarcoma
   G. Histiocytic sarcoma
   H. Blastic NK-cell lymphoma/leukemia.

5. **Lymph node with nodular infiltrate (Figure 13.5):**
   A. Reactive follicular hyperplasia
   B. Reactive lymph node with progressive transformation of germinal centers
   C. Reactive lymph node with mantle zone hyperplasia
   D. Castleman's disease
   E. Atypical follicular hyperplasia/proliferation
   F. Florid follicular hyperplasia, HIV-associated
   G. Follicular lymphoma
   H. B-small lymphocytic lymphoma with proliferation centers
   I. Mantle cell lymphoma
   J. Marginal zone B-cell lymphoma with follicle colonization
   K. Plasmablastic lymphoma associated with multicentric Castleman's disease
   L. Nodular lymphocyte-predominant Hodgkin lymphoma (NLPHL).

6. **Lymph node with paracortical/interfollicular infiltrate (Figure 13.6):**
   A. Peripheral T-cell lymphoma
   B. CD30⁺ T-cell lymphoma
   C. Anaplastic large cell lymphoma (ALK⁺)
   D. Diffuse large B-cell lymphoma with unusual interfollicular pattern
   E. Extramedullary myeloid tumor (granulocytic sarcoma)
   F. Castleman's disease, plasma cell type
   G. Plasma cell neoplasm
   H. Classical Hodgkin lymphoma
   I. Hairy cell leukemia
   J. Langerhans cell histiocytosis.

7. **Lymph node with blastic/blastoid infiltrate (Figure 13.7):**
   A. Mantle cell lymphoma, blastoid variant
   B. Immunoblastic lymphoma (diffuse large B-cell lymphoma, immunoblastic)
   C. Burkitt lymphoma
   D. Precursor T-lymphoblastic lymphoma
   E. Plasmablastic lymphoma
   F. Blastic NK-cell lymphoma/leukemia
   G. Precursor B-lymphoblastic lymphoma
   H. Extramedullary myeloid cell tumor (granulocytic sarcoma)
   I. Centroblastic lymphoma (diffuse large B-cell lymphoma, centroblastic).

8. **Lymph node with starry-sky pattern (Figure 13.8):**
   A. Burkitt lymphoma
   B. Mantle cell lymphoma, blastoid variant
   C. Plasmablastic lymphoma
   D. High-grade diffuse large B-cell lymphoma ('Burkitt-like')
   E. Peripheral T-cell lymphoma
   F. Follicular lymphoma, high grade.

9. **Lymph node with clear cell infiltrate (Figure 13.9):**
   A. Peripheral T-cell lymphoma
   B. Peripheral T-cell lymphoma with signet-ring cells
   C. Follicular lymphoma, signet-ring cell variant
   D. Langerhans cell histiocytosis
   E. Mast cell disease
   F. Rosai–Dorfman disease
   G. Angioimmunoblastic T-cell lymphoma
   H. Histiocytic sarcoma.

10. **Large cell infiltrate with anaplastic features (Figure 13.10):**
    A. Diffuse large B-cell lymphoma, anaplastic variant
    B. ALK⁺ positive large B-cell lymphoma
    C. Anaplastic large cell lymphoma
    D. Peripheral T-cell lymphoma
    E. Anaplastic plasma cell myeloma
    F. Hodgkin lymphoma, lymphocyte-depleted
    G. Poorly differentiated carcinoma (anaplastic carcinoma).

11. **Lymphoid infiltrate with large multilobated (multinucleated) cells with prominent nucleoli (Figure 13.11):**
    A. Hodgkin lymphoma
    B. Diffuse large B-cell lymphoma
    C. Peripheral T-cell lymphoma
    D. Anaplastic large cell lymphoma
    E. T-cell-rich large B-cell lymphoma
    F. EBV-associated lymphoproliferative disorder (post-transplant large B-cell lymphoma)
    G. Enteropathy-type T-cell lymphoma
    H. Nodular lymphocyte-predominant Hodgkin lymphoma
    I. EBV-associated lymphadenitis
    J. Multiple myeloma, anaplastic variant
    K. Cutaneous anaplastic large cell lymphoma
    L. Kimura disease
    M. CMV-associated lymphadenitis.

12. **Lymphoid infiltrate with numerous histiocytes (Figure 13.12):**
    A. Lennert's lymphoma
    B. Diffuse large B-cell lymphoma with granulomas
    C. Nodular lymphocyte-predominant Hodgkin lymphoma with granulomas
    D. Classical Hodgkin lymphoma
    E. Toxoplasmic lymphadenitis
    F. Sarcoidosis.

13. **Lymph node with plasma cell/plasmablastic infiltrate (Figure 13.13):**
    A. Castleman's disease, plasma cell type
    B. Castleman's disease, plasma cell type with monotypic (lambda⁺) plasma cells
    C. Lymphoplasmacytic lymphoma/Waldenstrom's macroglobulinemia
    D. Plasma cell myeloma
    E. Plasmablastic lymphoma
    F. B-small lymphocytic lymphoma with plasmacytic differentiation
    G. Marginal zone B-cell lymphoma with plasmacytic differentiation.

14. **Bone marrow with large cell infiltrate (Figure 13.14):**
    A. Diffuse large B-cell lymphoma
    B. Alveolar rhabdomyosarcoma
    C. Anaplastic large cell lymphoma

D. Precursor B-cell lymphoblastic leukemia
E. Plasma cell myeloma
F. Acute myeloid leukemia
G. Acute erythroid leukemia
H. Acute monocytic leukemia
I. Langerhans cell histiocytosis.

15. **Bone marrow with atypical megakaryocytosis (Figure 13.15):**
    A. Myelodysplastic syndrome (RA)
    B. Myelodysplastic syndrome (RAEB)
    C. Del 5(q) syndrome (5q⁻ syndrome)
    D. Chronic myelogenous leukemia
    E. Polycythemia vera
    F. Essential thrombocythemia
    G. Chronic idiopathic myelofibrosis
    H. Acute megakaryoblastic leukemia (AML-M7)
    I. Reactive megakaryocytosis.

16. **Bone marrow with reactive lymphoid aggregates (Figure 13.16).**

17. **Bone marrow with nodular lymphoid infiltrate (Figure 13.17):**
    A. B-chronic lymphocytic leukemia
    B. Diffuse large B-cell lymphoma
    C. Splenic marginal zone B-cell lymphoma
    D. Hodgkin lymphoma, classical
    E. Anaplastic large cell lymphoma
    F. Follicular lymphoma.

18. **Bone marrow with paratrabecular lymphoid infiltrate (Figure 13.18):**
    A. Follicular lymphoma
    B. Diffuse large B-cell lymphoma
    C. Mantle cell lymphoma.

19. **Bone marrow – discrepancy between the size of lymphocytes in primary lymphoma and the bone marrow involvement (Figure 13.19):**
    A. Bone marrow infiltrate composed of predominantly small lymphocytes
    B. Gastric large B-cell lymphoma.

20. **Bone marrow with diffuse lymphoid infiltrate (Figure 13.20):**
    A. B-chronic lymphocytic leukemia
    B. Lymphoplasmacytic lymphoma
    C. Mantle cell lymphoma
    D. Diffuse large B-cell lymphoma
    E. Hairy cell leukemia
    F. Immunoblastic lymphoma.

21. **Bone marrow – patterns of involvement by mature T-cell lymphoproliferative disorders (Figure 13.21):**
    A. Peripheral T-cell lymphoma – diffuse infiltrate
    B. Peripheral T-cell lymphoma – paratrabecular infiltrate
    C. T-cell prolymphocytic leukemia – interstitial infiltrate
    D. Angioimmunoblastic T-cell lymphoma – diffuse infiltrate with increased vascularity and fibrosis
    E. T-LGL leukemia – interstitial infiltrate
    F. Hepatosplenic gamma/delta T-cell lymphoma – diffuse infiltrate
    G. Hepatosplenic gamma/delta T-cell lymphoma – intrasinusoidal infiltrate
    H. Anaplastic large cell lymphoma – diffuse infiltrate
    I. Anaplastic large cell lymphoma – nodular infiltrate.

22. **Bone marrow with intrasinusoidal lymphoid infiltrate (Figure 13.22):**
    A. Hepatosplenic gamma/delta T-cell lymphoma
    B. Diffuse large B-cell lymphoma.

23. **Bone marrow with non-hematopoietic tumors (Figure 13.23):**
    A. Mucinous adenocarcinoma
    B. Breast carcinoma (lobular type)
    C. Prostate adenocarcinoma
    D. Malignant melanoma
    E. Neuroblastoma
    F. Small cell carcinoma
    G. Alveolar rhabdomyosarcoma
    H. Spindle-cell sarcoma (GIST).

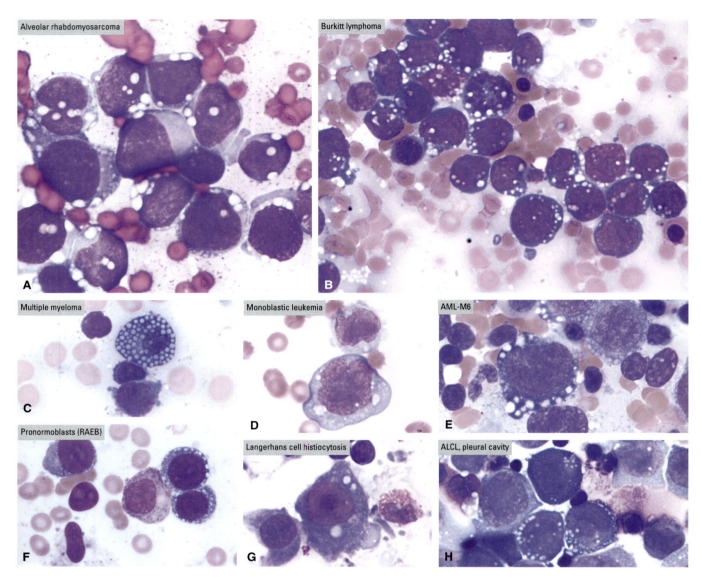

Figure 13.1   Differential diagnosis – vacuolated cells. (**A**) Alveolar rhabdomyosarcoma. (**B**) Burkitt lymphoma. (**C**) Plasma cell myeloma. (**D**) Monoblasts. (**E** and **F**) Pronormoblasts. (**G**) Langerhans cells. (**H**) Anaplastic large cell lymphoma

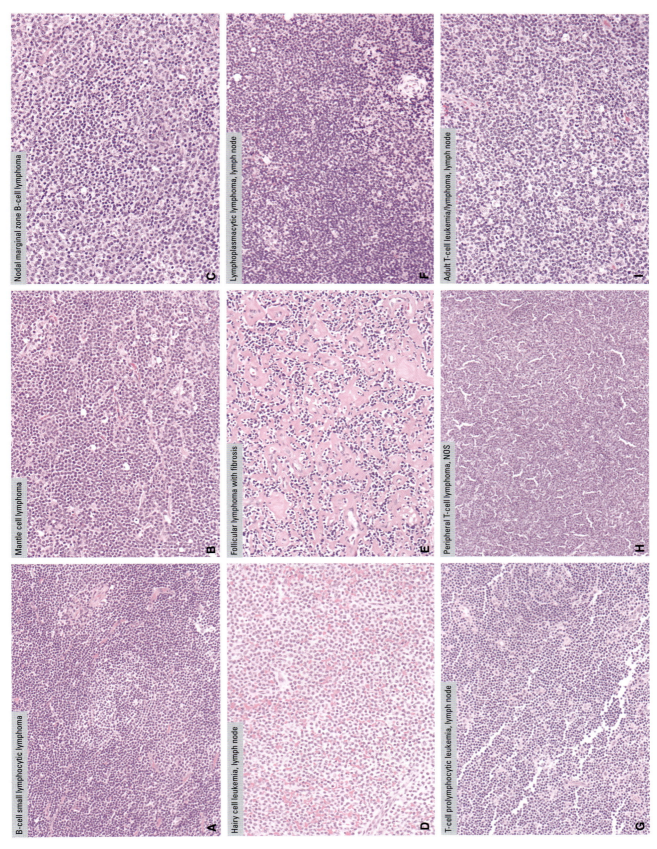

Figure 13.2 Lymph node. Differential diagnosis – diffuse small lymphocytic infiltrate. (**A**) B-small lymphocytic lymphoma. (**B**) Mantle cell lymphoma. (**C**) Marginal zone B-cell lymphoma. (**D**) Hairy cell leukemia. (**E**) Follicular lymphoma with fibrosis. (**F**) Lymphoplasmacytic lymphoma. (**G**) T-cell prolymphocytic leukemia. (**H**) Peripheral T-cell lymphoma, NOS (unspecified). (**I**) Adult T-cell leukemia/lymphoma

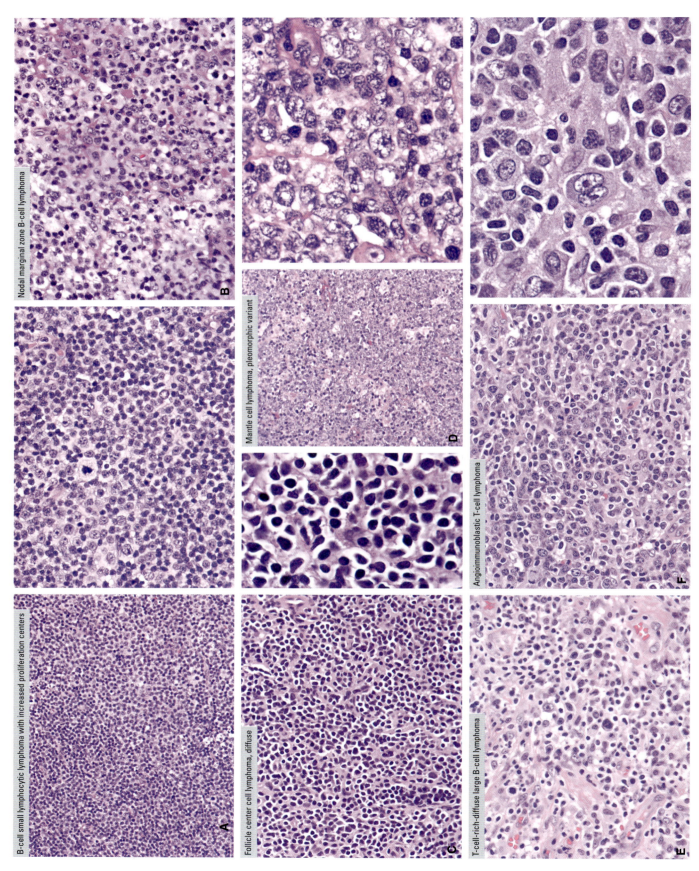

Figure 13.3   Lymph node. Differential diagnosis – diffuse mixed small and large cell infiltrate. (**A**) B-small lymphocytic lymphoma with increased proliferation centers. (**B**) Nodal marginal zone B-cell lymphoma with scattered large cells. (**C**) Diffuse follicle center cell lymphoma. (**D**) Mantle cell lymphoma, pleomorphic variant. (**E**) T-cell-rich large B-cell lymphoma. (**F**) Angioimmunoblastic T-cell lymphoma. (**G**) EBV-associated reactive hyperplasia. (**H**) Classical Hodgkin lymphoma, syncytial variant. (**I**) Mixed cellularity Hodgkin lymphoma. (**J**) Peripheral T-cell lymphoma. (**K**) Lennert's lymphoma. (**L**) Langerhans cell histiocytosis

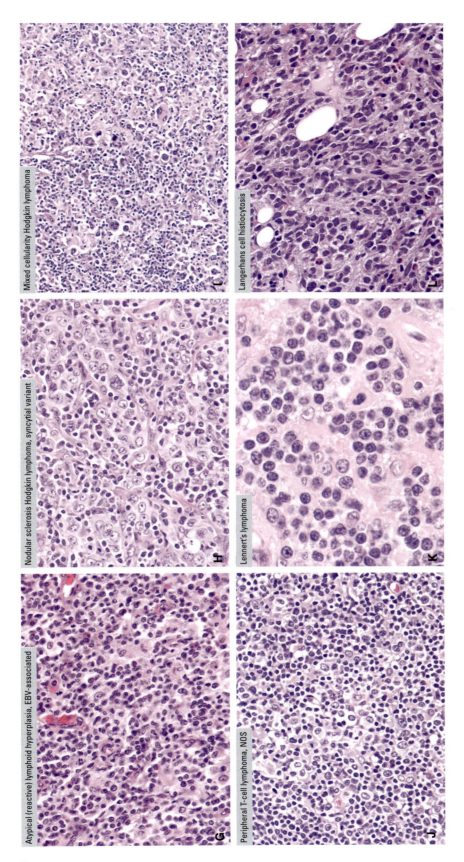

Figure 13.3   *(Continued)*

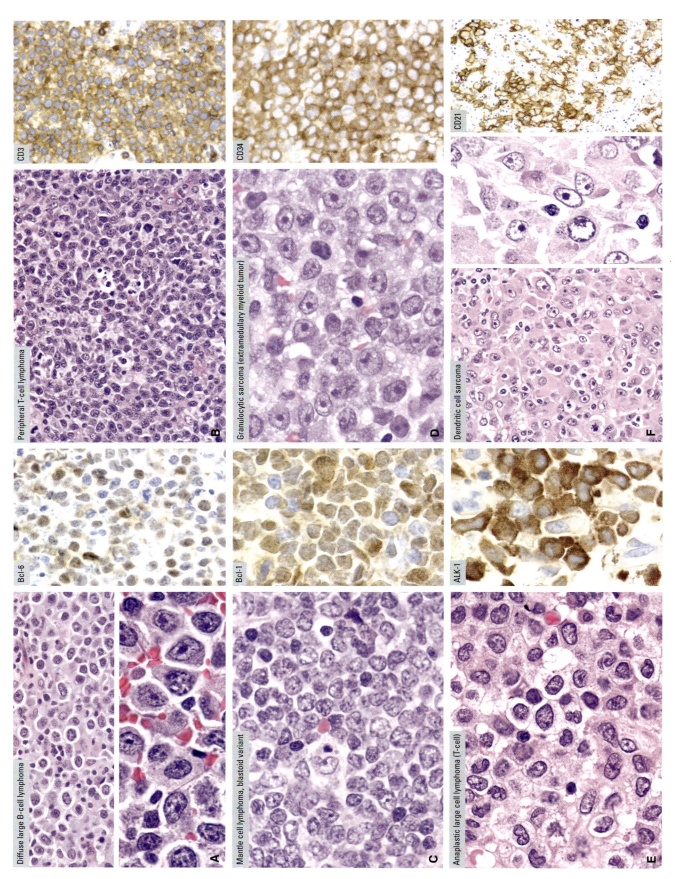

Figure 13.4 Lymph node. Differential diagnosis – diffuse large cell infiltrate. (**A**) Diffuse large B-cell lymphoma. (**B**) Peripheral T-cell lymphoma. (**C**) Mantle cell lymphoma, blastoid variant. (**D**) Granulocytic sarcoma. (**E**) Anaplastic large cell lymphoma. (**F**) Follicular dendritic cell sarcoma. (**G**) Histiocytic sarcoma. (**H**) Blastic NK-cell lymphoma/leukemia

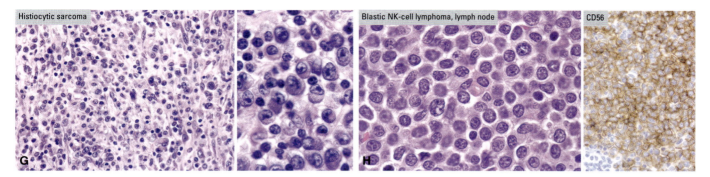

Figure 13.4   *(Continued)*

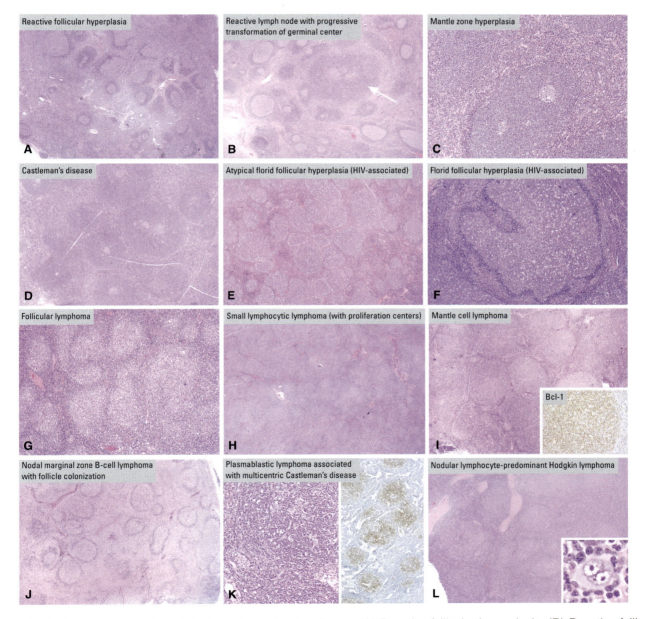

Figure 13.5   Lymph node. Differential diagnosis – nodular infiltrate. (**A**) Reactive follicular hyperplasia. (**B**) Reactive follicular hyperplasia with progressive transformation of germinal centers (PTGC). (**C**) Mantle zone hyperplasia. (**D**) Castleman's disease. (**E** and **F**) Atypical HIV-related florid follicular hyperplasia. (**G**) Follicular lymphoma. (**H**) Small lymphocytic lymphoma with proliferation centers. (**I**) Mantle cell lymphoma. (**J**) Nodal marginal zone B-cell lymphoma with follicle colonization. (**K**) Plasmablastic lymphoma with multicentric Castleman's disease. (**L**) Nodular lymphocyte-predominant Hodgkin lymphoma

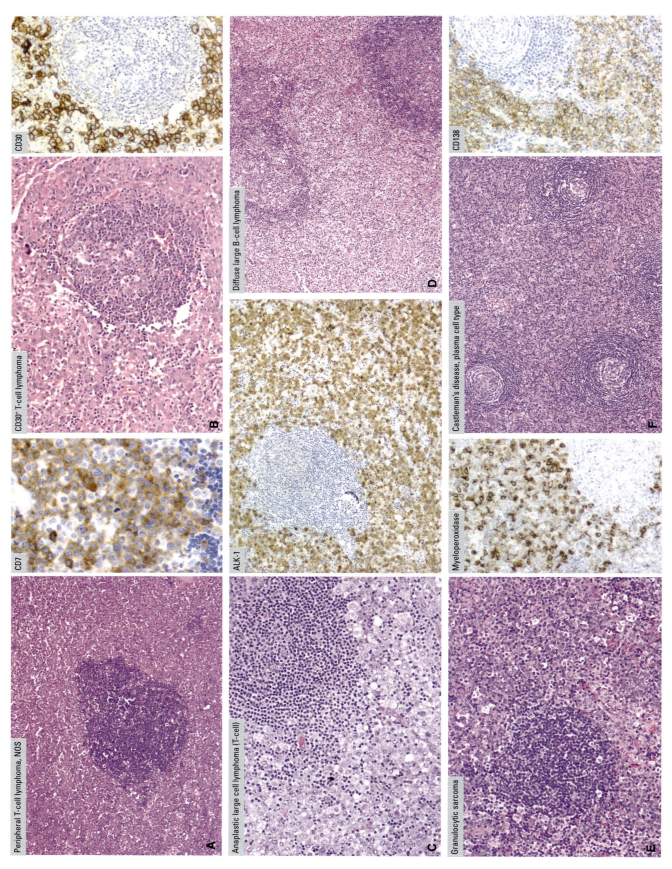

Figure 13.6   Lymph node. Differential diagnosis – paracortical/interfollicular infiltrate. (**A**) Peripheral T-cell lymphoma. (**B**) CD30⁺ peripheral T-cell lymphoma. (**C**) Anaplastic large cell lymphoma. (**D**) Diffuse large B-cell lymphoma with unusual interfollicular pattern. (**E**) Extramedullary myeloid tumor (granulocytic sarcoma). (**F**) Castleman's disease, plasma cell type. (**G**) Plasma cell neoplasm. (**H**) Hodgkin lymphoma (classical). (**I**) Hairy cell leukemia. (**J**) Langerhans cell histiocytosis

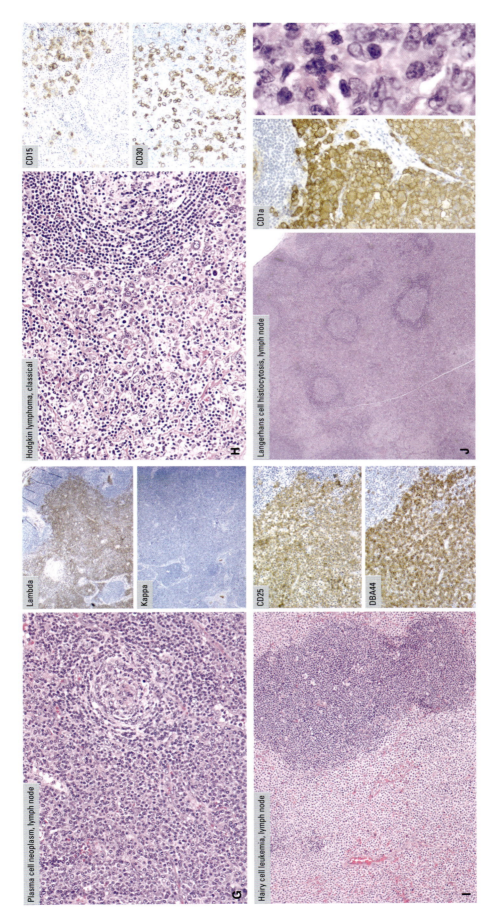

CD15

CD30

Hodgkin lymphoma, classical

H

CD1a

Langerhans cell histiocytosis, lymph node

J

Lambda

Kappa

Plasma cell neoplasm, lymph node

G

CD25

DBA44

Hairy cell leukemia, lymph node

I

Figure 13.6   (*Continued*)

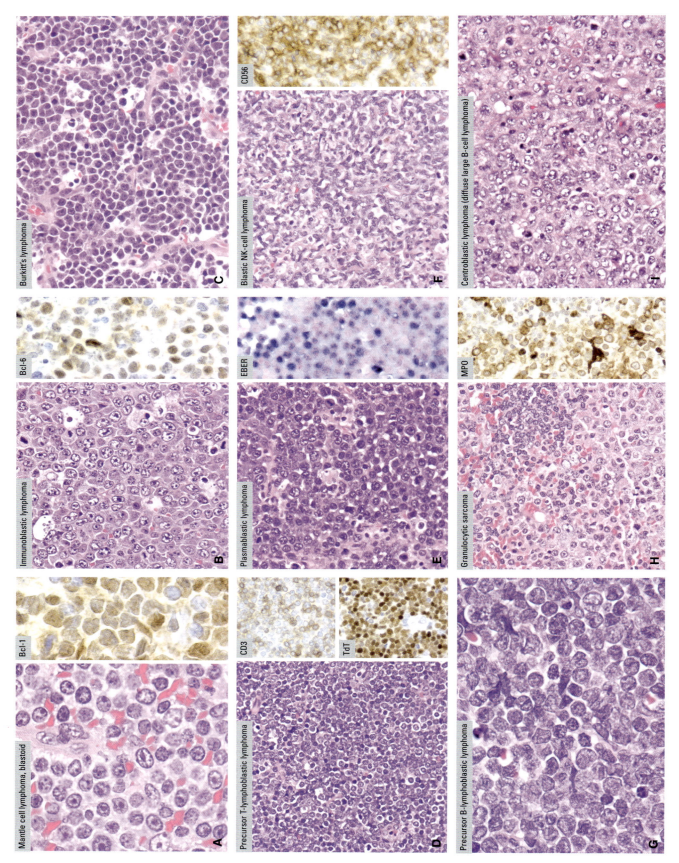

Figure 13.7   Lymph node. Differential diagnosis – blastic/blastoid infiltrate. (**A**) Mantle cell lymphoma, blastoid variant. (**B**) Immunoblastic lymphoma. (**C**) Burkitt lymphoma. (**D**) Precursor T-lymphoblastic lymphoma. (**E**) Plasmablastic lymphoma. (**F**) Blastic NK-cell lymphoma / leukemia. (**G**) Precursor B-lymphoblastic lymphoma. (**H**) Granulocytic sarcoma. (**I**) Centroblastic lymphoma

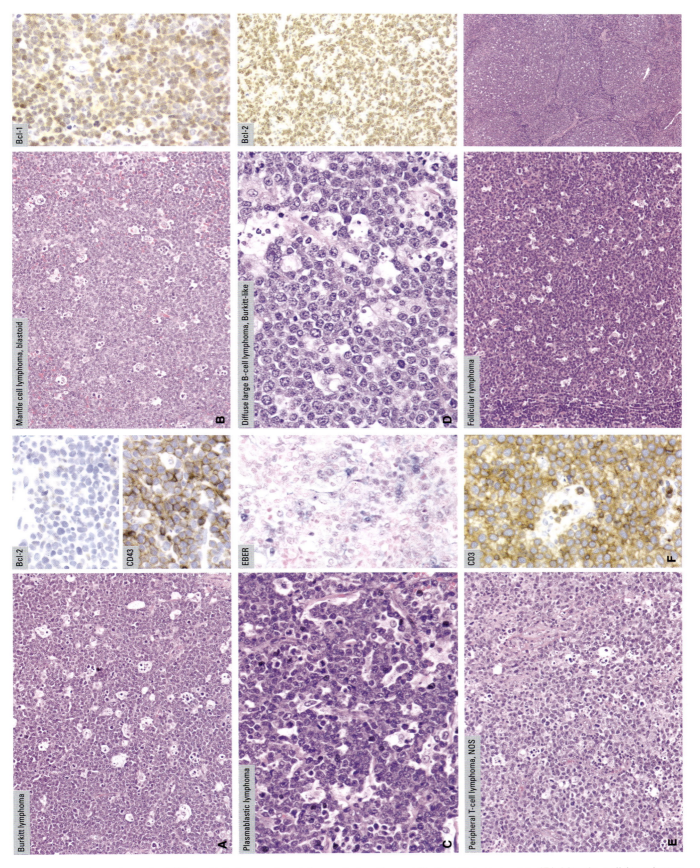

Figure 13.8   Lymph node. Differential diagnosis – 'starry-sky' pattern. (**A**) Burkitt lymphoma. (**B**) Mantle cell lymphoma. (**C**) Plasmablastic lymphoma. (**D**) Diffuse large B-cell lymphoma, Burkitt-like. (**E**) Peripheral T-cell lymphoma. (**F**) Follicular lymphoma with tingible-body macrophages

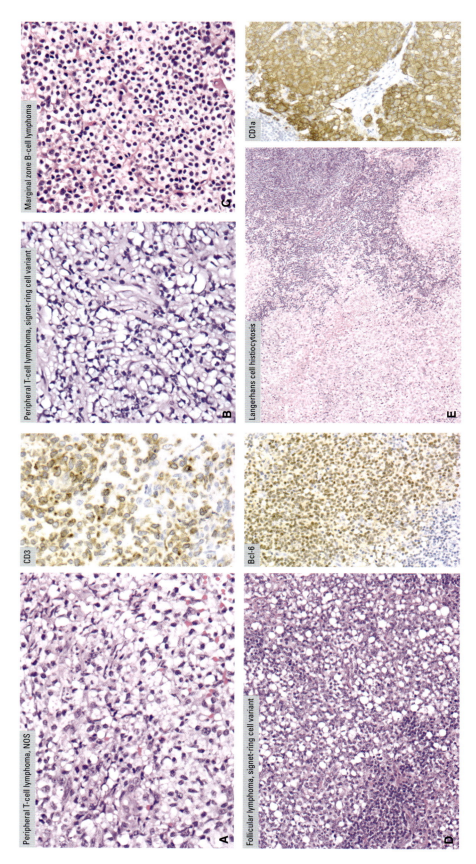

Figure 13.9   Lymph node. Differential diagnosis – clear cell infiltrate. (**A**) Peripheral T-cell lymphoma. (**B**) Peripheral T-cell lymphoma, signet-ring cell variant. (**C**) Marginal zone B-cell lymphoma. Follicular lymphoma, signet-ring cell variant. (**E**) Langerhans cell histiocytosis. (**F**) Mast cell disease. (**G**) Rosai–Dorfman disease. (**H**) Angioimmunoblastic T-cell lymphoma. (**I**) Histiocytic sarcoma

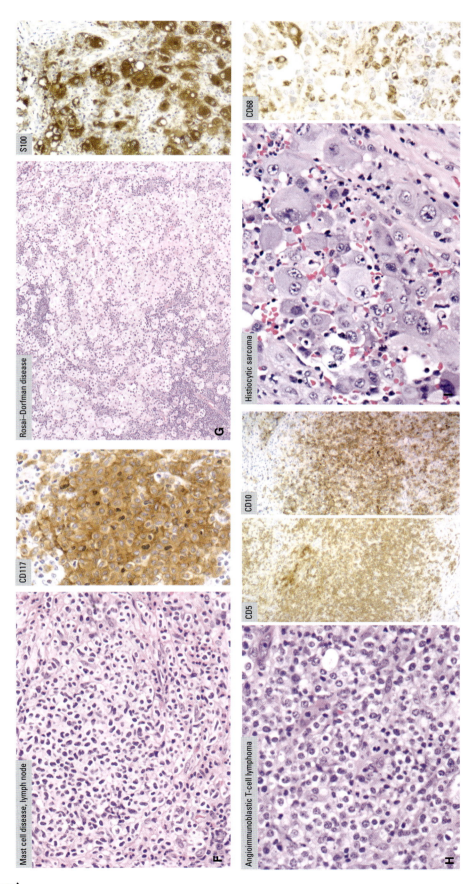

Figure 13.9   (*Continued*)

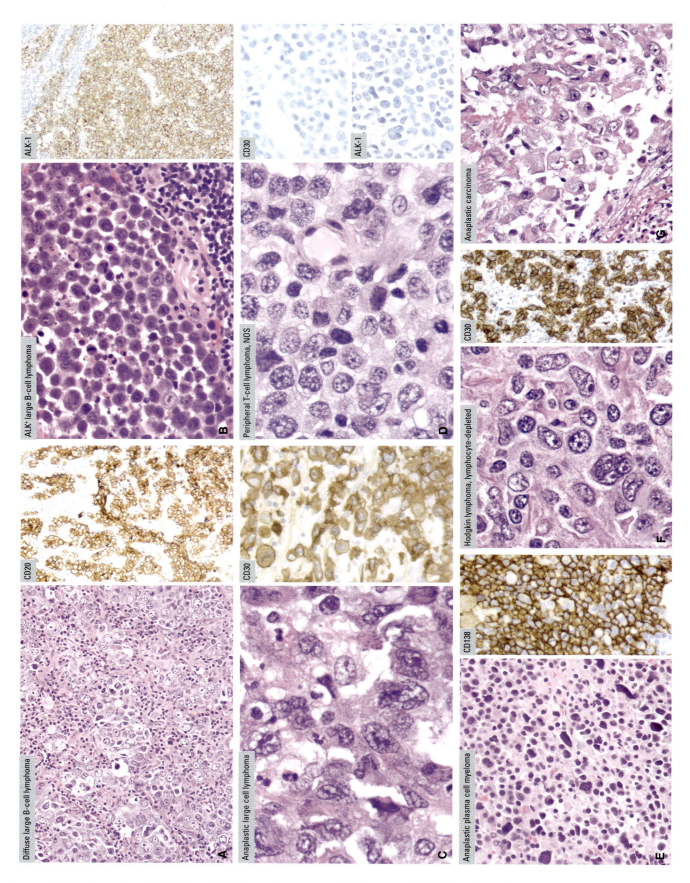

Figure 13.10   Lymph node. Differential diagnosis – anaplastic features. (**A**) Diffuse large B-cell lymphoma with anaplastic features. (**B**) ALK positive diffuse large B-cell lymphoma. (**C**) Anaplastic large cell lymphoma. (**D**) Peripheral T-cell lymphoma. (**E**) Plasma cell myeloma, anaplastic variant. (**F**) Hodgkin lymphoma, lymphocyte-depleted variant. (**G**) Anaplastic carcinoma

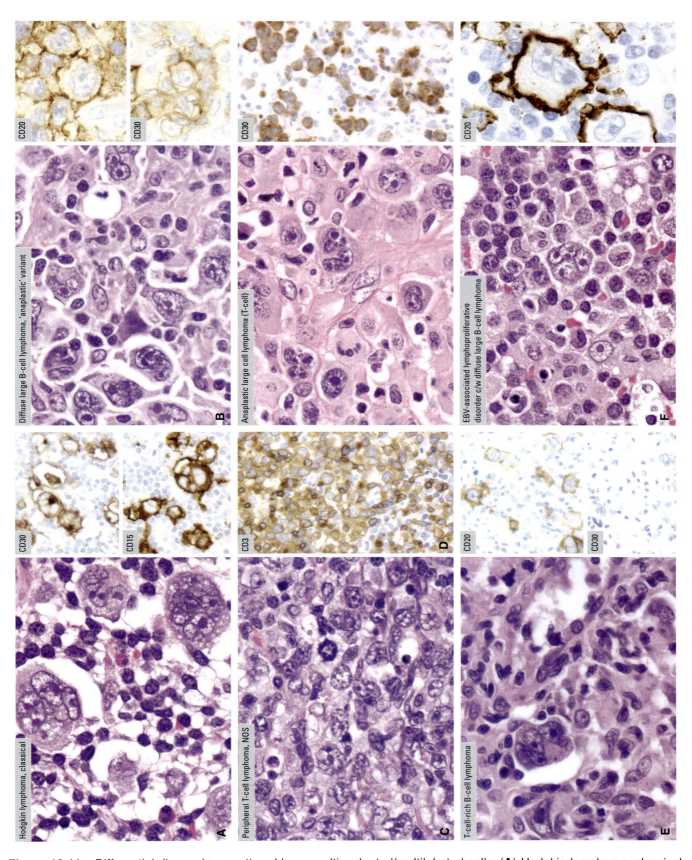

Figure 13.11   Differential diagnosis – scattered large multinucleated/multilobated cells. (**A**) Hodgkin lymphoma, classical. (**B**) Diffuse large B-cell lymphoma, anaplastic variant. (**C**) Peripheral T-cell lymphoma. (**D**) Anaplastic large cell lymphoma. (**E**) T-cell-rich, large B-cell lymphoma. (**F**) EBV-associated, large B-cell lymphoma. (**G**) Enteropathy-type, T-cell lymphoma. (**H**) Nodular lymphocyte-predominant Hodgkin lymphoma. (**I**) EBV-associated lymphadenitis. (**J**) Multiple myeloma, anaplastic variant. (**K**) Cutaneous anaplastic large cell lymphoma. (**L**) Kimura disease. (**M**) CMV-associated lymphadenitis

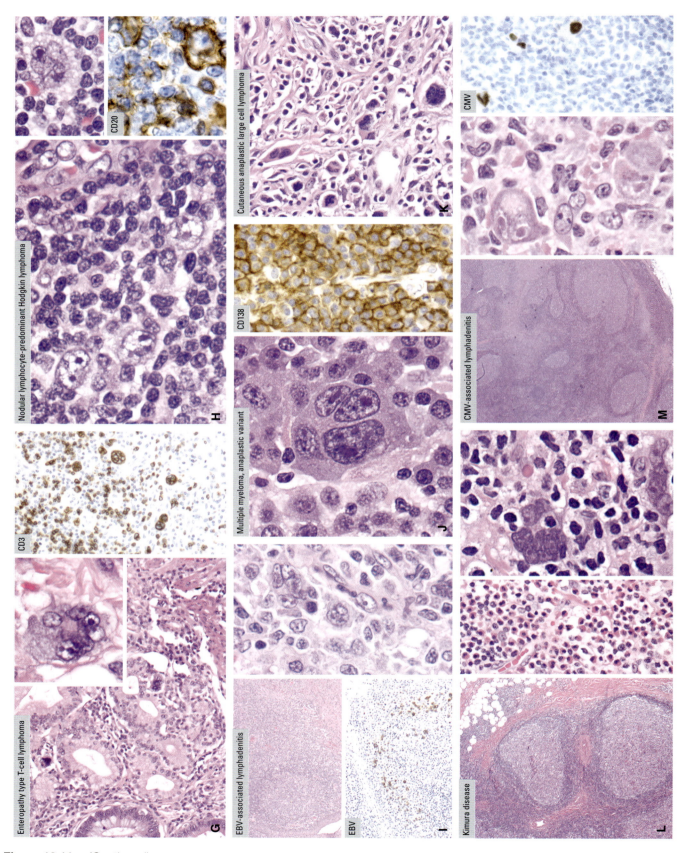

Figure 13.11   *(Continued)*

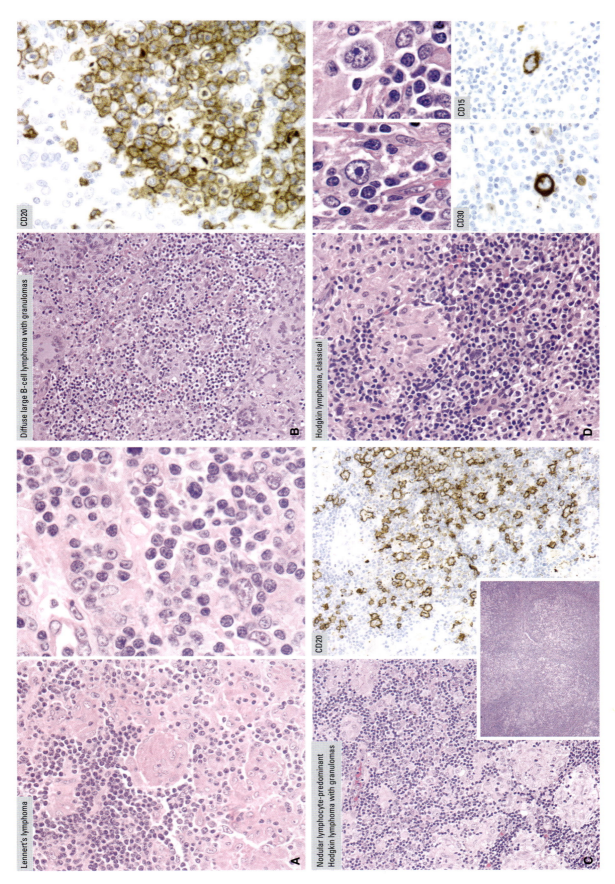

Figure 13.12   Lymph node. Differential diagnosis – histiocytic aggregates. (**A**) Lennert's lymphoma. (**B**) Diffuse large B-cell lymphoma with granulomas. (**C**) Nodular lymphocyte-predominant Hodgkin lymphoma with granulomas. (**D**) Hodgkin lymphoma, classical. (**E**) Toxoplasmosis. (**F**) Sarcoidosis

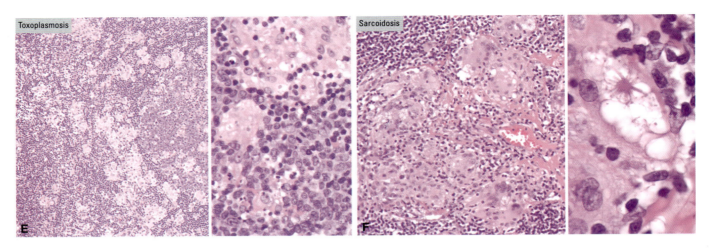

Figure 13.12   *(Continued)*

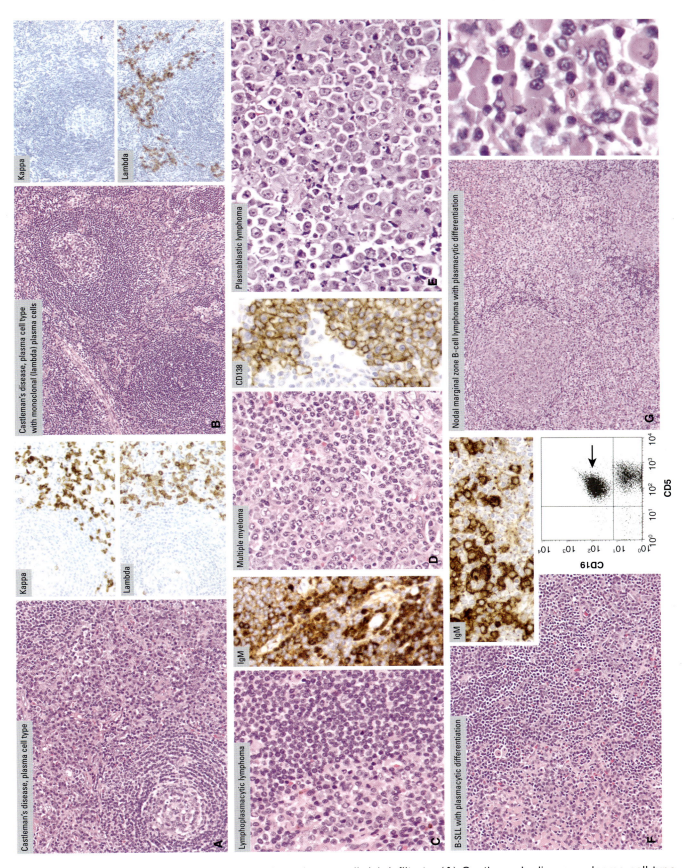

Figure 13.13   Lymph node. Differential diagnosis – plasma cell rich infiltrate. (**A**) Castleman's disease, plasma cell type. (**B**) Castleman's disease, plasma cell type with monoclonal (lambda) plasma cells. (**C**) Lymphoplasmacytic lymphoma. (**D**) Multiple myeloma. (**E**) Plasmablastic lymphoma. (**F**) Small lymphocytic lymphoma with plasmacytic differentiation. (**G**) Nodal marginal zone lymphoma with plasmacytic differentiation

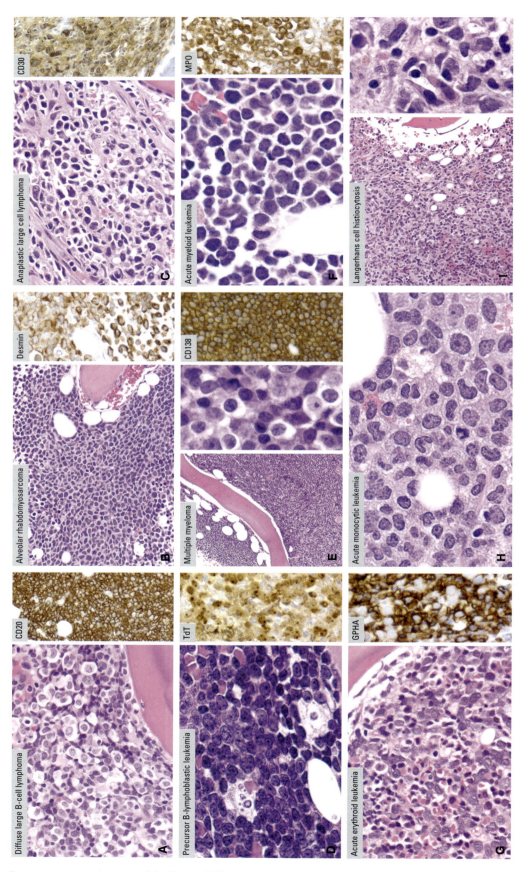

Figure 13.14   Bone marrow – large cell infiltrate (differential diagnosis). (**A**) Diffuse large B-cell lymphoma. (**B**) Alveolar rhabdomyosarcoma. (**C**) Anaplastic large cell lymphoma. (**D**) Precursor B-lymphoblastic leukemia. (**E**) Multiple myeloma. (**F**) Acute myeloid leukemia. (**G**) Acute erythroid leukemia. (**H**) Acute monocytic leukemia. (**I**) Langerhans cell histiocytosis

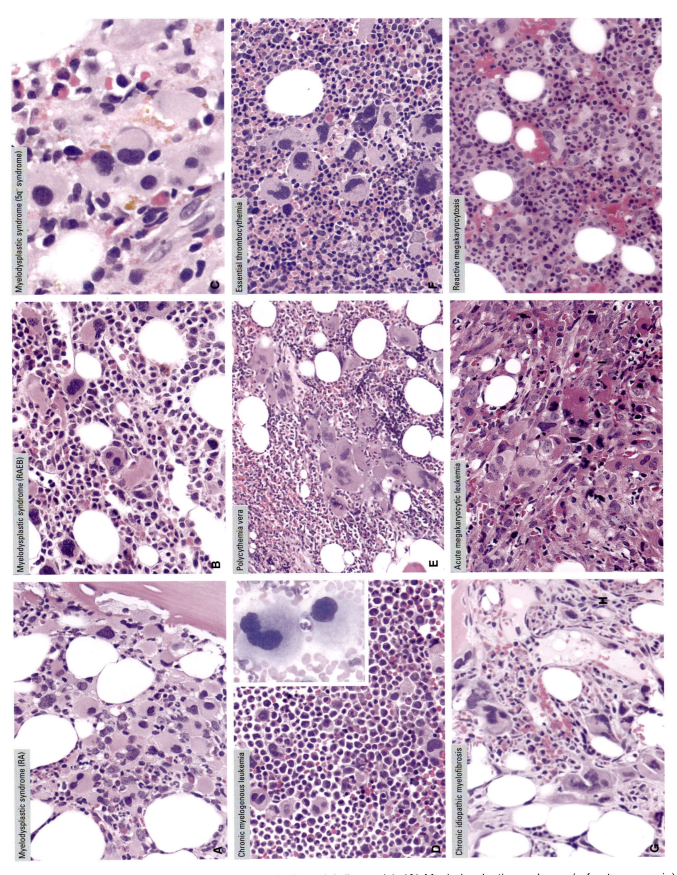

Figure 13.15   Bone marrow – megakaryocytosis (differential diagnosis). (**A**) Myelodysplastic syndrome (refractory anemia). (**B**) Myelodysplastic syndrome (refractory anemia with excess blasts). (**C**) Myelodysplastic syndrome (5q⁻ syndrome). (**D**) Chronic myelogenous leukemia. (**E**) Polycythemia vera. (**F**) Essential thrombocythemia. (**G**) Chronic idiopathic myelofibrosis. (**H**) Acute megakaryoblastic leukemia. (**I**) Reactive megakaryocytosis

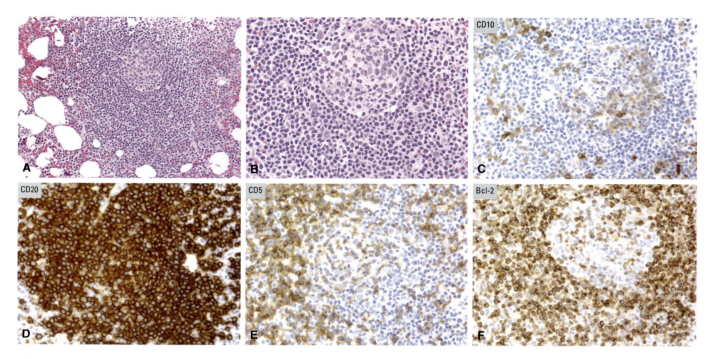

Figure 13.16   Bone marrow – reactive lymphoid aggregates. (**A** and **B**) Histology (**A**, low power; **B**, high power) showing well-demarcated lymphoid aggregate with germinal center. (**C–F**) Immunohistochemistry shows positive expression of germinal center cells with CD10 (**C**), B-cells with CD20 (**D**), T-cells with CD3 (**E**), and negative expression of germinal center cells with bcl-2 (**F**)

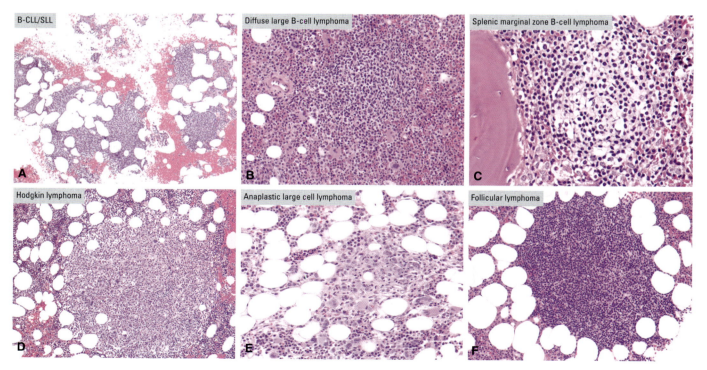

Figure 13.17   Bone marrow – nodular lymphoid infiltrate (differential diagnosis). (**A**) B-chronic lymphocytic leukemia/small lymphocytic lymphoma. (**B**) Diffuse large B-cell lymphoma. (**C**) Marginal zone B-cell lymphoma. (**D**) Classical Hodgkin lymphoma. (**E**) Anaplastic large cell lymphoma. (**F**) Follicular lymphoma

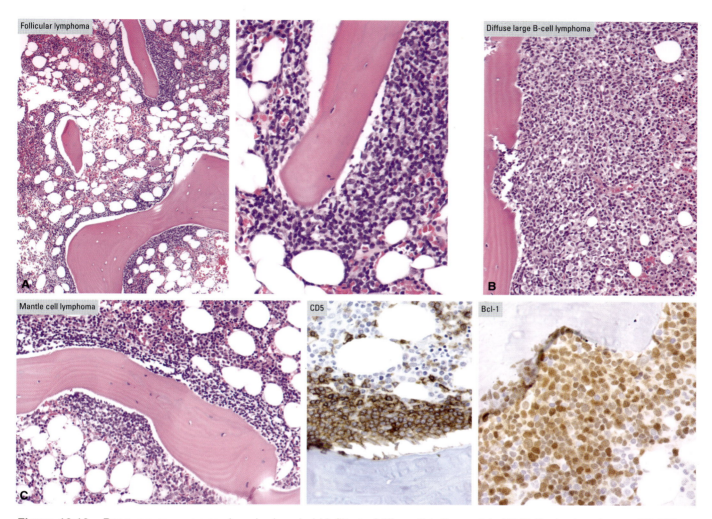

Figure 13.18 Bone marrow – paratrabecular lymphoid infiltrate (differential diagnosis). (**A**) Follicular lymphoma. (**B**) Diffuse large B-cell lymphoma. (**C**) Mantle cell lymphoma

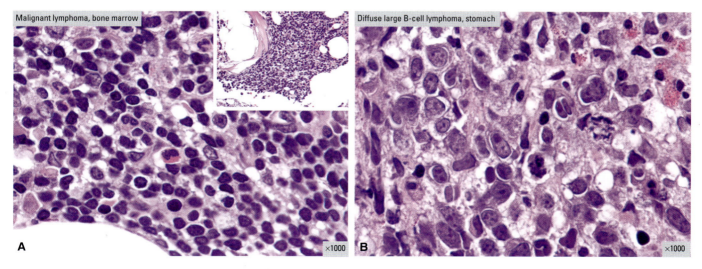

Figure 13.19 Bone marrow – discrepancy between size of lymphocytes of marrow infiltrate and primary site of lymphoma. (**A**) Malignant lymphoma involving the bone marrow. Small lymphoid cells predominate. (**B**) Stomach – large B-cell lymphoma

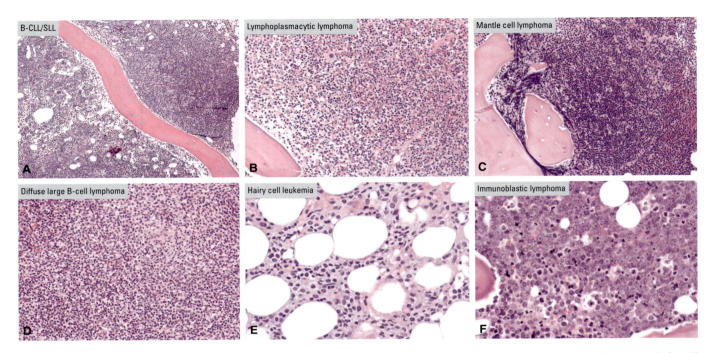

Figure 13.20   Bone marrow – diffuse B-cell lymphoid infiltrate (differential diagnosis). (**A**) B-chronic lymphocytic leukemia/small lymphocytic lymphoma. (**B**) Lymphoplasmacytic lymphoma. (**C**) Mantle cell lymphoma. (**D**) Diffuse large B-cell lymphoma. (**E**) Hairy cell leukemia. (**F**) Immunoblastic lymphoma

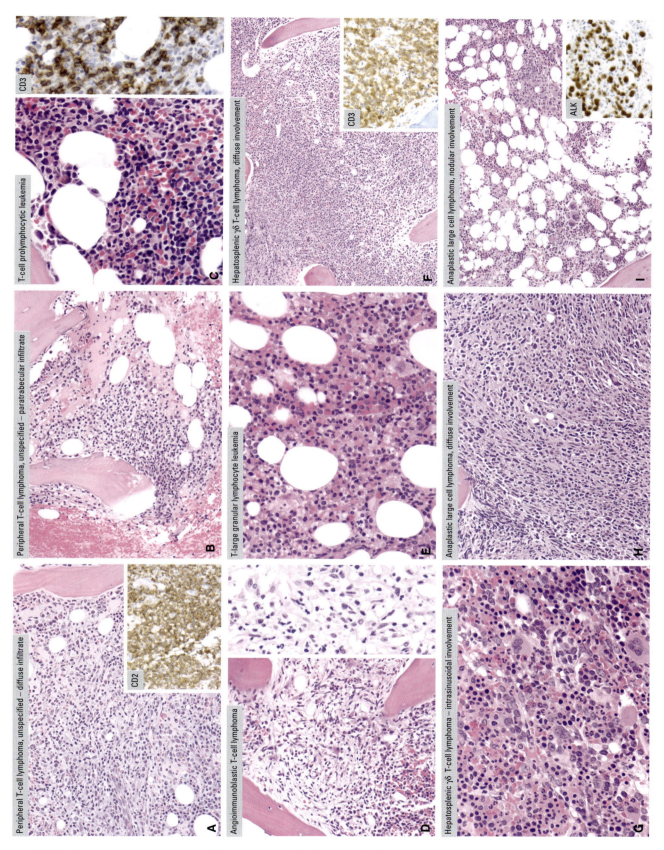

Figure 13.21   Bone marrow – patterns of bone marrow involvement by T-cell lymphoma (differential diagnosis). (**A**) Peripheral T-cell lymphoma unspecified – diffuse infiltrate. (**B**) Peripheral T-cell lymphoma, unspecified – paratrabecular infiltrate. (**C**) T-cell prolymphocytic leukemia. (**D**) Angioimmunoblastic T-cell lymphoma. (**E**) T-large granular lymphocyte leukemia. (**F**) Hepatosplenic γδ T-cell lymphoma – diffuse infiltrate. (**G**) Hepatosplenic γδ T-cell lymphoma – intrasinusoidal infiltrate. (**H**) Anaplastic large celllymphoma – diffuse infiltrate. (**I**) Anaplastic large cell lymphoma – nodular infiltrate

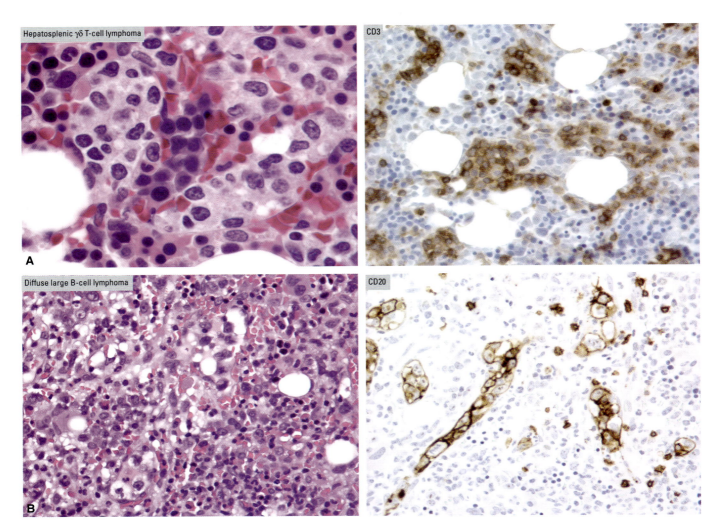

Figure 13.22   Bone marrow – intrasinusoidal infiltrate (differential diagnosis). (**A**) Hepatosplenic γδ T-cell lymphoma. (**B**) Diffuse large B-cell lymphoma

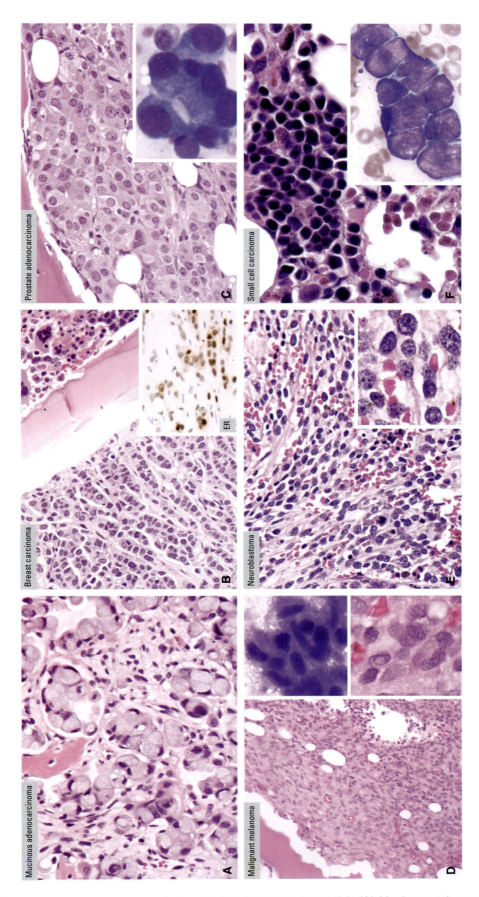

Figure 13.23   Bone marrow – non-hematopoietic tumors (differential diagnosis). **(A)** Mucinous adenocarcinoma. **(B)** Breast carcinoma. **(C)** Prostate adenocarcinoma. **(D)** Malignant melanoma. **(E)** Neuroblastoma. **(F)** Small cell carcinoma. **(G)** Alveolar rhabdomyosarcoma. **(H)** Spindle-cell sarcoma (GIST)

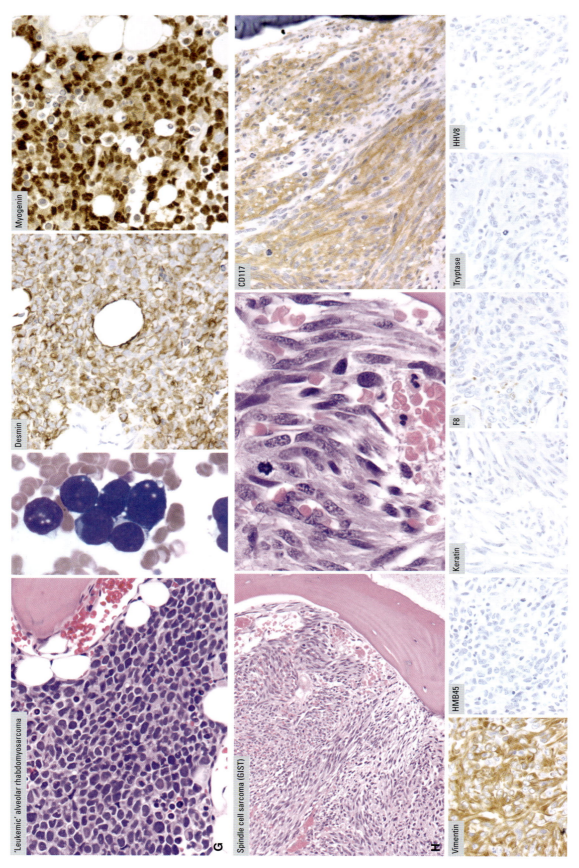

Figure 13.23   *(Continued)*

CHAPTER 14

Differential diagnosis – phenotype

1. **ALK-1⁺ neoplasms (Figure 14.1):**
   A. Anaplastic large cell lymphoma with cytoplasmic and nuclear ALK expression
   B. Anaplastic large cell lymphoma with cytoplasmic ALK expression
   C. Large B-cell lymphoma with ALK expression.

2. **Bcl-1⁺ neoplasms (Figure 14.2):**
   A. Mantle cell lymphoma
   B. Mantle cell lymphoma, blastoid variant
   C. Plasma cell myeloma
   D. Plasmablastic lymphoma
   E. Hairy cell leukemia, bone marrow
   F. Hairy cell leukemia, lymph node.

3. **Bcl-6⁺ neoplasms (Figure 14.3):**
   A. Follicular lymphoma
   B. Diffuse large B-cell lymphoma
   C. L&H cells in nodular lymphocyte-predominant Hodgkin lymphoma
   D. Primary effusion lymphoma
   E. Angioimmunoblastic T-cell lymphoma
   F. Burkitt lymphoma
   G. Reed–Sternberg and Hodgkin cells in classical Hodgkin lymphoma
   H. Anaplastic large cell lymphoma (T-cell).
   Not shown: precursor T-lymphoblastic lymphoma (subset), mantle cell lymphoma (rare cases), poorly differentiated carcinoma (subset).

4. **The CD4:CD8 ratio** – T-cell lymphoproliferative disorders with dual CD4/CD8 negativity (Figure 14.4):
   A. Peripheral T-cell lymphoma
   B. Anaplastic large cell lymphoma
   C. Precursor T-lymphoblastic lymphoma
   D. Hepatosplenic γδ T-cell lymphoma.

5. **The CD4:CD8 ratio** – neoplasms with CD4/CD8 ratio within normal range (Figure 14.5):
   A. Angioimmunoblastic T-cell lymphoma
   B. Classical Hodgkin lymphoma (reactive T-cells in Hodgkin lymphoma usually show predominance of CD4⁺ cells; occasional cases have normal, and rare cases have reversed CD4:CD8 ratio).

6. **The CD4:CD8 ratio** – neoplasms with dual CD4/CD8 expression (Figure 14.6):
   A. T-cell prolymphocytic leukemia
   B. Peripheral T-cell lymphoma
   C. Precursor T-lymphoblastic lymphoma
   D. Thymoma.

7. **The CD4:CD8 ratio** – predominance of CD4⁺ cells (Figure 14.7):
   A. Hodgkin lymphoma, classical
   B. Peripheral T-cell lymphoma
   C. Nodular lymphocyte-predominant Hodgkin lymphoma
   D. T-cell prolymphocytic leukemia.

8. **The CD4:CD8 ratio** – predominance of CD8⁺ cells (Figure 14.8):
   A. Peripheral T-cell lymphoma
   B. Hodgkin lymphoma, classical
   C. HIV-associated reactive lymph node
   D. Peripheral T-cell lymphoma, blood.

9. **The CD4:CD8 ratio** – comparison of CD4 and CD8 expression in thymic hyperplasia/thymoma versus precursor T-lymphoblastic lymphoma/leukemia (Figure 14.9). Benign immature thymocytes from either thymic hyperplasia or thymoma (Figure 14.9, upper panels; A–D) coexpress both CD4 and CD8.

The expression of CD4 and CD8 in thymic hyperplasia and thymoma is variable (with 'smeared-like' pattern), but the majority of cells display moderate expression of both antigens (Figure 14.9A and B). The immature cells from precursor T-lymphoblastic lymphoma/leukemia (lower panels; E–H) show coexpression of CD4 and CD8 without variability (Figure 14.9E and F). The pattern of expression of surface CD3 antigens helps to differentiate benign thymocytes from T-lymphoblasts[21]. The former display characteristic variable (smeared-like) expression of CD3 (Figure 14.9D), whereas T-lymphoblasts lack the variability of surface CD3 expression (Figure 14.9H).

10. **CD5⁺ neoplasms (Figure 14.10):**
    A. B-small lymphocytic lymphoma/chronic lymphocytic leukemia
    B. Mantle cell lymphoma
    C. *De novo* CD5⁺ diffuse large B-cell lymphoma
    D. Peripheral T-cell lymphoma
    E. Precursor T-lymphoblastic lymphoma/leukemia
    F. Benign B-cells in reactive lymph node in infant
    G. Intravascular large B-cell lymphoma
    H. Diffuse large B-cell lymphoma with CD5 and CD10 expression.
       Not shown: thymic carcinoma, (see Chapter 9), hairy cell leukemia (rare cases), and other mature T-cell lymphoproliferative disorders (see Chapter 3).

11. **CD10 expression (Figure 14.11):**
    A. Benign germinal centers
    B. Follicular lymphoma
    C. Burkitt lymphoma
    D. Diffuse large B-cell lymphoma
    E. Plasmablastic lymphoma
    F. Precursor B-lymphoblastic lymphoma/leukemia (B-ALL/LBL)
    G. Mantle cell lymphoma
    H. Hairy cell leukemia
    I. Angioimmunoblastic T-cell lymphoma
    J. Precursor T-lymphoblastic lymphoma/leukemia (T-ALL/LBL)
    K. Malignant melanoma
    L. Plasma cell myeloma
    M. Acute monocytic leukemia.

12. **CD15 expression (Figure 14.12):**
    A. Hodgkin lymphoma, classical
    B. Chronic myelomonocytic leukemia

    C. Acute myeloid leukemia
    D. Nodular lymphocyte-predominant Hodgkin lymphoma (rare cases)
    E. Anaplastic large cell lymphoma (rare cases)
    F. Peripheral T-cell lymphoma (rare cases).
       Not shown: granulocytes, subset of histiocytes.

13. **CD20⁺ neoplasms (Figure 14.13):**
    A. Diffuse large B-cell lymphoma
    B. T-cell/histiocyte-rich large B-cell lymphoma
    C. Diffuse large B-cell lymphoma, anaplastic variant
    D. Intravascular large B-cell lymphoma
    E. Hodgkin lymphoma, classical (subset)
    F. Nodular lymphocyte-predominant Hodgkin lymphoma (NLPHL)
    G. Plasma cell myeloma (subset)
    H. Lymphomatoid granulomatosis
    I. Peripheral T-cell lymphoma (unusual cases with aberrant CD20 expression).

14. **CD20⁻ B-cell neoplasms (Figure 14.14):**
    A. Diffuse large B-cell lymphoma (subset)
    B. Primary effusion lymphoma
    C. Diffuse large B-cell lymphoma with ALK expression
    D. Plasmablastic lymphoma.
       Not shown: B-cell lymphoma after Rituxan treatment.

15. **CD21 expression in hematolymphoid neoplasms (Figure 14.15):**
    A. Benign lymph node – regular cohesive pattern
    B. Follicular lymphoma – irregular pattern with preserved 'borders' of follicles
    C. Marginal zone lymphoma – prominent disruption of follicular dendritic cell meshwork
    D. Nodular lymphocyte-predominant Hodgkin lymphoma – prominent expansion of follicular dendritic cell with preserved nodularity
    E. Angioimmunoblastic T-cell lymphoma – expanded irregular pattern
    F. Follicular dendritic cell sarcoma – tumor cells are positive for CD21.

16. **CD23 expression (Figure 14.16):**
    A. Reactive germinal center with prominent polarization
    B. B-small lymphocytic lymphoma
    C. B-chronic lymphocytic leukemia
    D. Mantle cell lymphoma (unusual variant)
    E. Follicular dendritic cell sarcoma

F. Acute monocytic leukemia

G. Plasma cells (benign and neoplastic)

H. Follicular lymphoma (subset).

17. **CD25⁺ neoplasms (Figure 14.17):**
    A. Hairy cell leukemia, bone marrow
    B. Hairy cell leukemia, lymph node
    C. Adult T-cell lymphoma/leukemia
    D. Anaplastic large cell lymphoma
    E. Peripheral T-cell lymphoma.
    Not shown: subset of mature B- and T-cell lymphoproliferative disorders.

18. **CD30⁺ expression (Figure 14.18):**
    A. Activated B- and T-cells in reactive lymph node
    B. Diffuse large B-cell lymphoma (subset)
    C. Diffuse large B-cell lymphoma, anaplastic variant
    D. Hodgkin lymphoma, classical
    E. Primary mediastinal large B-cell lymphoma
    F. Anaplastic large cell lymphoma
    G. Extranodal T/NK-cell lymphoma, nasal type
    H. Enteropathy-type T-cell lymphoma
    I. Cutaneous anaplastic large cell lymphoma
    J. Plasma cell neoplasms (subset)
    K. EBV-associated high-grade lymphoma in patient with HIV.
    Not shown: embryonal cell carcinoma.

19. **CD45⁻ hematopoietic neoplasms (Figure 14.19):**
    A. Plasma cell myeloma
    B. Follicular dendritic cell sarcoma
    C. Anaplastic large cell lymphoma (subset)
    D. Hodgkin lymphoma, classical
    E. Plasmablastic lymphoma
    F. Precursor B-lymphoblastic lymphoma/leukemia (subset).

20. **CD45 versus side scatter – flow cytometric gating strategy of the bone marrow and peripheral blood (Figure 14.20).**

21. **CD45 versus side scatter – pattern recognition in flow cytometry analysis of the bone marrow and/or peripheral blood (Figure 14.21):**
    A. Normal (benign) sample
    B. Plasma cell myeloma with lack of CD45
    C. B-CLL with bright expression of CD45 and low side scatter
    D. Hairy cell leukemia with bright CD45 and increased side scatter
    E. Diffuse large B-cell lymphoma with moderate CD45 expression

F. Precursor B-lymphoblastic leukemia with moderate CD45

G. T-LGL leukemia with bright CD45 and low side scatter

H. Blastic NK-cell leukemia/lymphoma with moderate CD45 and low side scatter

I. Chronic myelomonocytic leukemia (CMML) with bright CD45 and increased side scatter

J. Chronic myeloid leukemia with prominent decrease of side scatter in granulocytes (compare with normal sample, A)

K. Acute myeloid leukemia with moderate CD45 and low side scatter

L. Acute myelomonocytic leukemia with increased blasts (green) and monocytic cells (blue)

M. Acute promyelocytic leukemia (APL) with high side scatter (green)

N. Acute promyelocytic leukemia (microgranular variant) with low side scatter (green)

O. Acute monocytic leukemia with bright CD45 and increased side scatter

P. Acute myeloid leukemia (non-APL) with unusual high side scatter

R. Metastatic small cell carcinoma with lack of CD45 and increased side scatter.

22. **CD56⁺ neoplasms (Figure 14.22):**
    A. Extranodal T/NK-cell lymphoma, nasal type
    B. Blastic NK-cell leukemia/lymphoma
    C. Subcutaneous panniculitis-like T-cell lymphoma
    D. Small cell carcinoma
    E. Precursor T-lymphoblastic leukemia/lymphoma
    F. Peripheral T-cell lymphoma
    G. Plasmablastic lymphoma
    H. Plasma cell myeloma
    I. Diffuse large B-cell lymphoma (rare cases)
    J. T-LGL leukemia
    K. Enteropathy-type T-cell lymphoma
    L. NK-LGL leukemia
    M. Acute myeloid leukemia (subset)
    N. Acute promyelocytic leukemia (rare cases)
    O. Acute monocytic leukemia.

23. **CD103⁺ neoplasms (Figure 14.23):**
    A. Hairy cell leukemia
    B. Hairy cell leukemia variant
    C. Enteropathy-type T-cell lymphoma.

24. **CD117⁺ neoplasms (Figure 14.24):**
    A. Acute myeloid leukemia
    B. Precursor T-lymphoblastic leukemia/lymphoma

C. Acute promyelocytic leukemia

D. Acute monocytic leukemia

E. Plasma cell myeloma

F. Small cell carcinoma

G. Peripheral T-cell lymphoma (rare cases)

H. Mast cell disease

I. Spindle-cell sarcoma (GIST).

Not shown: seminoma.

25. **EBV/EBER expression (Figure 14.25):**
   A. EBV-associated lymphadenitis
   B. Posttransplant polymorphic B-cell lymphoma
   C. Senile EBV⁺ large B-cell lymphoma
   D. Lymphomatoid granulomatosis
   E. Plasmablastic lymphoma
   F. Hodgkin lymphoma, classical
   G. Burkitt lymphoma (HIV⁺ patient)
   H. B-cells in angioimmunoblastic T-cell lymphoma
   I. Extranodal T/NK-cell lymphoma, nasal type
   J. Posttransplant T-cell lymphoma
   K. Methotrexate-induced, EBV-associated B-cell lymphoproliferative disorder
   L. Nasopharyngeal carcinoma.

26. **Epithelial membrane antigen (EMA) expression in hematopoietic neoplasms (Figure 14.26):**
   A. Plasma cell myeloma
   B. Nodular lymphocyte-predominant Hodgkin lymphoma
   C. Anaplastic large cell lymphoma
   D. Richter's syndrome (rare cases)
   E. Acute erythroid leukemia (subset).

27. **TCRγδ⁺ neoplasms (Figure 14.27):**
   A. γδ T-cell lymphoma, peripheral blood
   B. Enteropathy-type T-cell lymphoma

C. Subcutaneous, panniculitis-like T-cell lymphoma

D. γδ T-LGL leukemia.

28. **HHV-8⁺ lesions (Figure 14.28):**
   A. Primary effusion lymphoma
   B. Kaposi's sarcoma
   C. Castleman's disease (subset)
   D. Plasmablastic lymphoma associated with multicentric Castleman's disease.

29. **Ki-67 (MIB-1) expression (Figure 14.29):**
   A. Reactive lymph node with numerous Ki-67⁺ cells within germinal center
   B. Follicular lymphoma with scattered, haphazardly distributed Ki-67⁺ cells
   C. B-small lymphocytic lymphoma with occasional Ki-67⁺ cells
   D. Mantle cell lymphoma with rare Ki-67⁺ cells
   E. Diffuse large B-cell lymphoma (high grade) with numerous Ki-67⁺ cells (~70%)
   F. Burkitt lymphoma with virtually all cells expressing Ki-67.

30. **Pax-5 expression (Figure 14.30):**
   A. Diffuse large B-cell lymphoma
   B. Gastric large B-cell lymphoma with unusual lack of CD20
   C. Burkitt lymphoma
   D. Plasmablastic lymphoma (subset)
   E. Small cell carcinoma (subset)
   F. Precursor B-lymphoblastic lymphoma/leukemia
   G. Plasma cell neoplasm (subset)
   H. Hodgkin lymphoma, classical (dim expression)
   I. Nodular lymphocyte-predominant Hodgkin lymphoma.

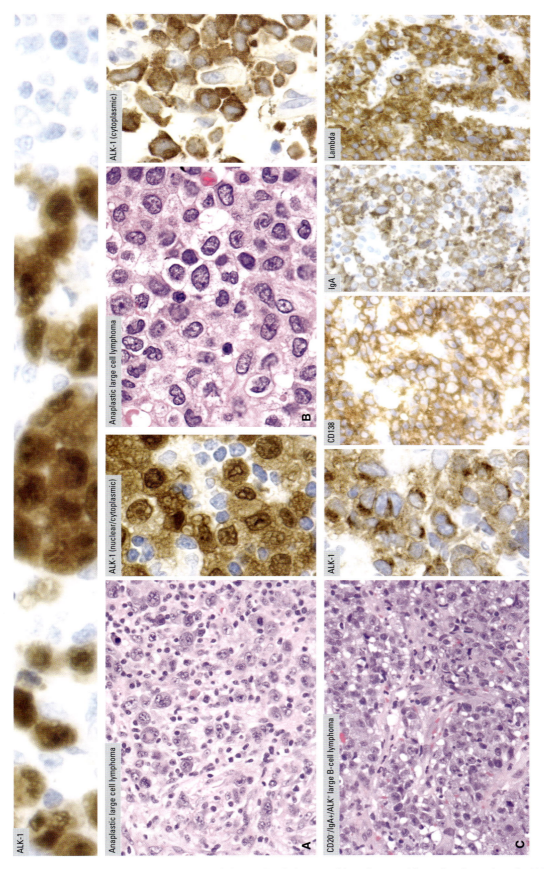

Figure 14.1 ALK-1 expression – differential diagnosis. (**A**) Anaplastic large cell lymphoma with nuclear/cytoplasmic ALK expression. (**B**) Anaplastic large cell lymphoma with cytoplasmic ALK expression. (**C**) Diffuse large B-cell lymphoma with ALK expression

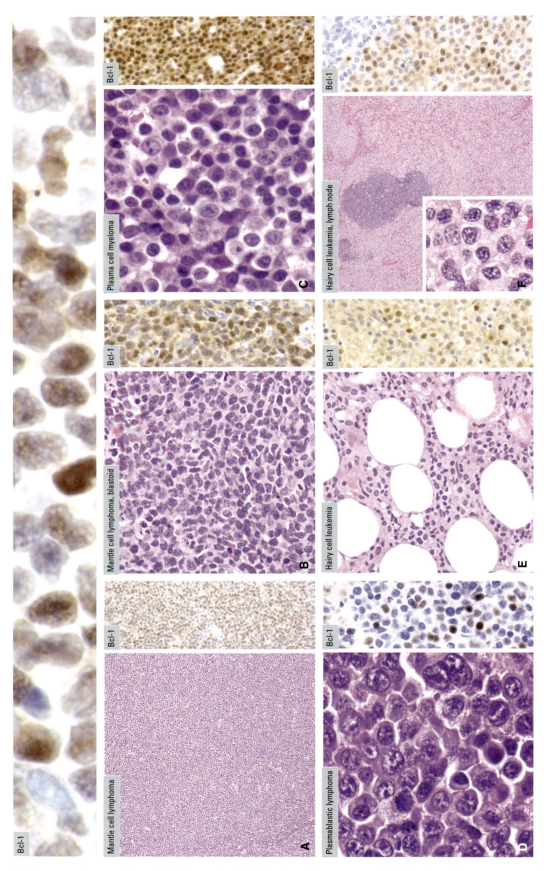

Figure 14.2   Bcl-1 expression – differential diagnosis. (**A**) Mantle cell lymphoma. (**B**) Mantle cell lymphoma, blastoid variant. (**C**) Plasma cell myeloma. (**D**) Plasmablastic lymphoma. (**E**) Hairy cell leukemia (bone marrow). (**F**) Hairy cell leukemia (lymph node)

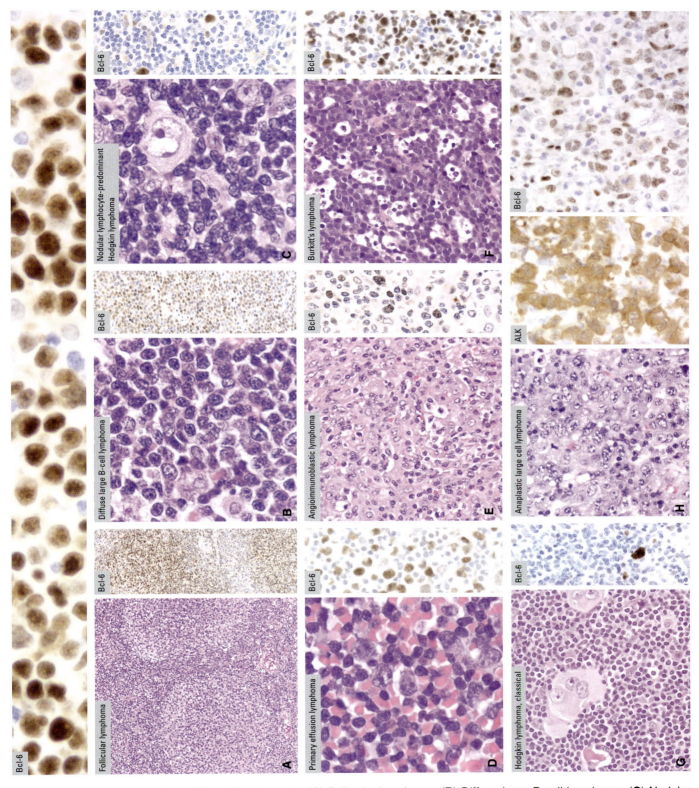

Figure 14.3   Bcl-6 expression – differential diagnosis. (**A**) Follicular lymphoma. (**B**) Diffuse large B-cell lymphoma. (**C**) Nodular lymphocyte-predominant Hodgkin lymphoma. (**D**) Primary effusion lymphoma. (**E**) Angioimmunoblastic T-cell lymphoma. (**F**) Burkitt lymphoma. (**G**) Classical Hodgkin lymphoma. (**H**) Anaplastic large cell lymphoma

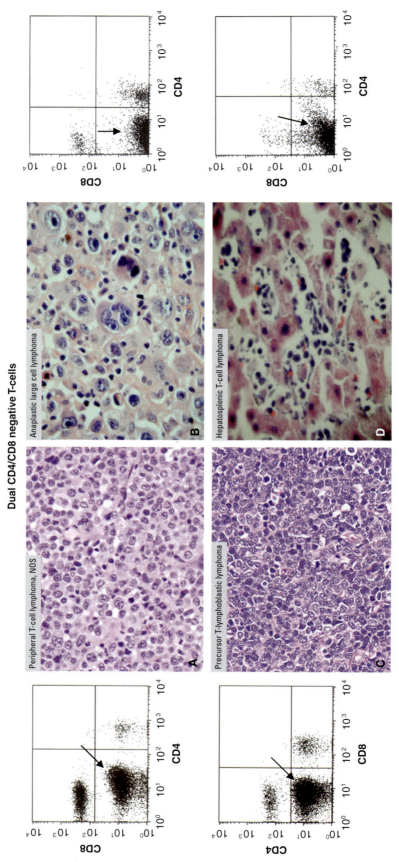

Figure 14.4   CD4/CD8: dual CD4/CD8 negative expression (differential diagnosis). (**A**) Peripheral T-cell lymphoma. (**B**) Anaplastic large cell lymphoma. (**C**) Precursor T-lymphoblastic lymphoma. (**D**) Hepatosplenic T-cell lymphoma

CD4 to CD8 ratio within normal range

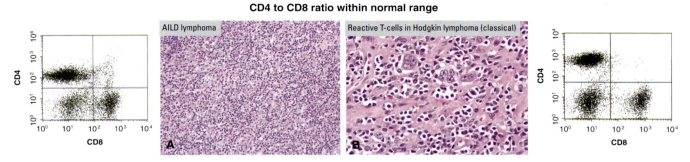

Figure 14.5 CD4/CD8: CD4:CD8 ratio within normal range (differential diagnosis). (**A**) Angioimmunoblastic T-cell lymphoma. (**B**) Reactive T-cells in Hodgkin lymphoma

Dual CD4/CD8 positive T-cells

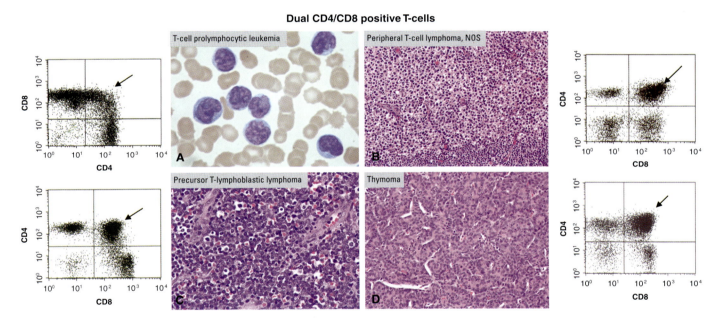

Figure 14.6 CD4/CD8: dual CD4/CD8 expression (differential diagnosis). (**A**) T-cell prolymphocytic leukemia. (**B**) Peripheral T-cell lymphoma. (**C**) Precursor T-lymphoblastic lymphoma. (**D**) Thymoma

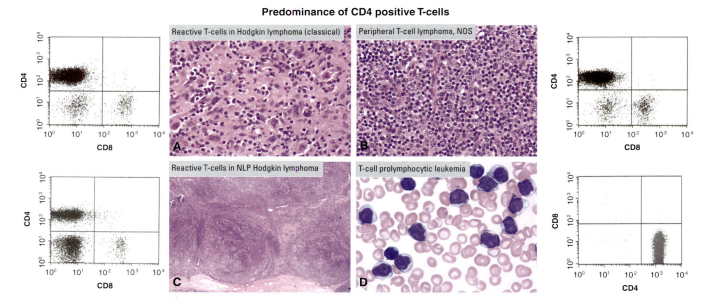

Figure 14.7   CD4/CD8: Predominance of CD4[+] T-cells (differential diagnosis). (**A**) Reactive T-cells in classical Hodgkin lymphoma. (**B**) Peripheral T-cell lymphoma. (**C**) Reactive T-cells in nodular lymphocyte-predominant Hodgkin lymphoma. (**D**) T-prolymphocytic leukemia

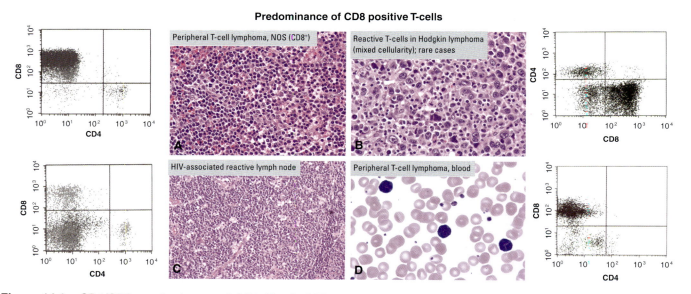

Figure 14.8   CD4/CD8: predominance of CD8[+] T-cells (differential diagnosis). (**A**) Peripheral T-cell lymphoma. (**B**) Reactive T-cells in classical Hodgkin lymphoma. (**C**) HIV-associated reactive lymphadenitis. (**D**) Peripheral T-cell lymphoma, blood

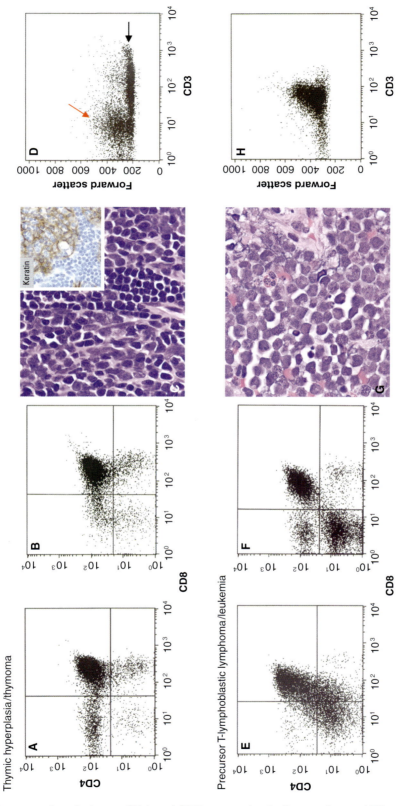

Figure 14.9   CD4/CD8: comparison between CD4 and CD8 expression in thymocytes and T-lymphoblasts. Thymocytes from both thymic hyperplasia and thymoma coexpress CD4 and CD8 (**A** and **B**). There is gradual transition of the expression of CD4 and CD8 from CD4+/CD8− cells to CD4−/CD8+ cells, with the majority of cells coexpressing both antigens. T-lymphoblasts which are dual CD4/CD8 positive show cohesive clusters of cells coexpressing both antigens (**E** and **F**). Residual (benign) small T-cells, when present, form separate minute populations of either CD4+ cells or CD8+ cells (**F**). Thymocytes display typical variable (smeared) expression of surface CD3 (**D**, black arrow). Additionally, there is a small population of larger T-cells, which are CD3− (**D**, red arrow). T-lymphoblasts show cohesive group of CD3+ cells (**H**). (**C**) Thymoma. (**G**) T-lymphoblastic lymphoma

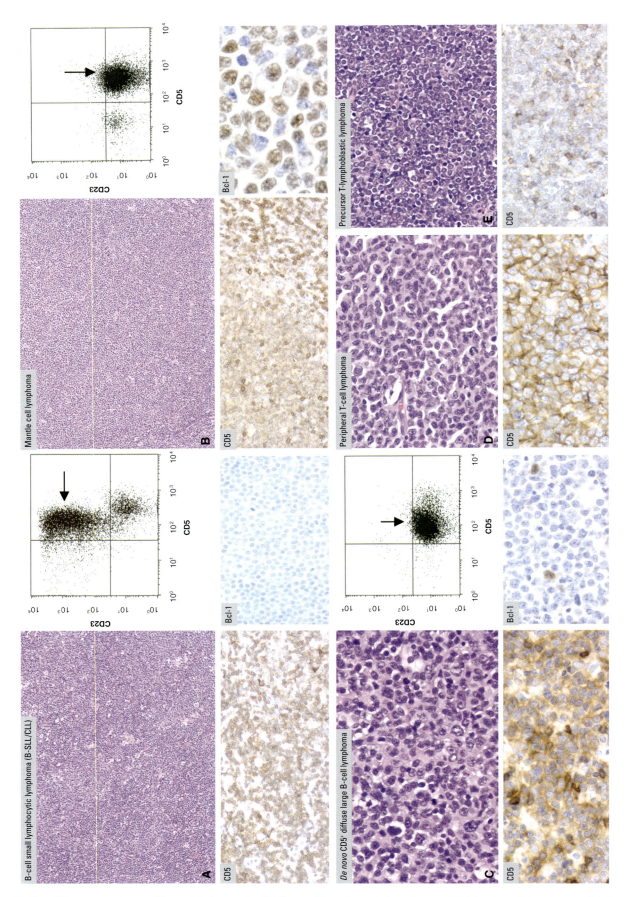

Figure 14.10 CD5 expression – differential diagnosis. (**A**) B-small lymphocytic lymphoma. (**B**) Mantle cell lymphoma. (**C**) *De novo* diffuse large B-cell lymphoma. (**D**) Peripheral T-cell lymphoma. (**E**) Precursor T-lymphoblastic lymphoma. (**F**) Benign B-cells in reactive lymph node infant. (**G**) Intavascular large B-cell lymphoma. (**H**) Diffuse large B-cell lymphoma with CD5 and CD10 expression

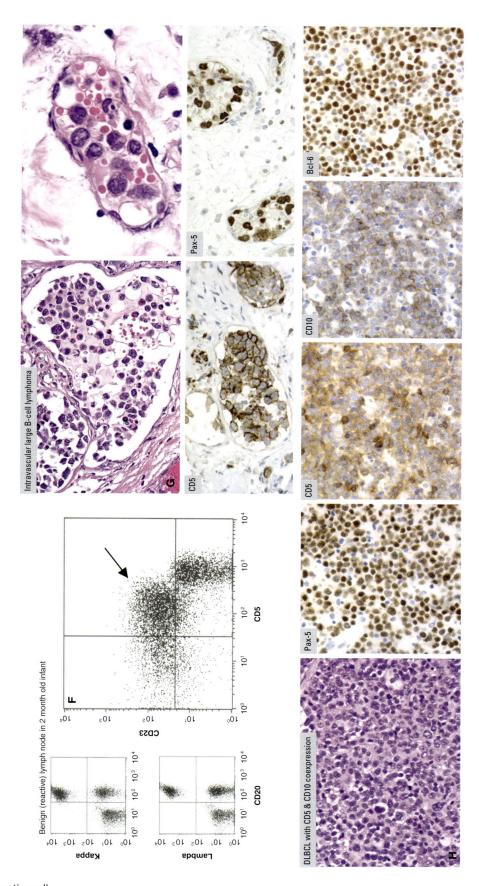

Figure 14.10 *(Continued)*

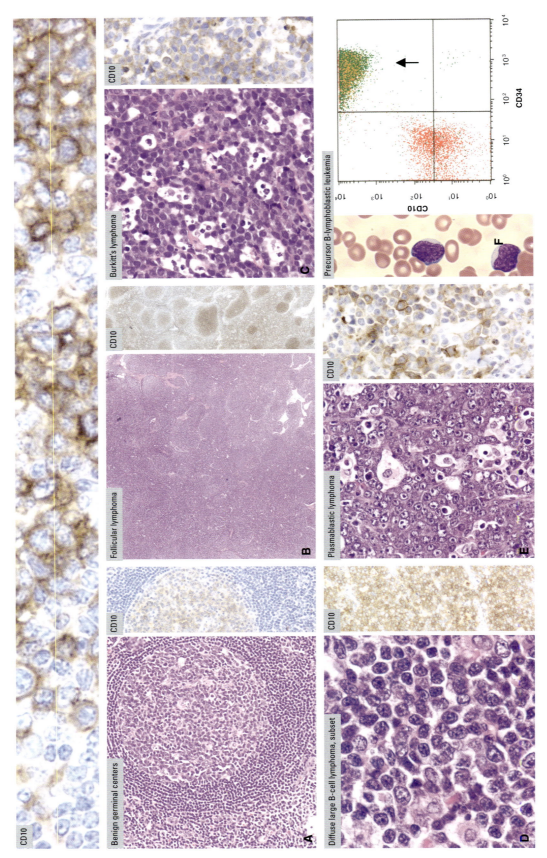

Figure 14.11   CD10 expression – differential diagnosis. (**A**) Benign germinal centers. (**B**) Follicular lymphoma. (**C**) Burkitt lymphoma. (**D**) Diffuse large B-cell lymphoma. (**E**) Plasmablastic lymphoma. (**F**) Precursor B-lymphoblastic lymphoma/leukemia. (**G**) Mantle cell lymphoma. (**H**) Hairy cell leukemia. (**I**) Angioimmunoblastic T-cell lymphoma. (**J**) Precursor T-lymphoblastic lymphoma/leukemia. (**K**) Malignant melanoma. (**L**) Multiple myeloma. (**M**) Acute monocytic leukemia

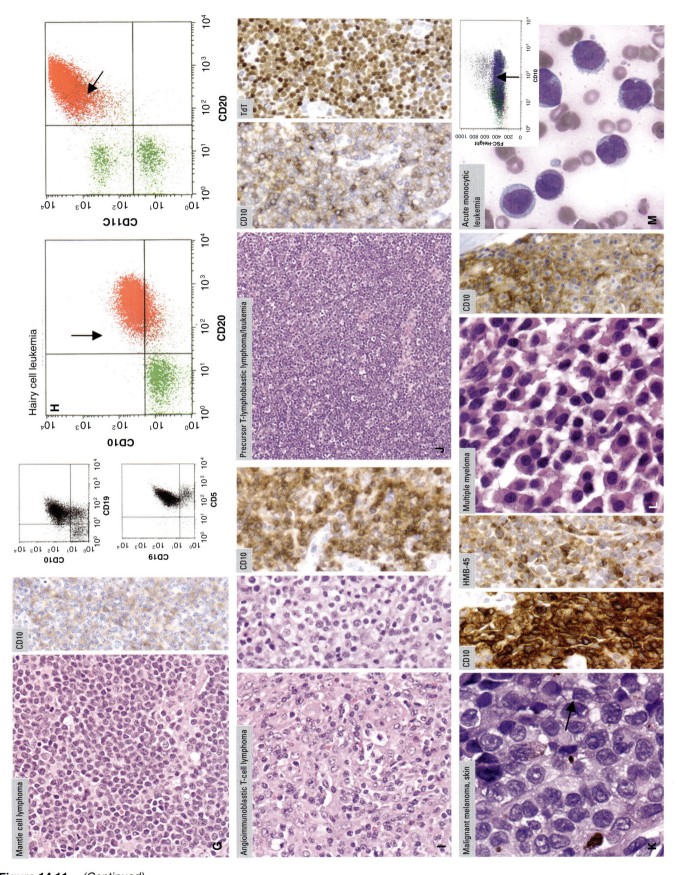

Figure 14.11   *(Continued)*

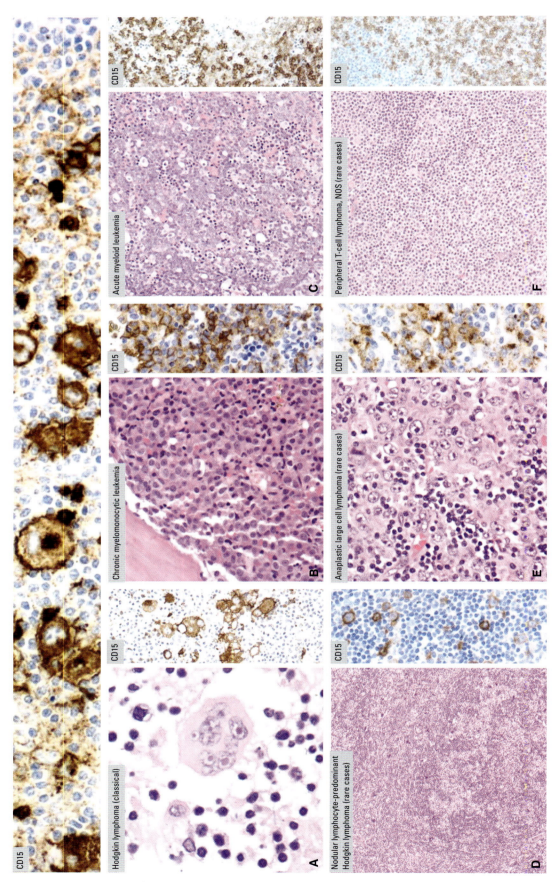

Figure 14.12   CD15 expression – differential diagnosis. (**A**) Hodgkin lymphoma (classical). (**B**) Chronic myelomonocytic leukemia. (**C**) Acute myeloid leukemia. (**D**) Nodular lymphocyte-predominant Hodgkin lymphoma (rare cases fixed in B5). (**E**) Anaplastic large cell lymphoma (rare cases). (**F**) Peripheral T-cell lymphoma (rare cases)

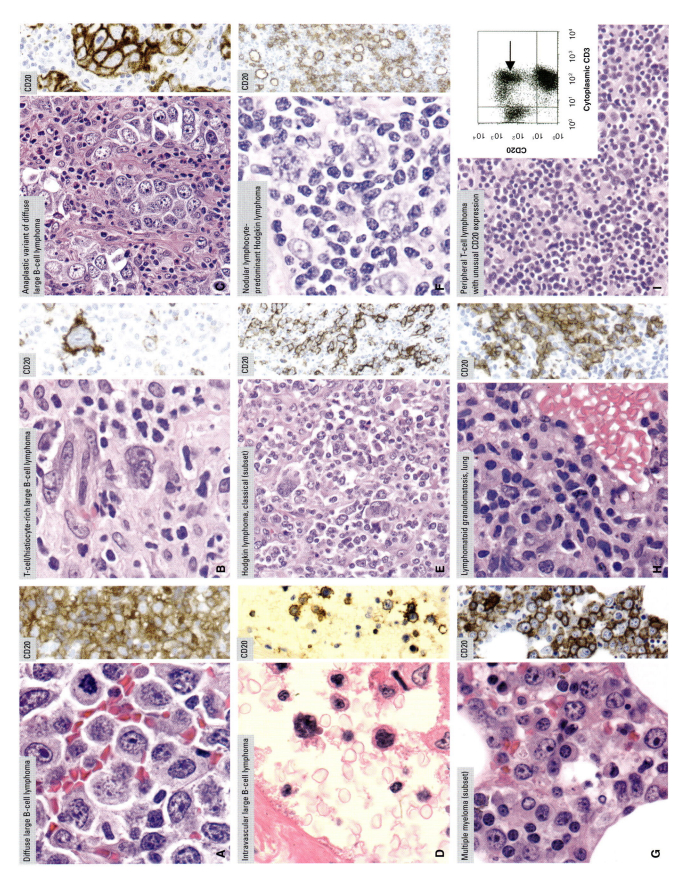

Figure 14.13 CD20 expression – differential diagnosis. (**A**) Diffuse large B-cell lymphoma. (**B**) T-cell/histiocyte-rich large B-cell lymphoma. (**C**) Anaplastic variant of diffuse large B-cell lymphoma. (**D**) Intravascular large B-cell lymphoma. (**E**) Classical Hodgkin lymphoma. (**F**) Nodular lymphocyte-predominant Hodgkin lymphoma. (**G**) Multiple myeloma. (**H**) Lymphomatoid granulomatosis, lung. (**I**) Peripheral T-cell lymphoma with unusual CD20 expression

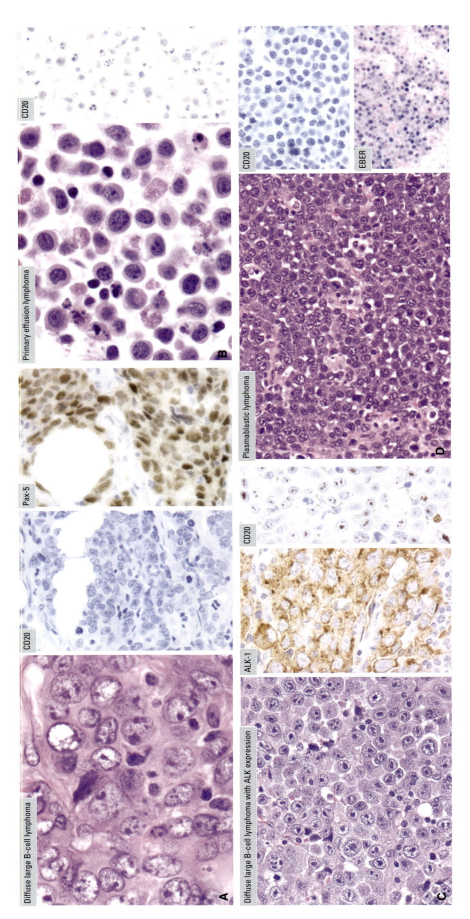

Figure 14.14   B-cell lymphomas with negative CD20 expression (differential diagnosis). (**A**) Diffuse large B-cell lymphoma (rare cases). (**B**) Primary effusion lymphoma. (**C**) Diffuse large B-cell lymphoma with ALK expression. (**D**) Plasmablastic lymphoma

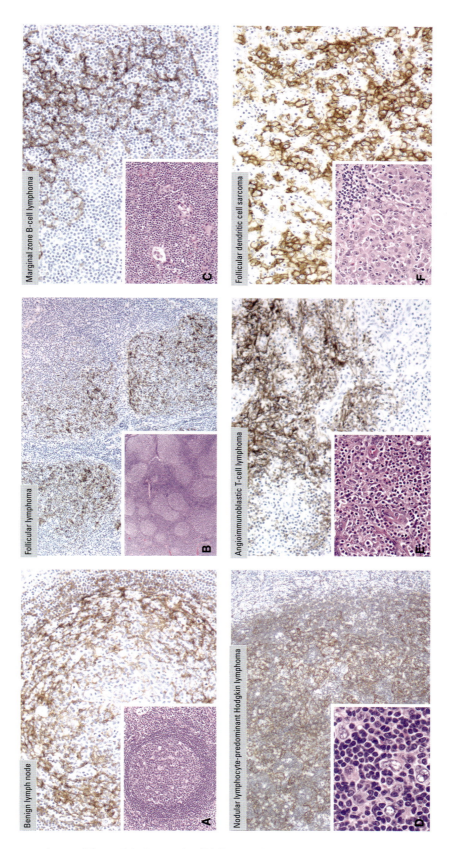

Figure 14.15 CD21 expression – differential diagnosis. (**A**) Benign lymph node: intact meshwork of follicular dendritic cells visualized by CD21 immunohistochemical staining. (**B**) Follicular lymphoma: neoplastic follicle with expanded, delicate follicular dendritic meshwork. (**C**) Marginal zone lymphoma: partially preserved residual follicles with focal distortion of dendritic cell meshwork. (**D**) Mantle cell lymphoma: positive staining of B-cells and follicular dendritic cells. (**E**) Angioimmunoblastic T-cell lymphoma: expanded and distorted pattern of follicular dendritic cell meshwork. Neoplastic T-cells are negative for CD21. (**F**) Follicular dendritic cell sarcoma

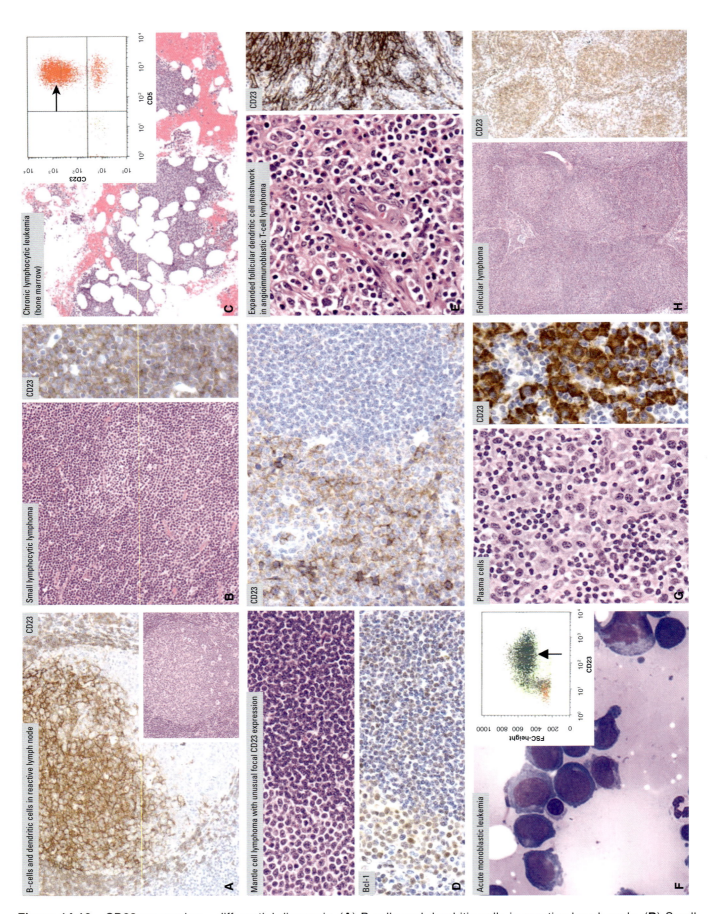

Figure 14.16   CD23 expression – differential diagnosis. (**A**) B-cells and dendritic cells in reactive lymph node. (**B**) Small lymphocytic lymphoma. (**C**) Chronic lymphocytic leukemia. (**D**) Mantle cell lymphoma (subset). (**E**) Follicular dendritic cell meshwork in angioimmunoblastic T-cell lymphoma. (**F**) Acute monoblastic leukemia. (**G**) Plasma cells. (**H**) Follicular lymphoma

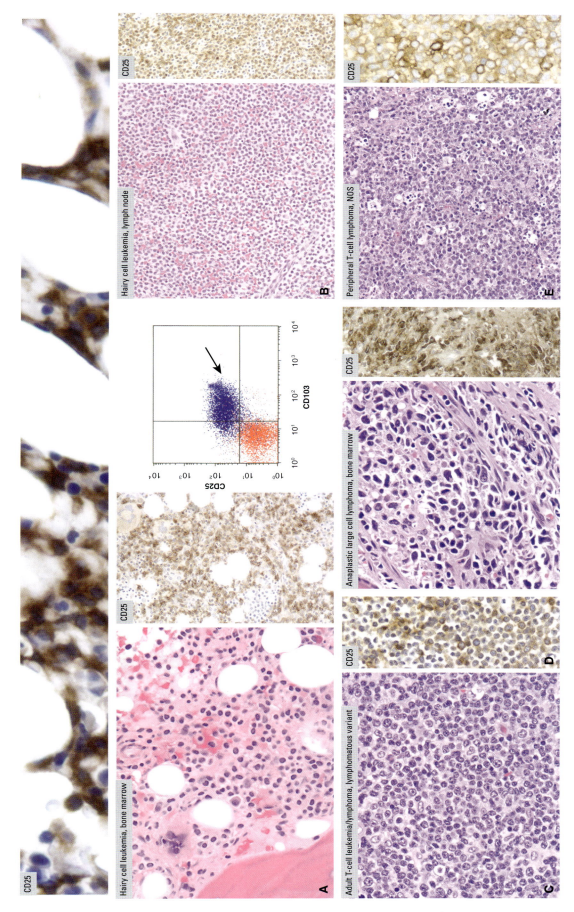

Figure 14.17   CD25 expression – differential diagnosis. (**A** and **B**) Hairy cell leukemia (**A**, bone marrow; **B**, lymph node). (**C**) Adult T-cell leukemia/lymphoma (lymph node). (**D**) Anaplastic large cell lymphoma. (**E**) Peripheral T-cell lymphoma

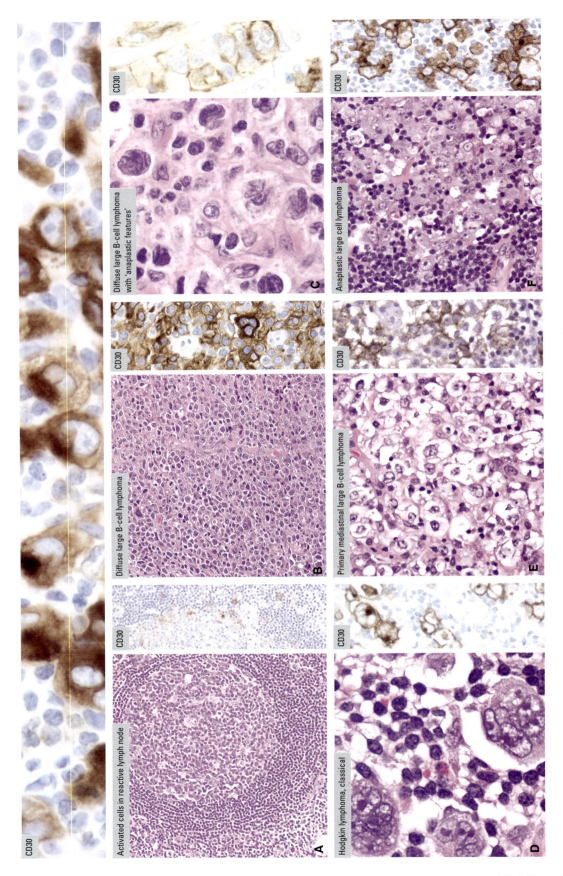

Figure 14.18 CD30 expression – differential diagnosis. (**A**) Activated cells in reactive lymph node. (**B**) Diffuse large B-cell lymphoma. (**C**) Diffuse large B-cell lymphoma, anaplastic variant. (**D**) Classical Hodgkin lymphoma. (**E**) Primary mediastinal large B-cell lymphoma. (**F**) Anaplastic large cell lymphoma. (**G**) NK/T-cell lymphoma, nasal type. (**H**) Enteropathy-type T-cell lymphoma. (**I**) Cutaneous anaplastic large cell lymphoma. (**J**) Plasma cell myeloma. (**K**) EBV-associated high-grade lymphoma in HIV⁺ patient

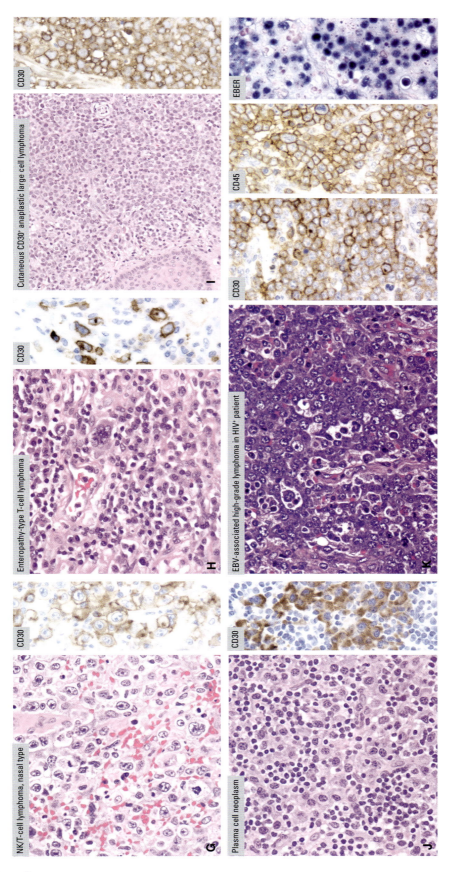

Figure 14.18   *(Continued)*

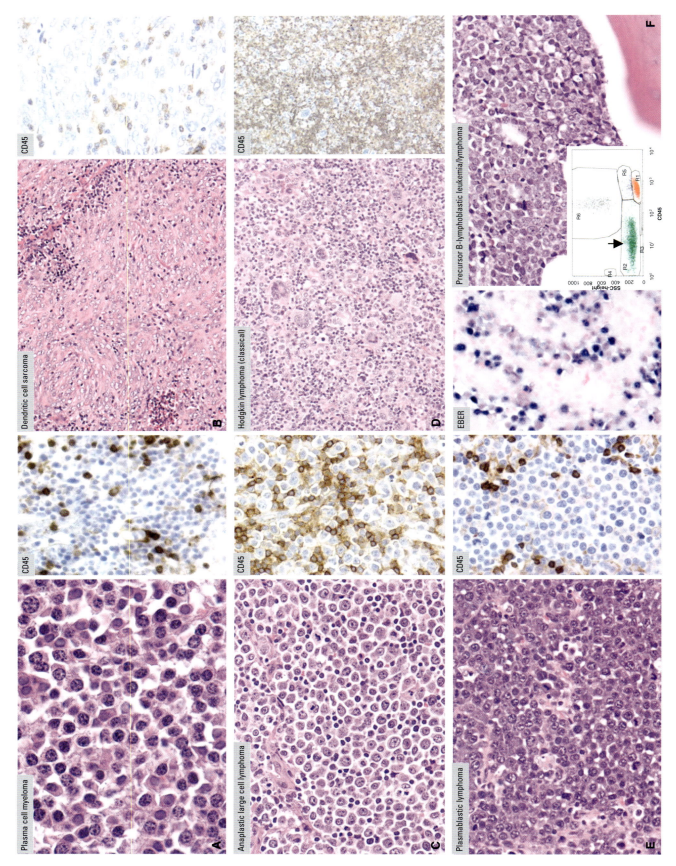

Figure 14.19   CD45: hematopoietic tumors with negative CD45 expression (differential diagnosis). (**A**) Plasma cell myeloma. (**B**) Dendritic cell sarcoma. (**C**) Anaplastic large cell lymphoma. (**D**) Classical Hodgkin lymphoma. (**E**) Plasmablastic lymphoma. (**F**) Precursor B-lymphoblastic leukemia/lymphoma

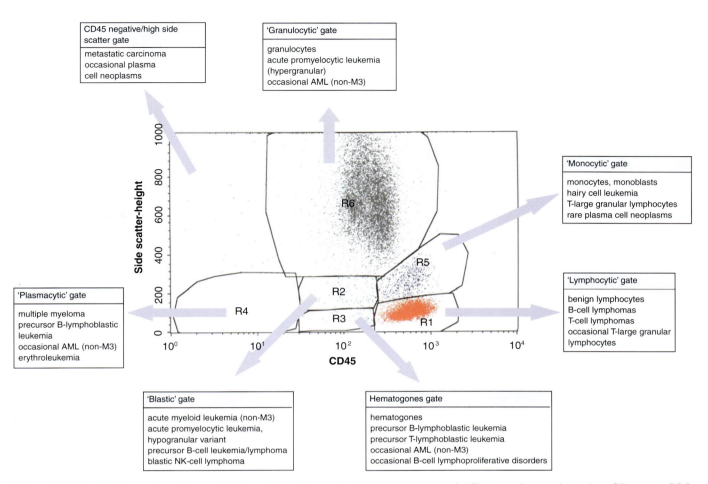

CD45 negative/high side scatter gate

metastatic carcinoma
occasional plasma
cell neoplasms

'Granulocytic' gate

granulocytes
acute promyelocytic leukemia
(hypergranular)
occasional AML (non-M3)

'Monocytic' gate

monocytes, monoblasts
hairy cell leukemia
T-large granular lymphocytes
rare plasma cell neoplasms

'Lymphocytic' gate

benign lymphocytes
B-cell lymphomas
T-cell lymphomas
occasional T-large granular
lymphocytes

'Plasmacytic' gate

multiple myeloma
precursor B-lymphoblastic
leukemia
occasional AML (non-M3)
erythroleukemia

'Blastic' gate

acute myeloid leukemia (non-M3)
acute promyelocytic leukemia,
hypogranular variant
precursor B-cell leukemia/lymphoma
blastic NK-cell lymphoma

Hematogones gate

hematogones
precursor B-lymphoblastic leukemia
precursor T-lymphoblastic leukemia
occasional AML (non-M3)
occasional B-cell lymphoproliferative disorders

Figure 14.20 CD45 versus orthogonal side scatter – flow cytometry. Localization of different cell types based on CD45 and SSC properties (scheme)

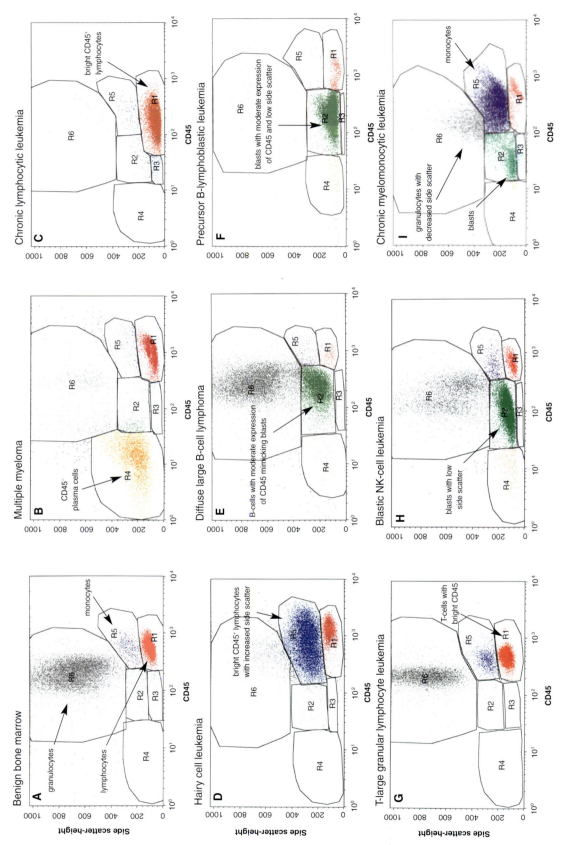

Figure 14.21 CD45 versus orthogonal side scatter – flow cytometry. (**A**) Benign sample of the bone marrow. (**B**) Multiple myeloma. (**C**) Chronic lymphocytic leukemia. (**D**) Hairy cell leukemia. (**E**) Diffuse large B-cell lymphoma. (**F**) Precursor B-lymphoblastic leukemia. (**G**) T-LGL leukemia. (**H**) Blastic NK-cell leukemia/lymphoma. (**I**) Chronic myelomonocytic leukemia. (**J**) CML (accelerated phase). (**K**) Acute myeloid leukemia. (**L**) Acute myelomonocytic leukemia. (**M**) Acute promyelocytic leukemia (hypergranular variant). (**N**) Acute promyelocytic leukemia (hypogranular variant). (**O**) Acute monocytic leukemia. (**P**) Acute myeloid leukemia with unusual side scatter. (**R**) Metastatic small cell carcinoma

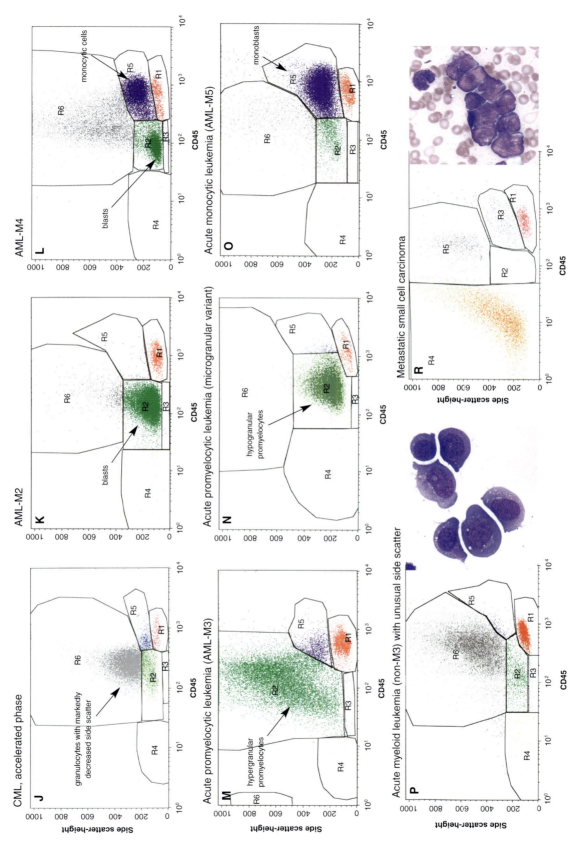

Figure 14.21   *(Continued)*

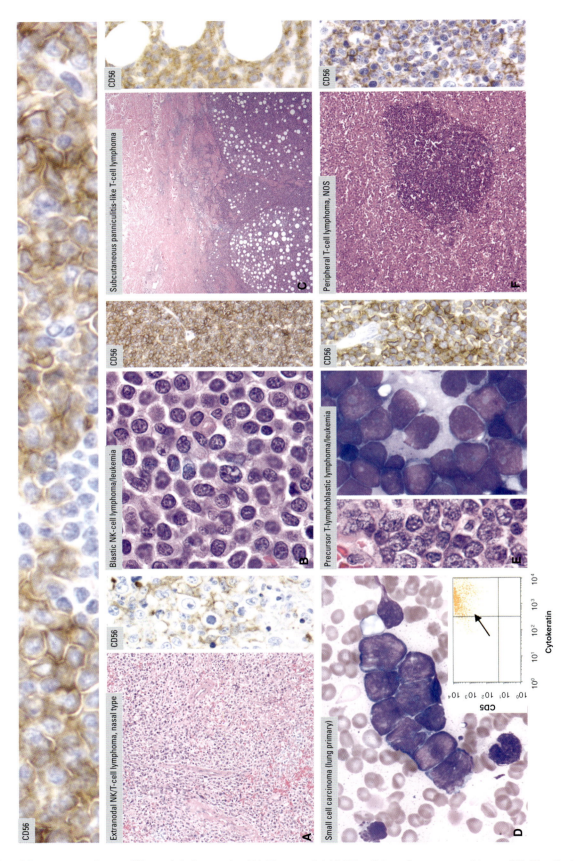

Figure 14.22   CD56 expression – differential diagnosis. (**A**) Extranodal NK/T-cell lymphoma, nasal type. (**B**) Blastic NK-cell lymphoma/leukemia. (**C**) Subcutaneous panniculitis-like T-cell lymphoma. (**D**) Small cell carcinoma. (**E**) Precursor T-lymphoblastic lymphoma/leukemia. (**F**) Peripheral T-cell lymphoma, NOS. (**G**) Plasmablastic lymphoma. (**H**) Multiple myeloma. (**I**) Large B-cell lymphoma (CD10+). (**J**) T-LGL leukemia. (**K**) Enteropathy-type T-cell lymphoma. (**L**) NK-LGL leukemia. (**M**) Acute myeloid leukemia. (**N**) Acute promyelocytic leukemia. (**O**) Acute monocytic leukemia

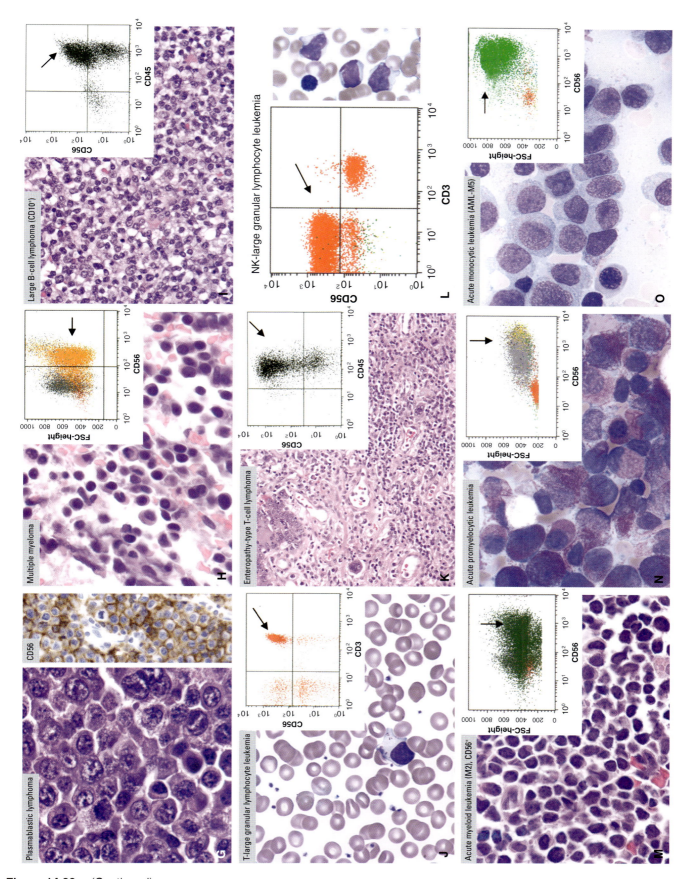

Figure 14.22 *(Continued)*

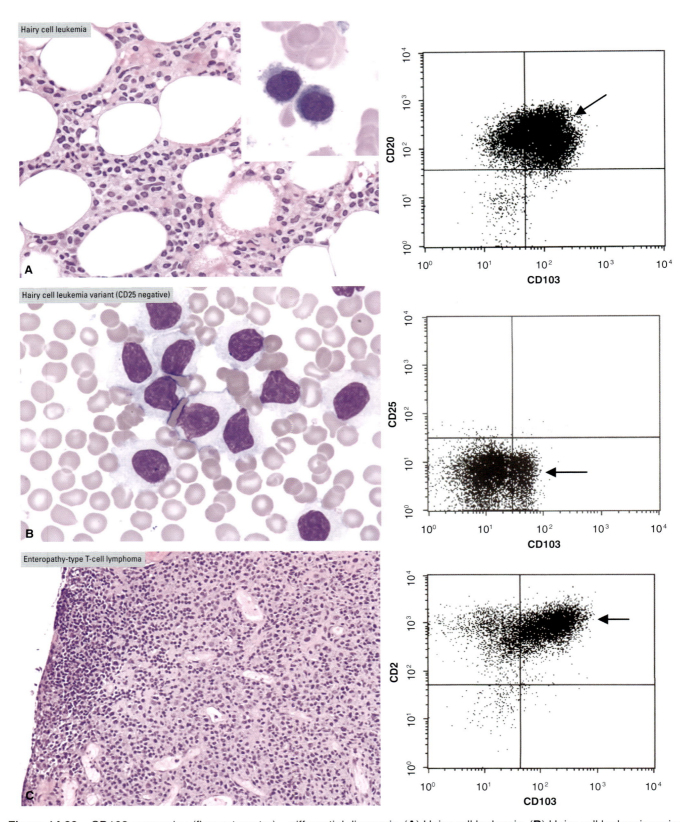

Figure 14.23 CD103 expression (flow cytometry) – cifferential diagnosis. (**A**) Hairy cell leukemia. (**B**) Hairy cell leukemia variant (CD25−). (**C**) Enteropathy-type T-cell lymphoma

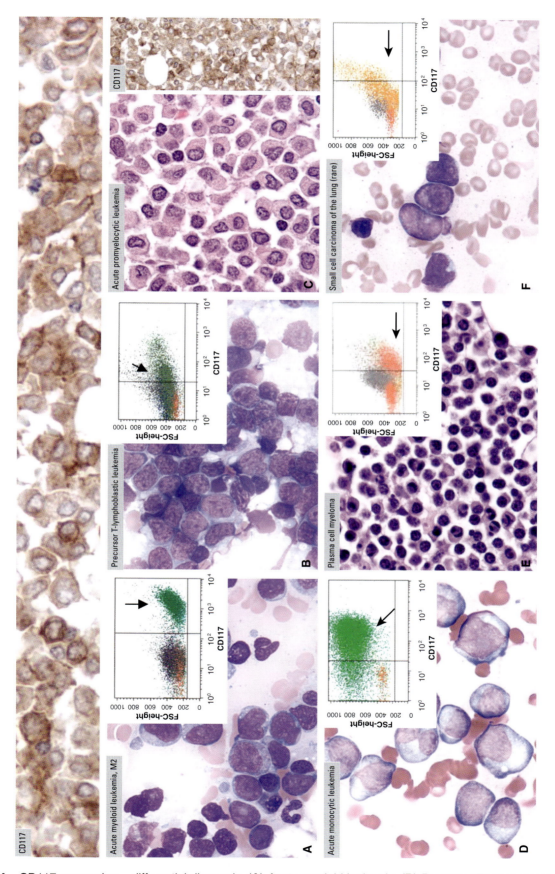

Figure 14.24   CD117 expression – differential diagnosis. (**A**) Acute myeloid leukemia. (**B**) Precursor T-lymphoblastic leukemia. (**C**) Acute promyelocytic leukemia. (**D**) Acute monoblastic leukemia. (**E**) Plasma cell myeloma. (**F**) Small cell carcinoma. (**G**) Peripheral T-cell lymphoma (CD8+). (**H**) Mast cell disease. (**I**) Spindle-cell sarcoma (GIST)

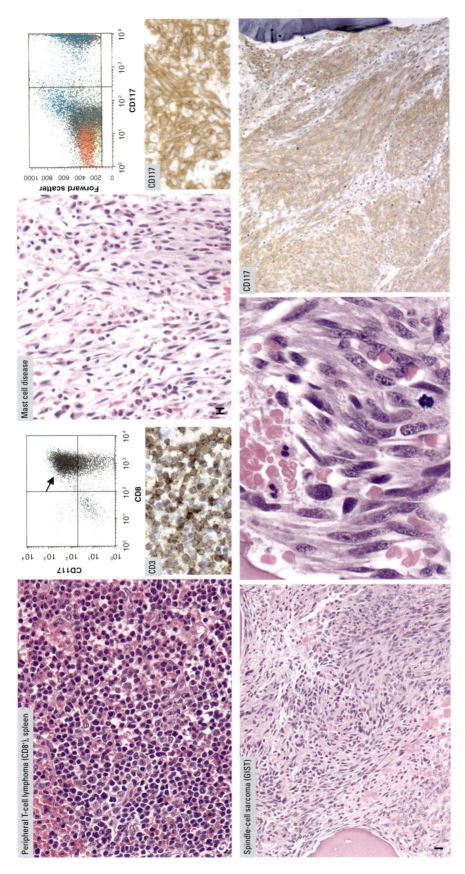

Figure 14.24 *(Continued)*

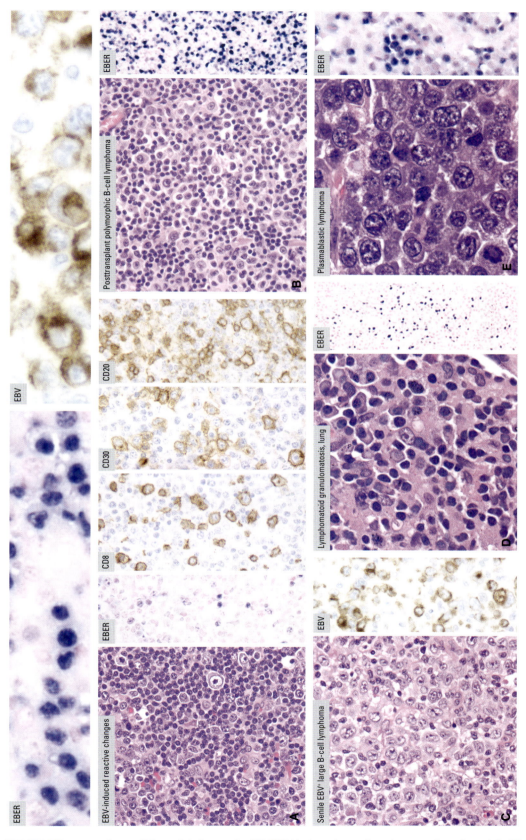

Figure 14.25   EBV/EBER expression – differential diagnosis. (**A**) EBV-induced reactive changes (lymph node). (**B**) Posttransplant polymorphic B-cell lymphoma. (**C**) Senile EBV⁺ large B-cell lymphoma. (**D**) Lymphomatoid granulomatosis, lung. (**E**) Plasmablastic lymphoma. (**F**) Hodgkin lymphoma, classical. (**G**) Burkitt lymphoma (HIV⁺ patient). (**H**) B-cells in angioimmunoblastic T-cell lymphoma. (**I**) NK/T-cell lymphoma, nasal type. (**J**) Posttransplant T-cell lymphoma. (**K**) Methotrexate-induced, EBV-associated B-cell lymphoproliferative disorder. (**L**) Nasopharyngeal carcinoma

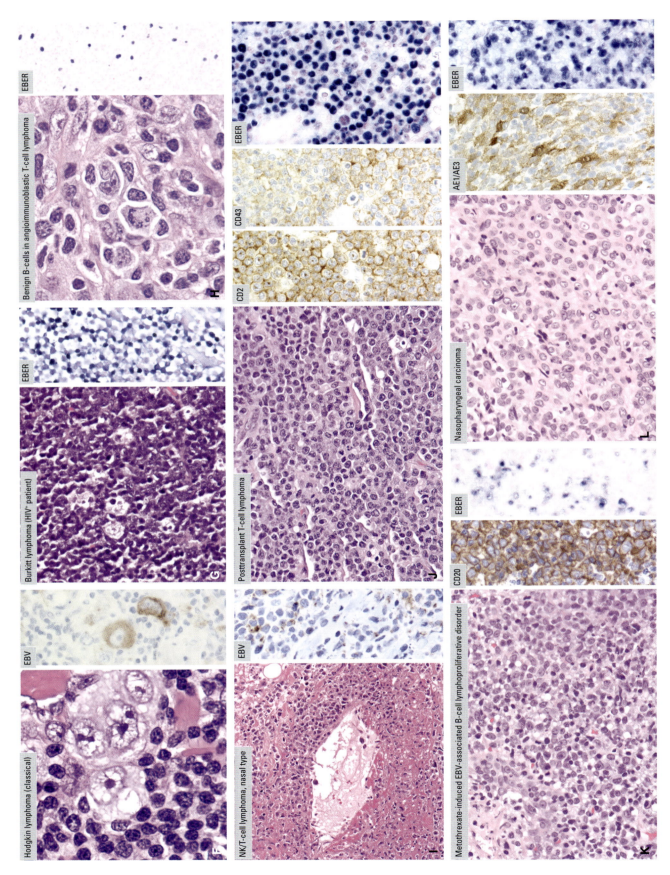

Figure 14.25   (*Continued*)

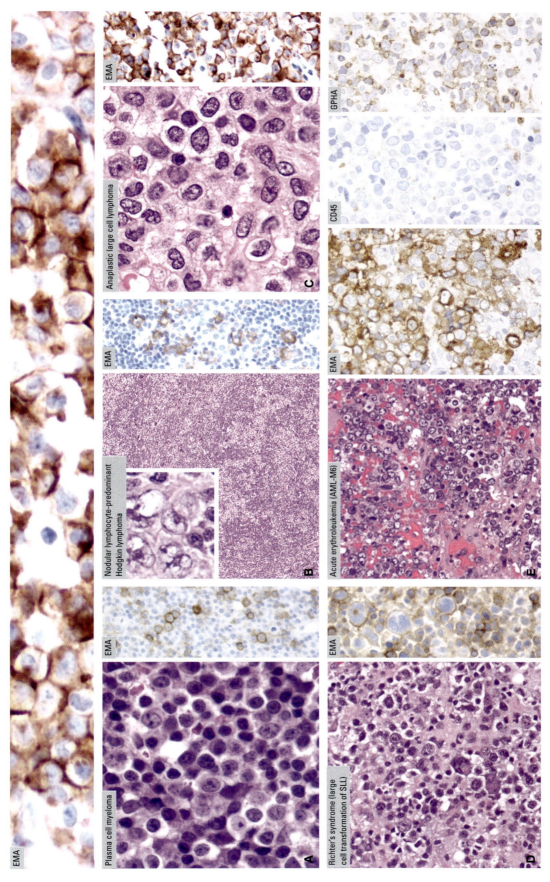

Figure 14.26 EMA expression – differential diagnosis. (**A**) Plasma cell myeloma. (**B**) Nodular lymphocyte-predominant Hodgkin lymphoma. (**C**) Anaplastic large cell lymphoma. (**D**) Richter's syndrome (large cell transformation of SLL/CLL). (**E**) Acute erythroid leukemia

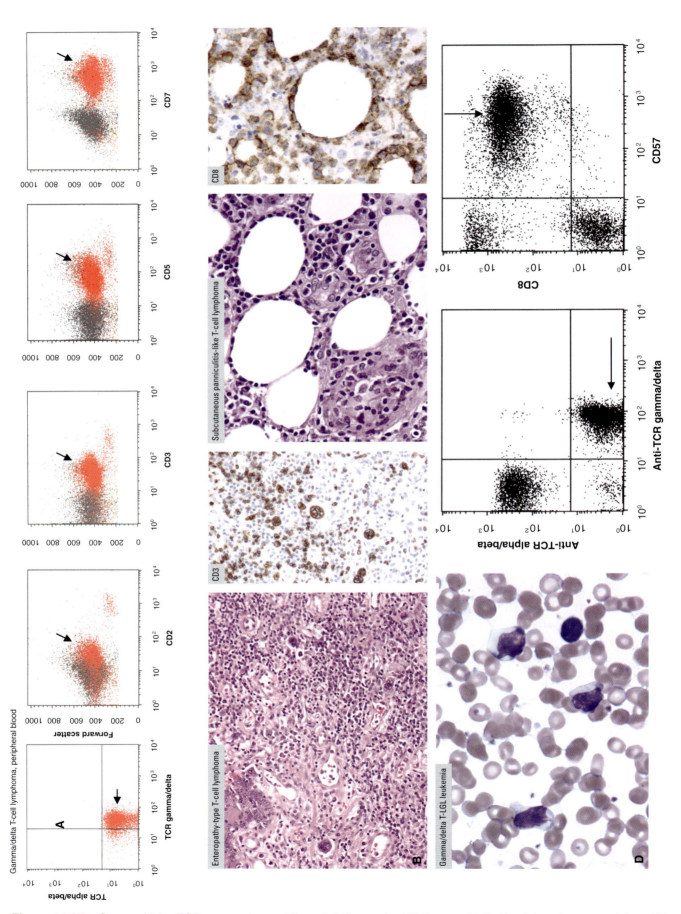

Figure 14.27 Gamma/delta TCR expression – differential diagnosis. (**A**) Gamma/delta T-cell lymphoma, peripheral blood. (**B**) Enteropathy-type T-cell lymphoma. (**C**) Subcutaneous panniculitis-like T-cell lymphoma. (**D**) Gamma/delta LGL leukemia

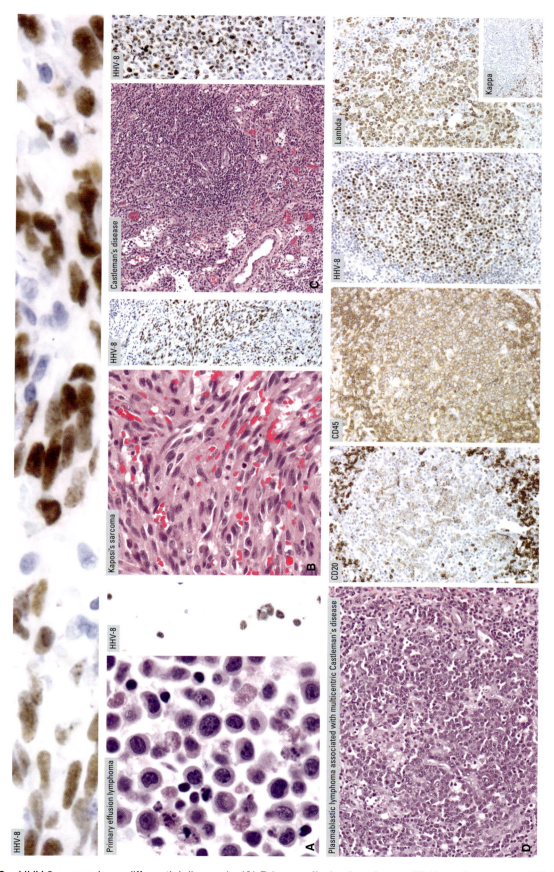

Figure 14.28   HHV-8 expression – differential diagnosis. (**A**) Primary effusion lymphoma. (**B**) Kaposi's sarcoma. (**C**) Castleman's disease. (**D**) Plasmablastic lymphoma associated with multicentric Castleman's disease

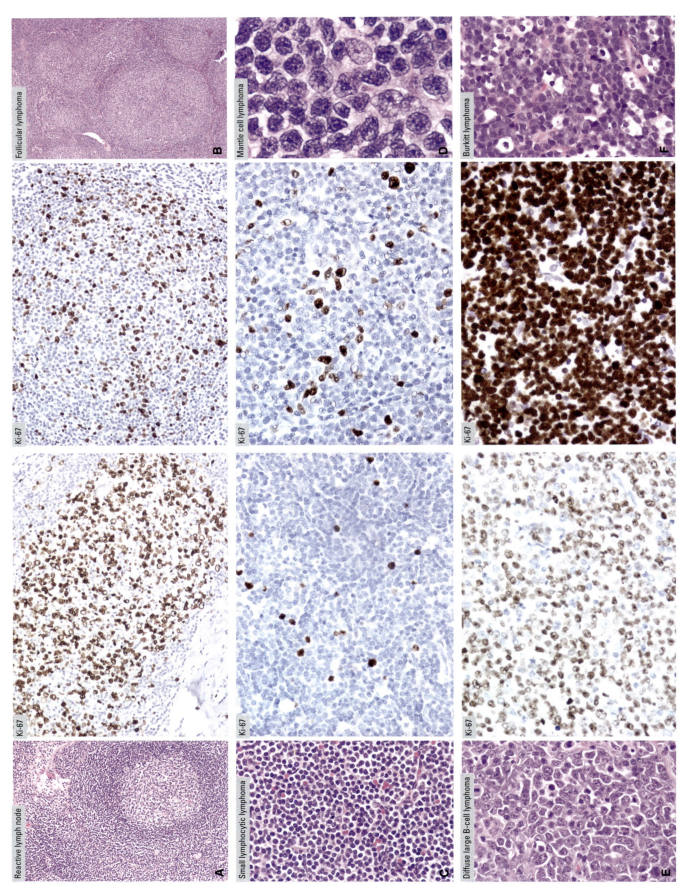

Figure 14.29   Ki-67 (MIB-1) expression (pattern) – differential diagnosis. (**A**) Reactive lymph node. (**B**) Follicular lymphoma. (**C**) Small lymphocytic lymphoma. (**D**) Mantle cell lymphoma. (**E**) Diffuse large B-cell lymphoma. (**F**) Burkitt lymphoma

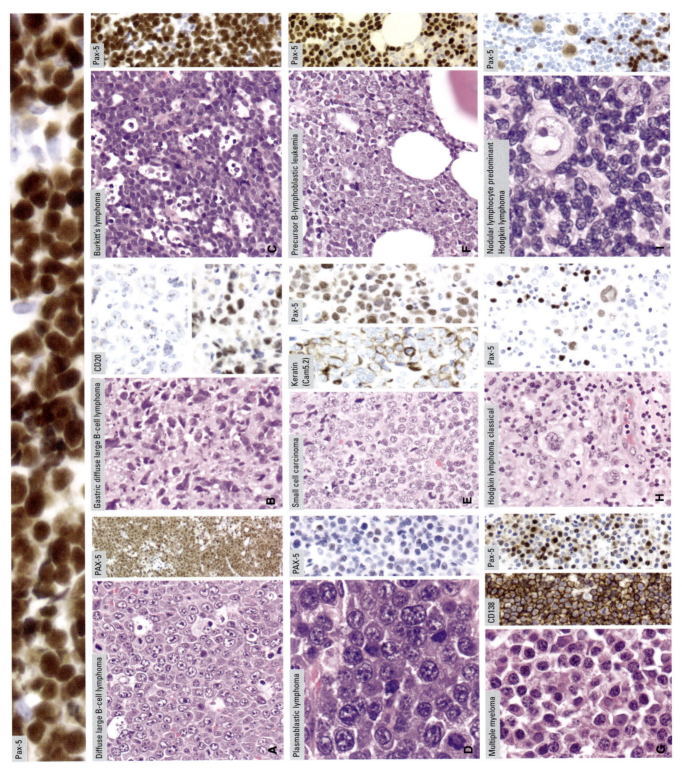

Figure 14.30   Pax-5 expression – differential diagnosis. (**A**) Diffuse large B-cell lymphoma. (**B**) Gastric large B-cell lymphoma (CD20⁻). (**C**) Burkitt lymphoma. (**D**) Plasmablastic lymphoma. (**E**) Small cell carcinoma. (**F**) Precursor B-lymphoblastic lymphoma/leukemia. (**G**) Multiple myeloma. (**H**) Classical Hodgkin lymphoma. (**I**) Nodular lymphocyte-predominant Hodgkin lymphoma

CHAPTER 15

Differential diagnosis – localization

1. **Body cavity:**
   - Anaplastic large cell lymphoma (Figure 15.1)
   - Diffuse large B-cell lymphoma (Figure 15.2)
   - Diffuse large B-cell lymphoma with anaplastic features (Figure 15.3)
   - Plasma cell neoplasm (Figure 15.4)
   - Primary effusion lymphoma (Figure 15.5)
   - Primary effusion lymphoma with aberrant expression of CD3 (Figure 15.6)
   - T-cell prolymphocytic leukemia (Figure 15.7).

2. **Lung:**
   - Anaplastic large cell lymphoma (Figure 15.8)
   - Diffuse large B-cell lymphoma (Figure 15.9)
   - Hodgkin lymphoma, classical (Figure 15.10)
   - Langerhans cell histiocytosis (Figure 15.11)
   - Marginal zone B-cell lymphoma (Figure 15.12)
   - Extranodal T/NK-cell lymphoma, nasal type (Figure 15.13)
   - Nodular lymphoid hyperplasia (Figure 15.14).

3. **Mediastinum:**
   - Diffuse large B-cell lymphoma (Figure 15.15)
   - Hodgkin lymphoma (classical) within hyperplastic thymus (Figure 15.16)
   - Nodular lymphocyte-predominant Hodgkin lymphoma (Figure 15.17)
   - Plasmacytoma (Figure 15.18)
   - Precursor T-lymphoblastic lymphoma (Figure 15.19)
   - Thymic hyperplasia (Figure 15.20)
   - Thymoma with predominance of epithelial elements (Figure 15.21)
   - Thymoma with predominance of lymphoid elements (Figure 15.22).

4. **Salivary gland:**
   - Benign sialadenitis with lymphoepithelial lesions (Figure 15.23)
   - Benign lymphoepithelial cyst (Figure 15.24)
   - Warthin's tumor (Figure 15.25)
   - B-small lymphocytic lymphoma/chronic lymphocytic leukemia (Figure 15.26)
   - Marginal zone B-cell lymphoma (Figure 15.27)
   - Follicular lymphoma (Figure 15.28)
   - Diffuse large B-cell lymphoma (Figure 15.29).

5. **Skin:**
   - Reactive lymphoid infiltrate (Figure 15.30)
   - B-small lymphocytic lymphoma with plasmacytic differentiation (Figure 15.31)
   - Marginal zone B-cell lymphoma (Figure 15.32)
   - Mantle cell lymphoma (Figure 15.33)
   - Follicular lymphoma (Figure 15.34)
   - Diffuse large B-cell lymphoma (Figure 15.35)
   - Plasmacytoma (Figure 15.36)
   - Mycosis fungoides (Figure 15.37)
   - Primary cutaneous anaplastic large cell lymphoma (Figure 15.38)
   - Rosai–Dorfman disease (Figure 15.39)
   - Poorly differentiated carcinoma with T-cell-rich infiltrate (Figure 15.40).

6. **Spleen:**
   - Gross characteristics of splenic tumors (Figure 15.41)
   - B-small lymphocytic lymphoma/chronic lymphocytic leukemia (Figure 15.42)
   - Splenic marginal zone B-cell lymphoma (Figure 15.43)
   - Mantle cell lymphoma (Figure 15.44)

- Follicular lymphoma (Figure 15.45)
- Diffuse large B-cell lymphoma (Figure 15.46)
- Peripheral T-cell lymphoma (Figure 15.47)
  - A. Normal spleen
  - B, C. Spleen with congestion
  - D–F. Three examples of peripheral T-cell lymphoma, unspecified
- Hepatosplenic T-cell lymphoma (Figure 15.48)
- Extranodal T/NK-cell lymphoma, nasal type (Figure 15.49)
- Hodgkin lymphoma, classical (Figure 15.50)
- Myeloid metaplasia in patient with chronic idiopathic myelofibrosis (Figure 15.51)
- Blast crisis (extramedullary myeloid tumor) in patient with history of chronic myeloproliferative disorder (Figure 15.52)
- Hemophagocytic syndrome (Figure 15.53).

7. **Stomach:**
   - Chronic active gastritis with *H. pylori* (Figure 15.54)
   - Marginal zone B-cell lymphoma with lymphoepithelial lesions and aberrant expression of CD43 (Figure 15.55)
   - Mantle cell lymphoma (Figure 15.56)
   - Follicular lymphoma (Figure 15.57)
   - Diffuse large B-cell lymphoma (Figure 15.58)
   - Burkitt lymphoma (Figure 15.59)
   - Monotypic plasma cell infiltrate (plasmacytoma versus plasma cell component of MALT lymphoma) (Figure 15.60)
   - Diffuse large B-cell lymphoma with ALK expression (Figure 15.61)
   - Anaplastic large B-cell lymphoma (Figure 15.62)
   - Peripheral T-cell lymphoma, unspecified (Figure 15.63).

8. **Small and large intestine:**
   - Mantle cell lymphoma, duodenum (Figure 15.64)
   - Follicular lymphoma, duodenum (Figure 15.65)
   - Benign lymphoid infiltrate, terminal ileum (Figure 15.66; note CD43 expression by benign B-cells)
   - Follicular lymphoma, terminal ileum and rectum (Figure 15.67)
   - Marginal zone B-cell lymphoma, large intestine (Figure 15.68)
   - Lymphomatous polyposis, large intestine (Figure 15.69)
   - Mantle cell lymphoma, appendix (Figure 15.70)
   - Diffuse large B-cell lymphoma imitating grossly lymphomatous polyposis, large intestine (Figure 15.71)
   - Burkitt lymphoma, large intestine (Figure 15.72)
   - Peripheral T-cell lymphoma, small intestine (Figure 15.73)
   - Enteropathy-type T-cell lymphoma, small intestine (Figure 15.74)

     - A–C. Enteropathy-type T-cell lymphoma with diffuse monomorphic lymphoid infiltrate
     - D–H. Enteropathy-type T-cell lymphoma with focal 'anaplastic' features and Reed–Sternberg-like cells

   - Extranodal T/NK-cell lymphoma, nasal type; small intestine (Figure 15.75)
   - Anaplastic large cell lymphoma (15.76)
   - Hodgkin lymphoma, classical; large intestine (Figure 15.77)
   - Langerhans cell histiocytosis, large intestine (Figure 15.78)
   - Extramedullary myeloid tumor (granulocytic sarcoma), small intestine (Figure 15.79).

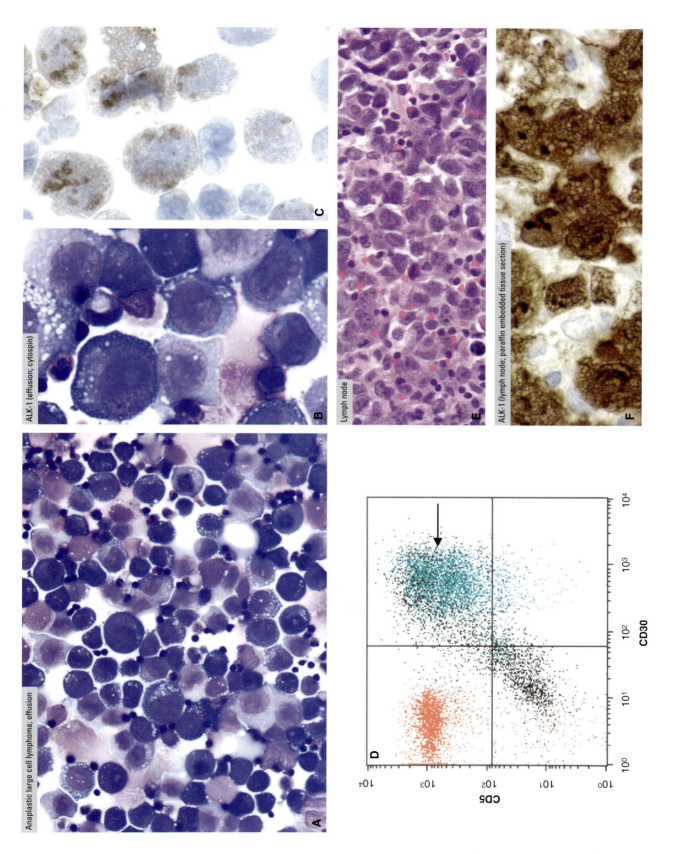

Figure 15.1   Pleural effusion – anaplastic large cell lymphoma. (**A**) Cytospin preparation shows numerous malignant cells with large nuclei, dense cytoplasm with occasional vacuoles. (**B**) High magnification shows detailed cytologic features. (**C**) Immunohistochemical staining with ALK-1 (effusion). (**D**) Flow cytometry shows T-cells coexpressing CD30 (arrow). (**E**) Histologic section of the lymph node from the same patient shows diffuse large cell infiltrate. (**F**) Tumor cells show nuclear, nucleolar and cytoplasmic staining with ALK-1

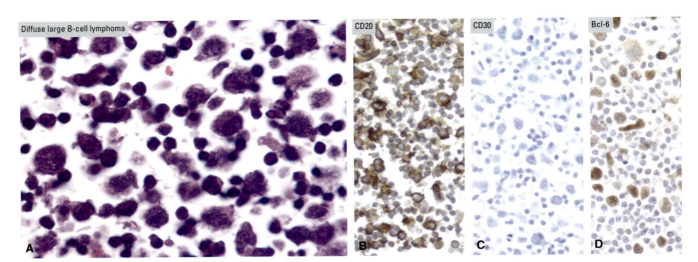

Figure 15.2   Pleural effusion – diffuse large B-cell lymphoma. (**A**) Cytology shows large pleomorphic cells. (**B–D**) Immunohistochemistry. Lymphomatous cells are positive for CD20 (**B**) and bcl-6 (**D**). CD30 is negative (**C**)

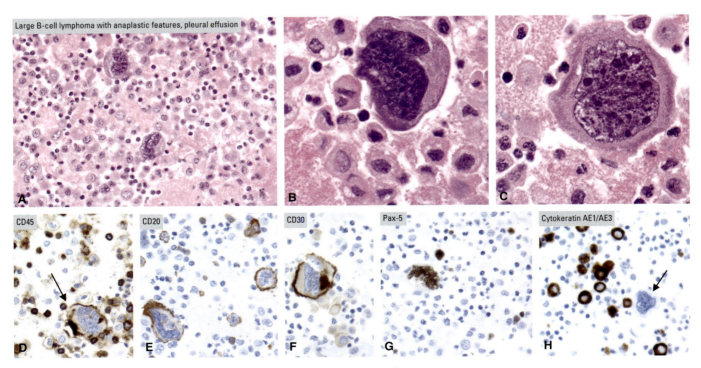

Figure 15.3   Pleural effusion – diffuse large B-cell lymphoma with anaplastic features. (**A–C**) Section from cell block preparation shows lymphoid cells with scattered, large, highly pleomorphic cells with irregular nuclei and several nucleoli. (**D–H**) Immunohistochemistry. Tumor cells are positive for CD45 (**D**), CD20 (**E**), CD30 (**F**), Pax-5 (**G**) and are negative for cytokeratin (**H**, arrow). Mesothelial cells express cytokeratin

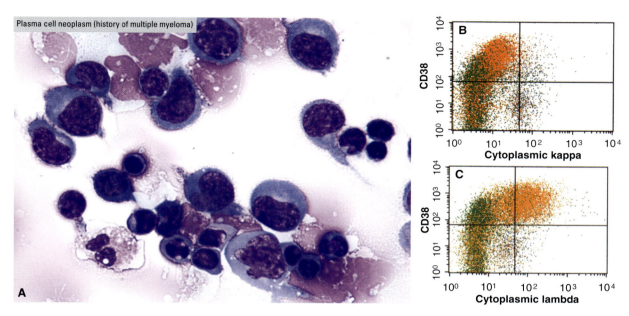

Figure 15.4 Pleural effusion – plasma cell neoplasm. (**A**) Cytospin preparation shows numerous atypical plasma cells. (**B** and **C**) Flow cytometry. Plasma cells are clonal with cytoplasmic lambda expression (**C**)

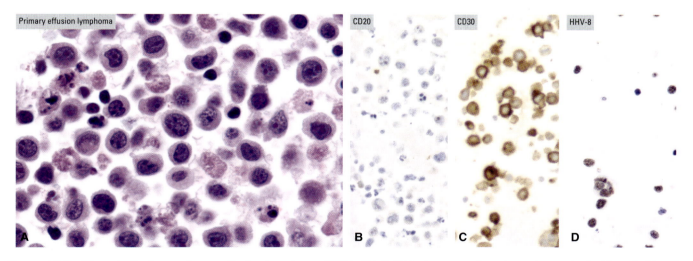

Figure 15.5 Pleural effusion – primary effusion lymphoma (PEL). (**A**) Cell block preparation shows large atypical lymphoid cells. (**B–D**) Immunohistochemistry. Tumor cells are negative for CD20 (**B**), positive for CD30 (**C**) and positive for HHV-8 (**D**)

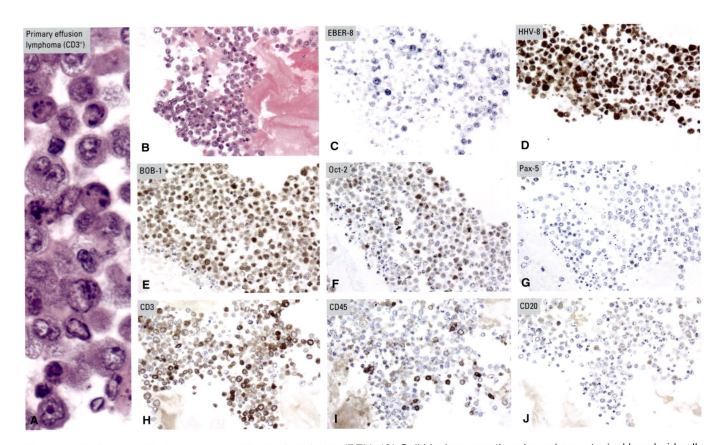

Figure 15.6 Pleural effusion – primary effusion lymphoma (PEL). (**A**) Cell block preparation shows large atypical lymphoid cells with prominent pleomorphism. (**B**) Low magnification (compare with immunohistochemical staining). (**C–J**) Immunohistochemical staining: tumor cells are positive for EBER (**C**), HHV-8 (**D**), BOB-1 (**E**), OCT-2 (**F**), CD3 (**H**) and CD45 (**I**). Pax-5 and CD20 are not expressed (**G** and **J**, respectively). Aberrant expression of CD3 is not unusual in PEL

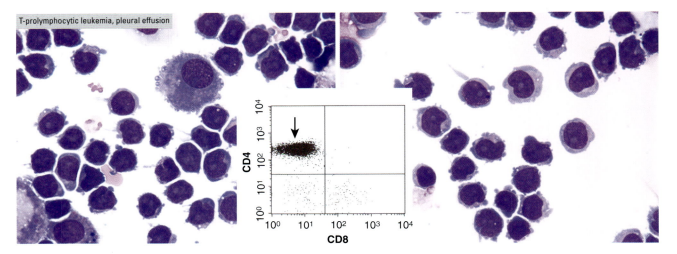

Figure 15.7 Pleural effusion – T-cell prolymphocytic leukemia. Small lymphocytes with irregular nuclear outlines are present. Inset: flow cytometry shows restricted CD4 expression (arrow)

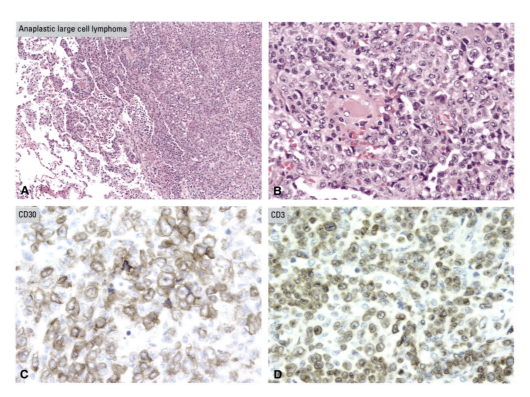

Figure 15.8   Lung – anaplastic large cell lymphoma. (**A**) Low magnification shows a dense lymphoid infiltrate within lung parenchyma. (**B**) Higher magnification shows predominance of large cells. (**C** and **D**) Immunohistochemistry: tumor cells are positive for CD30 (**C**) and CD3 (**D**)

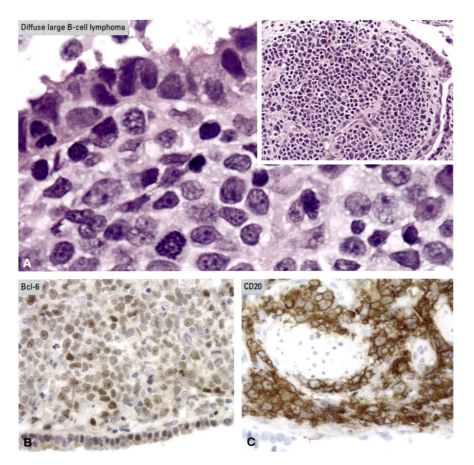

Figure 15.9   Lung – diffuse large B-cell lymphoma. Diffuse large cell lymphoid infiltrate (**A**). Tumor cells are positive for bcl-6 (**B**) and CD20 (**C**)

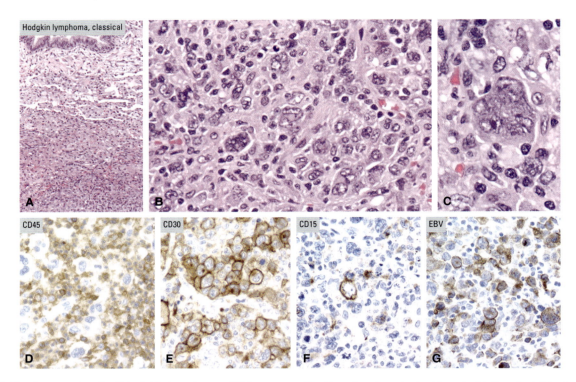

Figure 15.10 Lung – classical Hodgkin lymphoma. (**A**) Low magnification showing atypical lymphohistiocytic infiltrate. (**B** and **C**) Higher magnifications show polylobated cells with macronucleoli (Reed–Sternberg cells). Large tumor cells are negative for CD45 (**D**) and positive for CD30 (**E**), CD15 (**F**) and EBV (**G**)

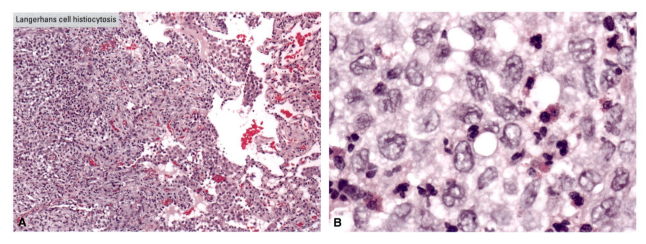

Figure 15.11 Lung – Langerhans cell histiocytosis. Large cell infiltrate with irregular nuclei and pale cytoplasm. (**A**, low magnification; **B**, high magnification)

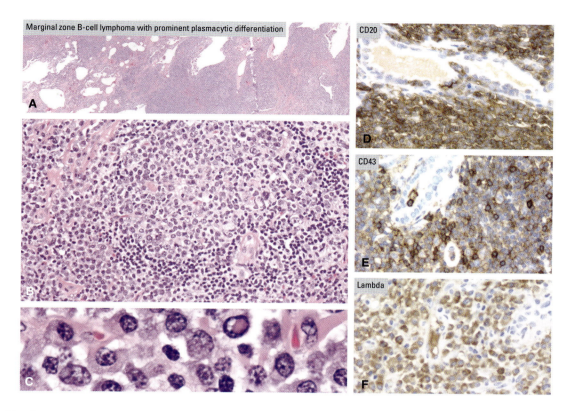

Figure 15.12   Lung – marginal zone B-cell lymphoma. (**A**) Low magnification shows dense lymphocytic infiltrate. (**B** and **C**) Higher magnifications show a mixed population of small lymphocytes and plasma cells. Dutcher bodies are present. (**D–F**) Immunohistochemistry: lymphomatous cells are positive for CD20 (**D**), CD43 (**E**) and lambda (**F**)

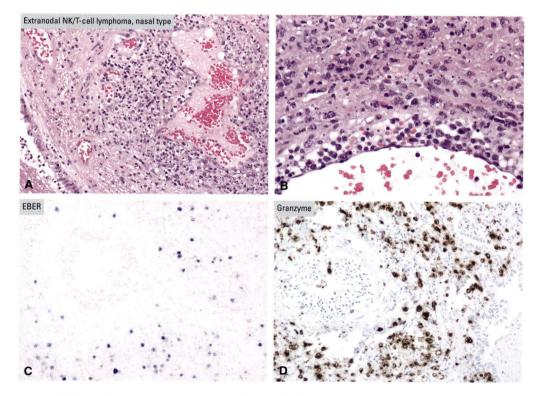

Figure 15.13   Lung – T/NK-cell lymphoma, nasal type. (**A** and **B**) Atypical pleomorphic lymphoid infiltrate with necrosis and numerous apoptotic cells. Tumor cells express EBER (**C**) and granzyme (**D**)

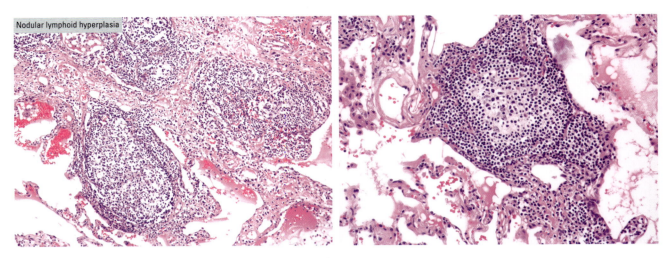

Figure 15.14 Lung – reactive lymphoid infiltrate (hyperplasia)

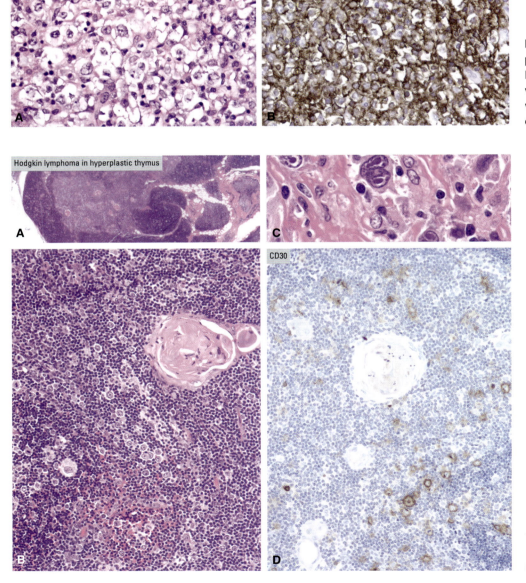

Figure 15.15 Mediastinum – primary mediastinal large B-cell lymphoma. (**A**) Histology with typical large lymphoid cells with clear cytoplasm. (**B**) Tumor cells express CD20

Figure 15.16 Mediastinum – Hodgkin lymphoma (classical) within hyperplastic thymus (**A–C**, histology; **D**, CD30 staining)

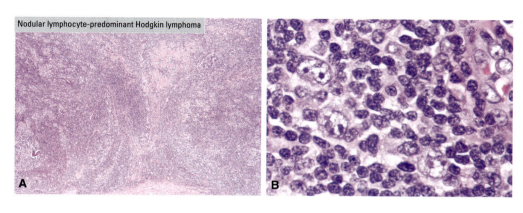

Figure 15.17 Mediastinum – nodular lymphocyte-predominant Hodgkin lymphoma (**A** and **B**; low and high magnification with typical histologic features)

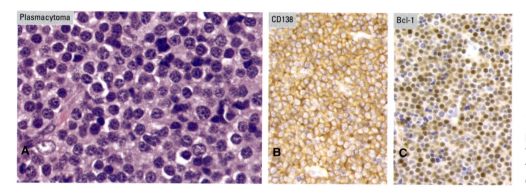

Figure 15.18 Mediastinum – plasmacytoma. (**A**) Histology with atypical plasma cell infiltrate. Tumor cells are positive for CD138 (**B**) and bcl-1 (**C**)

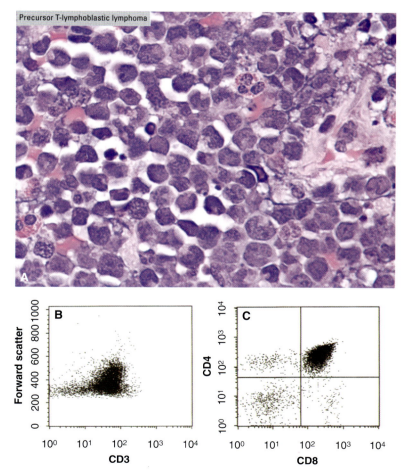

Figure 15.19 Mediastinum – precursor T-lymphoblastic lymphoma (T-ALL/LBL). (**A**) Histology. (**B** and **C**) Flow cytometry showing expression of CD3 (**B**) and dual positive expression of CD4 and CD8 (**C**)

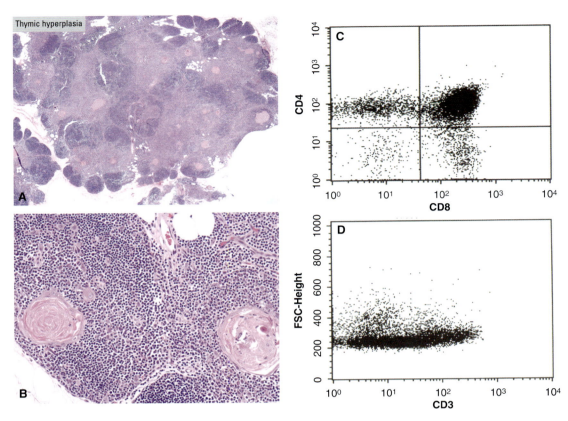

Figure 15.20   Mediastinum – thymic hyperplasia. (**A** and **B**) Histology. Flow cytometry shows dual positive expression of CD4 and CD8 (**C**) and characteristic variable expression of surface CD3 (**D**)

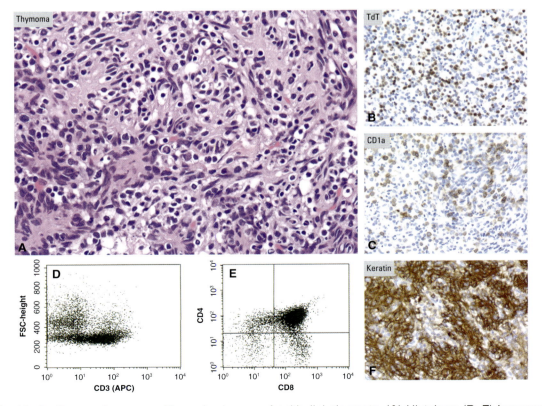

Figure 15.21   Mediastinum – thymoma with predominance of epithelial elements. (**A**) Histology. (**B–F**) Immunophenotyping. Benign thymocytes are positive for TdT (**B**), CD1a (**C**), CD3 (**D**) and CD4/CD8 (**E**). Epithelial component is positive for cytokeratin (**F**). Variable expression of surface CD3 (**D**) distinguishes benign immature thymocytes from precursor T-lymphoblastic lymphoma

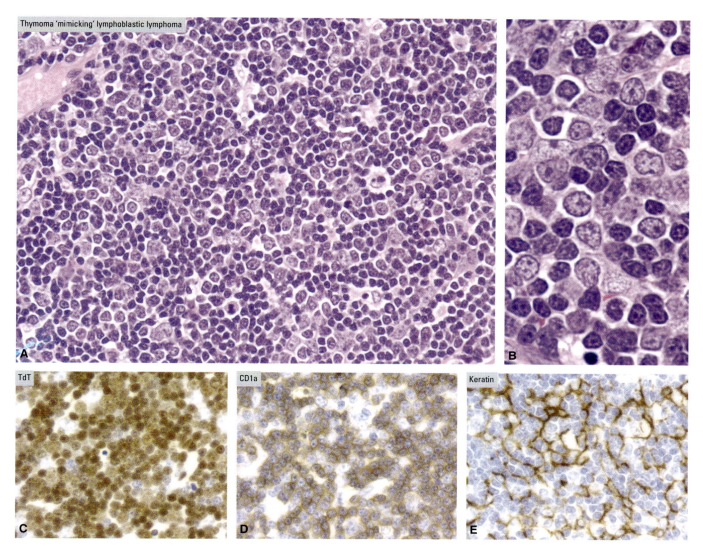

Figure 15.22 Mediastinum – thymoma with predominance of lymphoid elements. (**A** and **B**) Histology. (**C–E**) Immunohistochemistry. Thymocytes are positive for TdT (**C**) and CD1a (**D**), and rare epithelial elements are positive for cytokeratin (**E**)

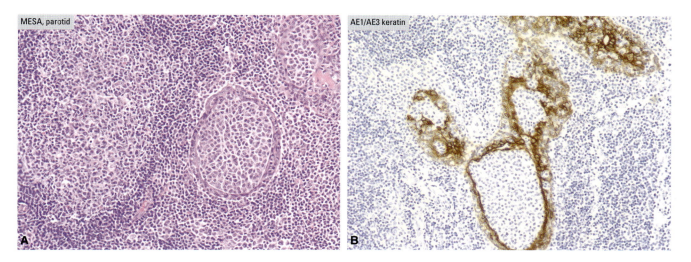

Figure 15.23   Salivary gland – myoepithelial sialadenitis. (**A**) Histology section showing dense lymphoid infiltrate with formation of follicles and prominent lymphoepithelial lesions. (**B**) Staining with cytokeratin shows lymphoepithelial lesions

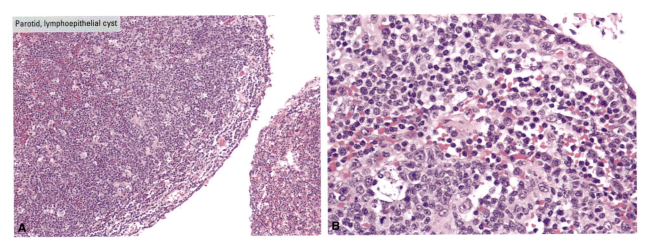

Figure 15.24 Salivary gland – lymphoepithelial cyst (**A** and **B**, low and intermediate magnification). Prominent lymphoid infiltrate composed of small to medium-sized lymphocytes without atypia

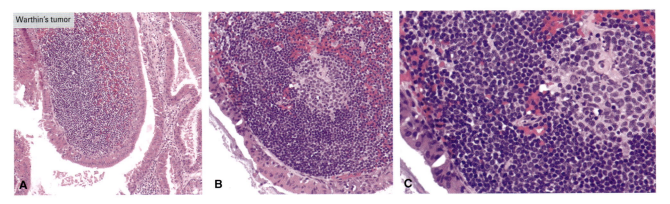

Figure 15.25 Salivary gland – Warthin's tumor. (**A–C**) Cystic spaces lined by glandular epithelium with oncocytic changes. Stroma shows dense lymphoid infiltrate with formation of germinal centers

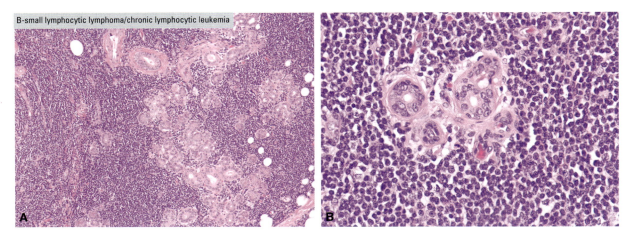

Figure 15.26 Salivary gland – B-small lymphocytic lymphoma. Salivary gland structures are infiltrated by small lymphocytes with compact chromatin and round nuclei. (**A**, low magnification; **B**, intermediate magnification)

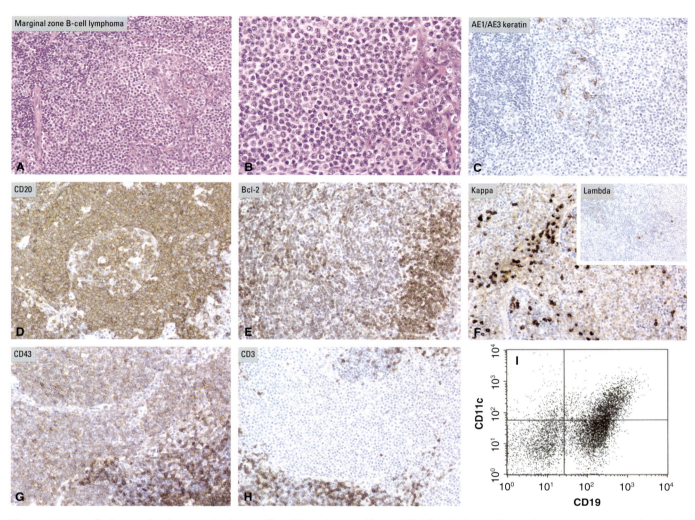

Figure 15.27 Salivary gland – marginal zone B-cell lymphoma. (**A** and **B**) Histologic sections show a monotonous lymphoid infiltrate with prominent lymphoepithelial lesions. Lymphocytes are small to medium-sized with pale to clear cytoplasm. (**C–H**) Immunohistochemistry: lymphoepithelial lesions are highlighted by cytokeratin staining (**C**). Lymphomatous cells are positive for CD20 (**D**), bcl-2 (**E**) and CD43 (**G**), and are negative for CD3 (**H**). Plasma cells are monoclonal with kappa restriction (**F**). (**I**) Flow cytometry shows partial expression of CD11c by neoplastic B-cells

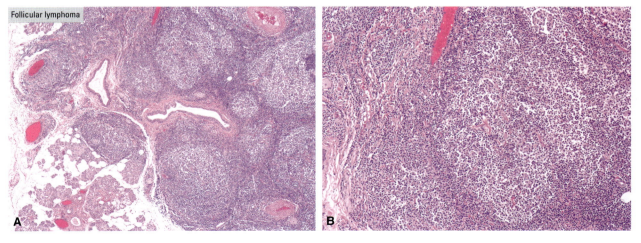

Figure 15.28 Salivary gland – follicular lymphoma. (**A** and **B**) Histology shows lymphoid infiltrate with nodular architecture. Neoplastic nodules are large and irregular

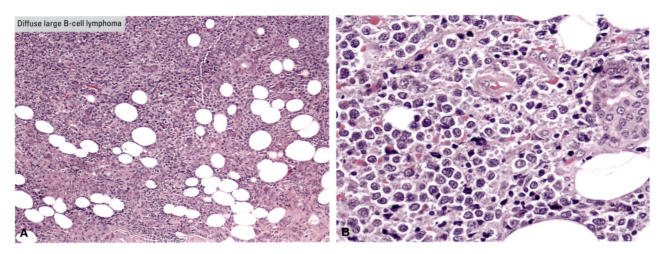

Figure 15.29   Salivary gland – diffuse large B-cell lymphoma. (**A** and **B**) Large cell lymphoid infiltrate

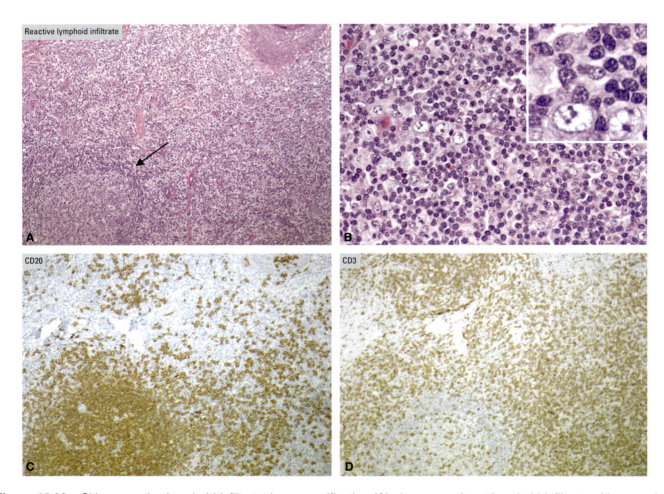

Figure 15.30   Skin – reactive lymphoid infiltrate. Low magnification (**A**) shows prominent lymphoid infiltrate with secondary follicle (arrow). Higher magnification (**B**) shows pleomorphism of the infiltrate, which is composed of mixed population of small and medium-sized lymphocytes with occasional large activated cells (inset). Immunohistochemical staining reveals presence of B- and T-lymphocytes (**C** and **D**)

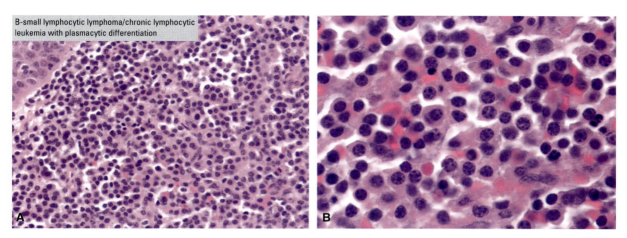

Figure 15.31   Skin – B-small lymphocytic lymphoma with plasmacytic differentiation (**A**, low magnification; **B**, high magnification). The phenotype of B-cells (CD5⁺/CD23⁺) differentiates B-SLL/CLL from other low-grade lymphomas with plasmacytic differentiation (e.g., marginal zone lymphoma and lymphoplasmacytic lymphoma)

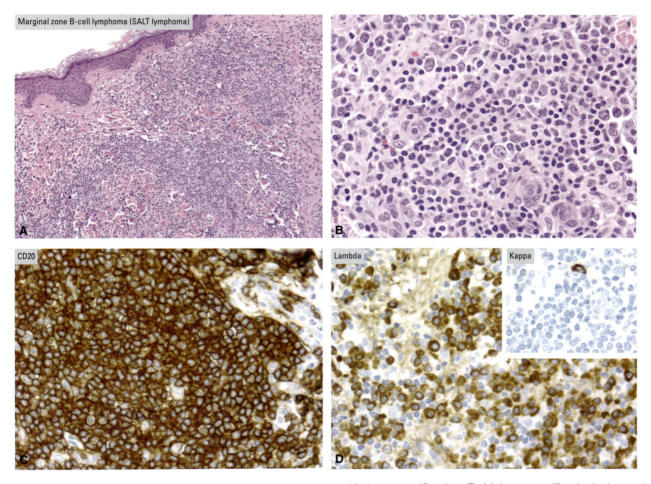

Figure 15.32   Skin – marginal zone B-cell lymphoma. Histology (**A**, low magnification; **B**, higher magnification) shows dense lymphoid infiltrate composed of small and medium-sized lymphocytes with numerous plasma cells. Immunohistochemistry reveals predominance of B-cells (**C**) and monotypic lambda⁺ plasma cells (**D**; inset: kappa)

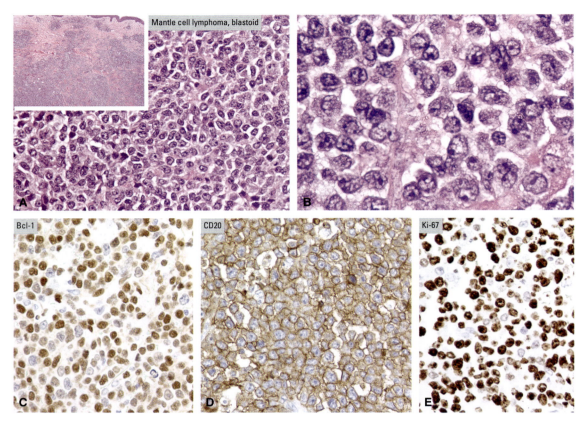

Figure 15.33   Skin – mantle cell lymphoma. (**A** and **B**) Histology shows dense lymphoid infiltrate composed of medium to large cells with irregular nuclei. (**C–E**) Immunohistochemistry reveals expression of bcl-1 (**C**), CD20 (**D**) and high Ki-67⁺ proliferation fraction (**E**)

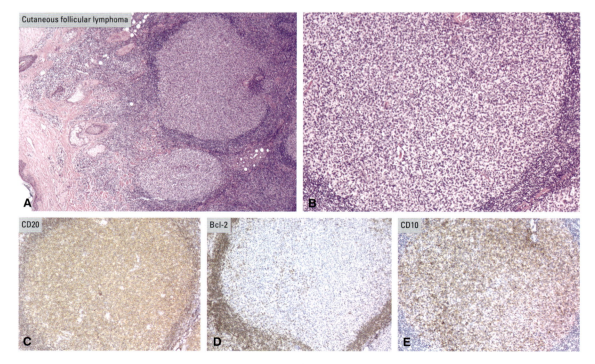

Figure 15.34   Skin – follicular lymphoma (FL). (**A** and **B**) Histology shows prominent nodular lymphoid infiltrate within dermis. Nodules are composed of larger lymphocytes with paler cytoplasm when compared to surrounding small benign lymphocytes. Lymphomatous cells express CD20 (**C**) and CD10 (**E**) and lack bcl-2 expression (**D**). Lack of bcl-2 expression is observed more often in cutaneous FL than in its nodal counterpart

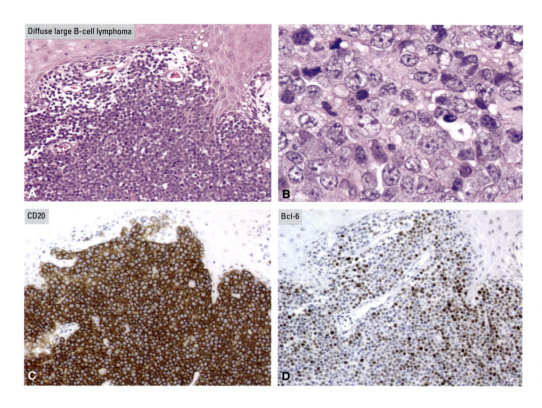

Figure 15.35 Skin – diffuse large B-cell lymphoma. Histologic section shows large cell lymphoid infiltrate composed of centroblasts (**A** and **B**). Tumor cells are positive for CD20 (**C**) and bcl-6 (**D**)

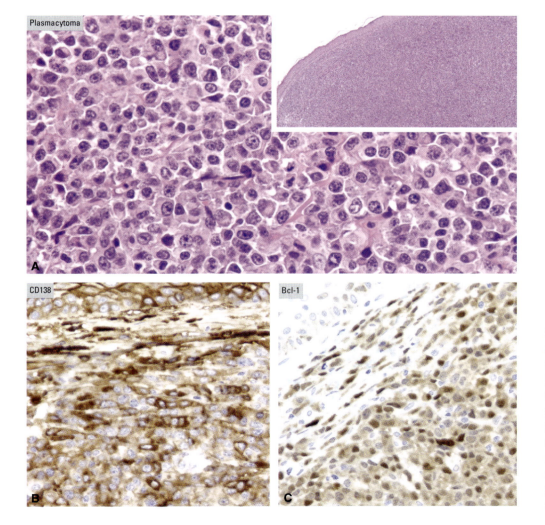

Figure 15.36 Skin – plasmacytoma. (**A**) Dense plasmacytic infiltrate within dermis. Plasma cells are positive for CD138 (**B**) and bcl-1 (**C**). The phenotype and lack of B-lymphocytes distinguishes (in most cases) extramedullary plasmacytoma from marginal zone B-cell lymphoma with prominent plasmacytic differentiation

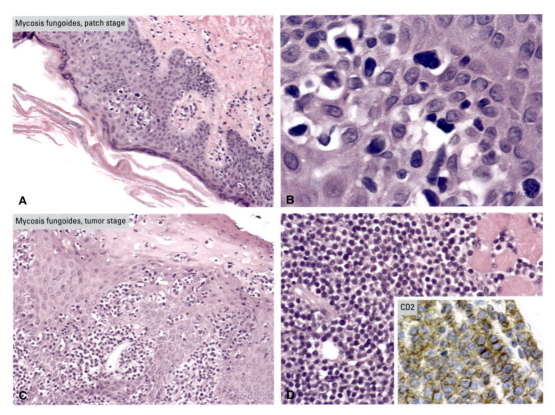

Figure 15.37   Skin – mycosis fungoides (MF). Early (**A** and **B**) and advanced (**C** and **D**) MF; see Figures 3.25 and 3.26 (Chapter 3) for details

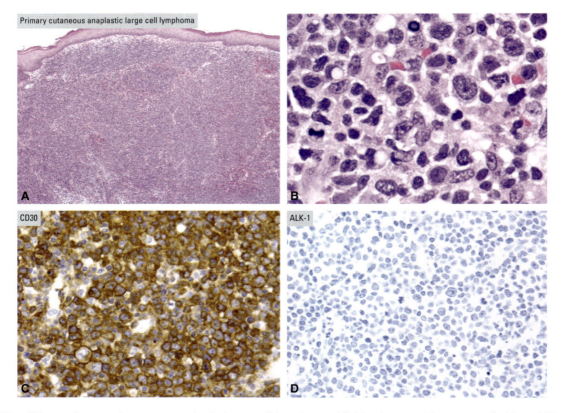

Figure 15.38   Skin – primary cutaneous anaplastic large cell lymphoma. Highly pleomorphic tumor cells (**A** and **B**) are positive for CD30 (**C**) and negative for ALK-1 (**D**)

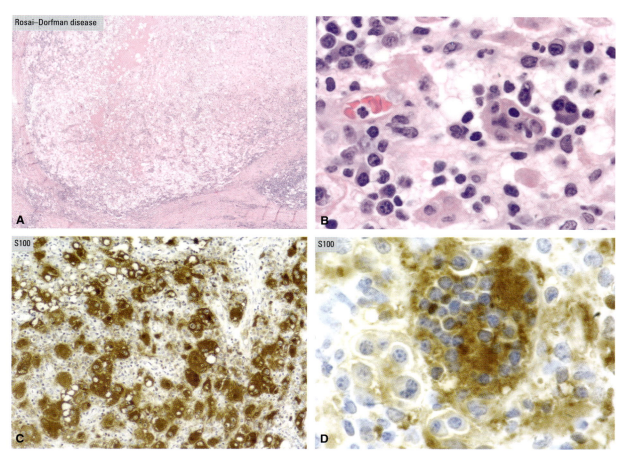

Figure 15.39   Skin – Rosai–Dorfman disease. Dense histiocytic infiltrate (**A**) with emperipolesis (**B** and **D**). Atypical histiocytes are positive for S100 (**C** and **D**)

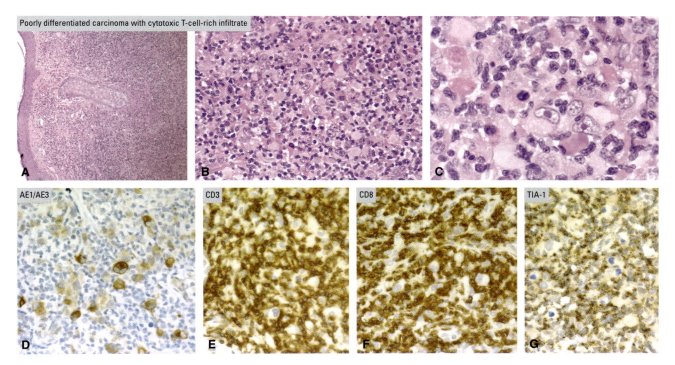

Figure 15.40   Skin – poorly differentiated carcinoma with T-cell-rich infiltrate. (**A–C**) Dense lymphoid infiltrate with scattered large atypical cells (**C**) imitating lymphoma or lymphomatoid papulosis. Immunohistochemistry (**D–G**) reveals cytokeratin$^+$ neoplastic cells (**D**) and reactive lymphoid cells composed predominantly of cytotoxic T-cells expressing CD3 (**E**), CD8 (**F**) and TIA-1 (**G**)

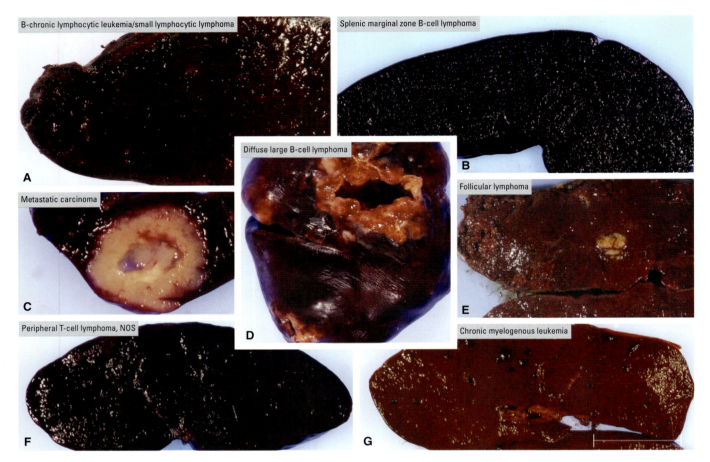

Figure 15.41 Spleen – gross characteristics of splenic tumors. (**A**) B-chronic lymphocytic leukemia/small lymphocytic lymphoma. (**B**) Marginal zone B-cell lymphoma. (**C**) Metastatic carcinoma. (**D**) Diffuse large B-cell lymphoma. (**E**) Follicular lymphoma. (**F**) Peripheral T-cell lymphoma. (**G**) Chronic myelogenous leukemia

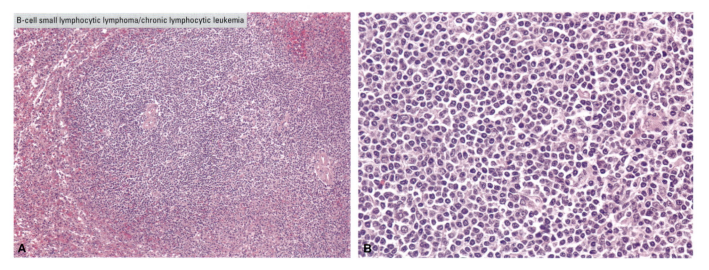

Figure 15.42 Spleen – B-cell small lymphocytic lymphoma/chronic lymphocytic leukemia. (**A** and **B**) Prominent white pulp with predominance of small lymphocytes

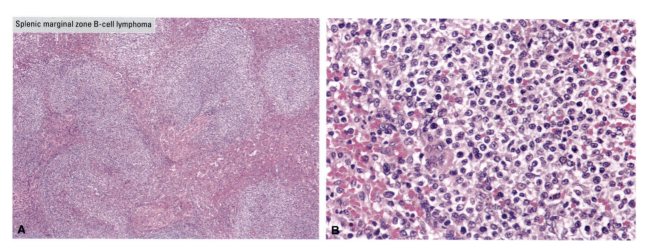

Figure 15.43   Spleen – marginal zone B-cell lymphoma. (**A** and **B**) Histologic sections show prominent white pulp. The majority of lymphocytes have clear cytoplasm

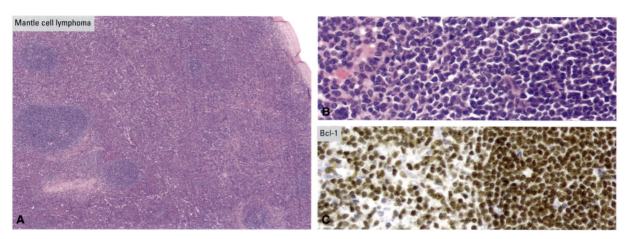

Figure 15.44   Spleen – mantle cell lymphoma. (**A** and **B**) Histology section. (**C**) Positive expression of bcl-1

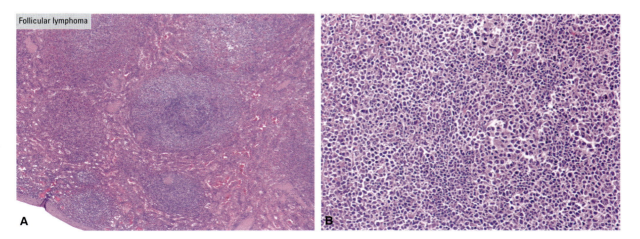

Figure 15.45   Spleen – follicular lymphoma. (**A**) Prominent white pulp. (**B**) Lymphoid nodules are composed of mixed population of lymphocytes. Medium-sized lymphocytes predominate

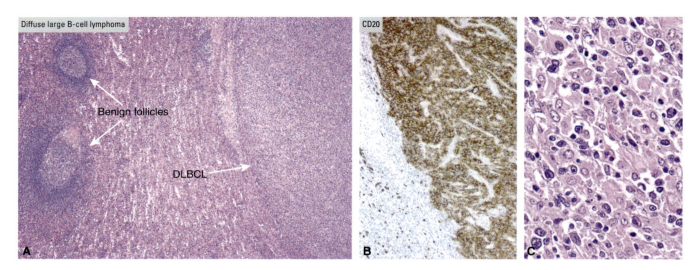

Figure 15.46 Spleen – diffuse large B-cell lymphoma. Partial replacement of the splenic parenchyma with large cell infiltrate (**A**, low magnification; **B**, expression of CD20; **C**, large magnification)

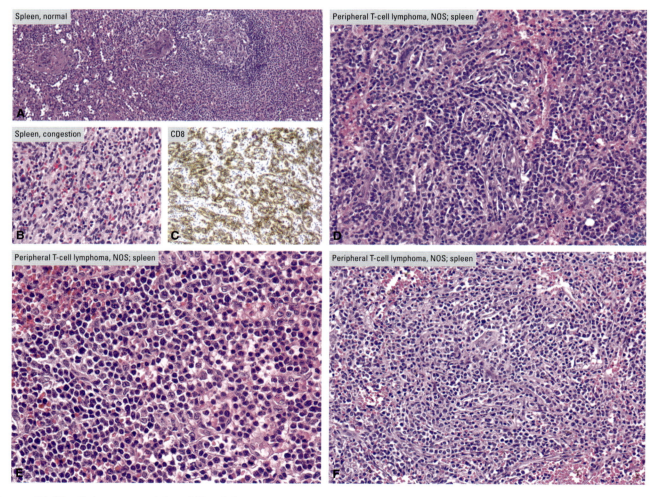

Figure 15.47 Spleen – peripheral T-cell lymphoma. (**A**) Benign spleen. (**B**) Benign spleen with congestion (**C**, CD8 immunostaining). (**D–F**) Three examples of peripheral T-cell lymphoma, unspecified, involving the spleen

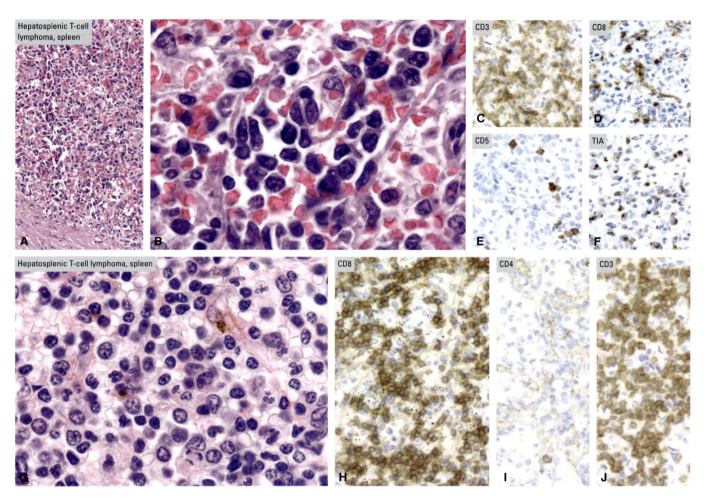

Figure 15.48   Spleen – hepatosplenic T-cell lymphomas. (**A–F**) Case no. 1. (**A**) Low magnification shows clusters of atypical lymphoid cells. (**B**) High magnification shows intrasinusoidal distribution of neoplastic cells. (**C–F**) Immunohistochemistry: tumor cells are positive for CD3 (**C**), CD8 (**D**) and TIA (**F**). CD5 is negative (**E**). (**G–J**) Case no. 2. (**G**) Atypical lymphoid infiltrate. (**H–J**) Immunohistochemistry: lymphomatous cells are positive for CD8 (**H**) and CD3 (**J**). CD4 is negative (**I**)

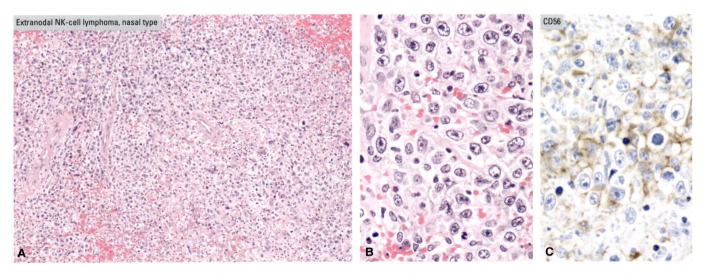

Figure 15.49   Spleen – extranodal NK/T-cell lymphoma, nasal type. (**A** and **B**) Diffuse large cell lymphoid infiltrate with prominent nucleoli. Neoplastic cells express CD56 (**C**)

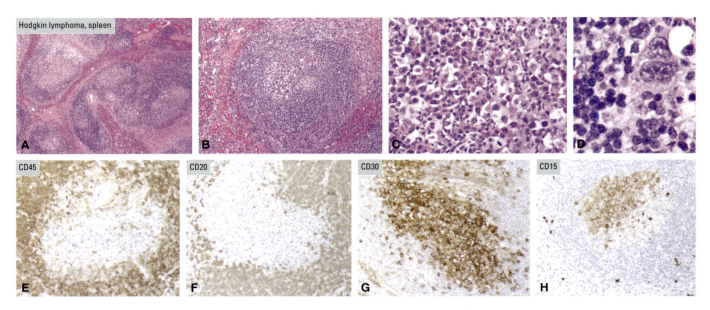

Figure 15.50 Spleen – Hodgkin lymphoma (classical). (**A** and **B**) Low magnification shows lymphoid nodules composed of small lymphocytes and large cells in the center. (**C** and **D**) Higher magnification shows large cells with multilobated nuclei and macronucleoli. (**E–H**) Immunohistochemistry: large neoplastic cells are negative for CD45 (**E**) and CD20 (**F**) and are positive for CD30 (**G**) and CD15 (**H**). Small lymphocytes have reversed immunostaining pattern

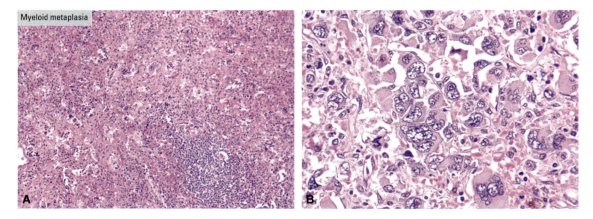

Figure 15.51 Spleen – myeloid metaplasia. (**A**) Low power shows extensive extramedullary hematopoiesis. (**B**) High magnification shows numerous atypical megakaryocytes

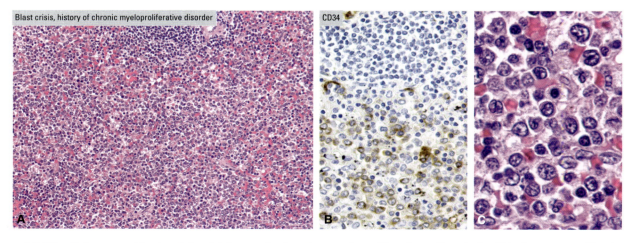

Figure 15.52 Spleen – blast crisis (history of chronic myeloproliferative disorder). (**A**) Low magnification. (**B**) Immunohistochemical staining with CD34. (**C**) High magnification

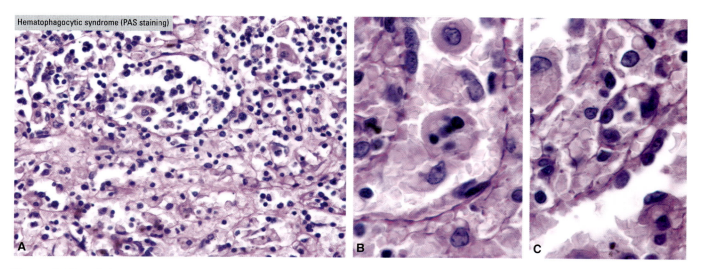

Figure 15.53   Spleen – hemophagocytic syndrome. (**A**) Low magnification shows numerous histiocytes within vascular spaces. (**B** and **C**) High magnification shows histiocytes with engulfed red cells and lymphocytes

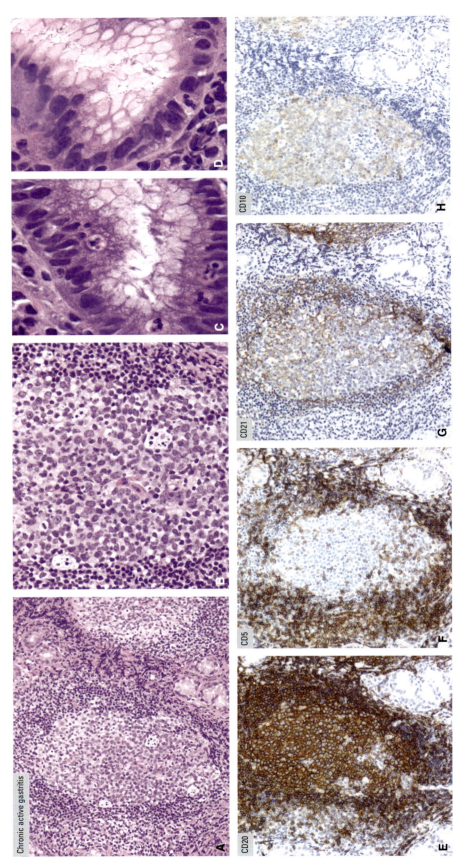

Figure 15.54   Stomach – chronic active 'follicular' gastritis. (**A**) Prominent lymphoid infiltrate within lamina propria with formation of germinal centers. (**B**) Higher magnification shows details of reactive germinal centers. Tingible-body macrophages are present. (**C** and **D**) High magnification shows granulocytes and numerous *H. pylori*. (**E–H**) Immunohistochemistry: mixed B- and T-cell infiltrate is present (**E** and **F**). Follicular dendritic cell meshwork is not distorted (**G**). Germinal center cells are CD10+ (**H**)

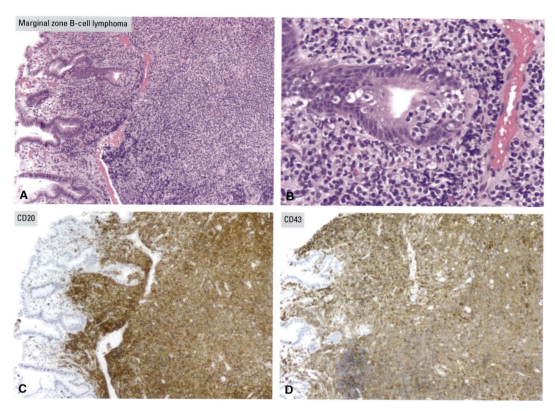

Figure 15.55   Stomach – marginal zone B-cell lymphoma (MALT lymphoma). (**A**) Low magnification shows a dense small lymphocytic infiltrate. (**B**) Higher magnification shows prominent lymphoepithelial lesions. (**C** and **D**) Immunohistochemistry: neoplastic CD20⁺ (**C**) B-cells display aberrant expression of CD43 (**D**)

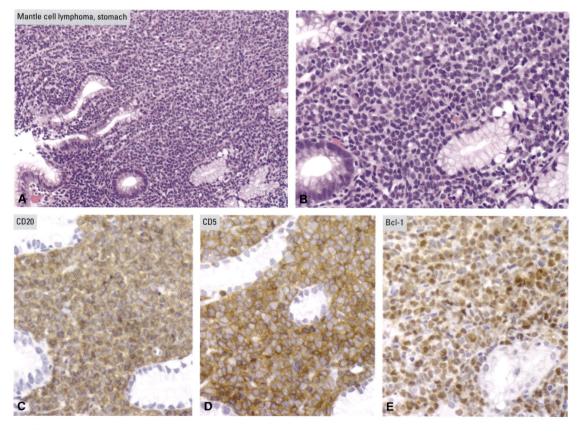

Figure 15.56   Stomach – mantle cell lymphoma. (**A** and **B**) Dense lymphoid infiltrate. (**C–E**) Immunohistochemistry: lymphomatous cells are positive for CD20 (**C**), CD5 (**D**) and bcl-1 (**E**)

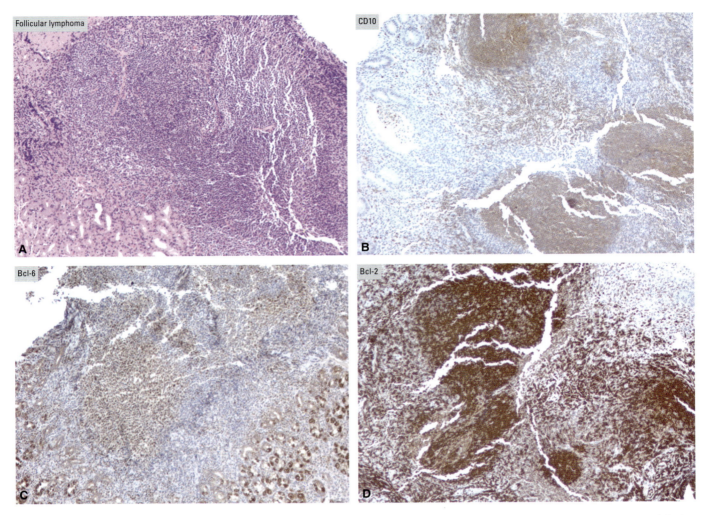

Figure 15.57 Stomach – follicular lymphoma. (**A**) Nodular lymphoid infiltrate. (**B–D**) Immunohistochemistry: neoplastic follicles are positive for CD10 (**B**), bcl-6 (**C**) and bcl-2 (**D**)

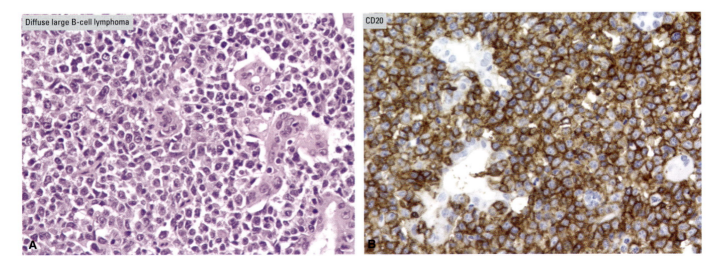

Figure 15.58 Stomach – diffuse large B-cell lymphoma. (**A**) Histology. (**B**) Positive expression of CD20

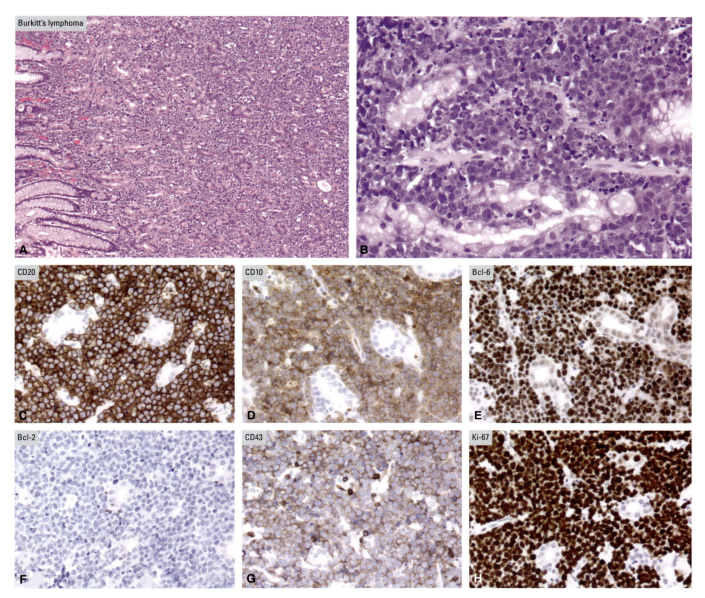

Figure 15.59 Stomach – Burkitt lymphoma. (**A**) Low magnification shows lymphoid infiltrate within lamina propria. (**B**) High magnification shows medium-sized lymphocytes with high nuclear: cytoplasmic ratio, and minimal pleomorphism. Numerous apoptotic cells are noted. (**C–H**) Immunohistochemistry: lymphomatous cells are positive for CD20 (**C**), CD10 (**D**), bcl-6 (**E**) and CD43 (**G**), and are negative for bcl-2 (**F**). Proliferation fraction determined by Ki-67 (MIB-1) staining approaches 100% (**H**)

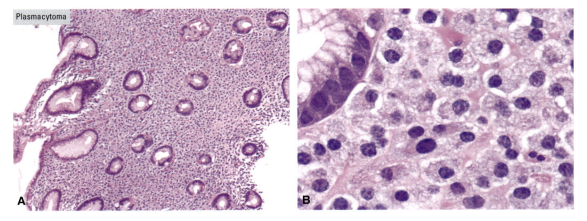

Figure 15.60 Stomach – monotypic plasma cell infiltrate (**A**, low magnification; **B**, high magnification). Differential diagnosis includes extramedullary plasma cell tumor and MALT lymphoma with extensive plasmacytic differentiation. Location favors the latter

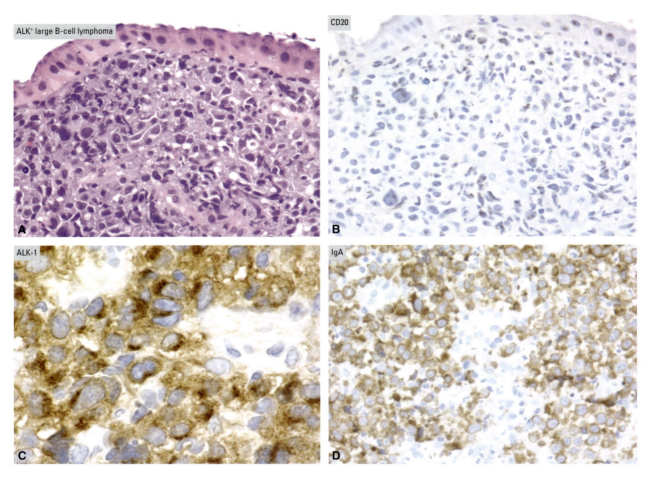

Figure 15.61 Stomach – diffuse large B-cell–lymphoma with ALK expression. (**A**) Histology. Diffuse large cell lymphoid infiltrate. (**B–D**) Immunohistochemistry: neoplastic B-cells are negative for CD20 (**B**) and are positive for ALK-1 (**C**) and IgA (**D**)

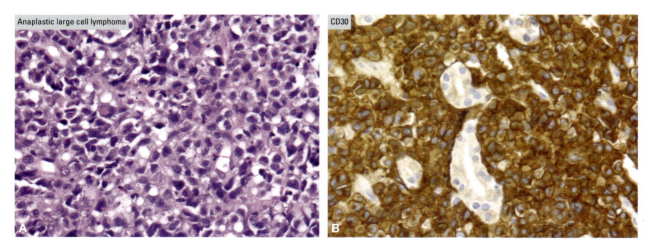

Figure 15.62 Stomach – anaplastic large cell lymphoma. (**A**) Diffuse pleomorphic lymphoid infiltrate. (**B**) Tumor cells are strongly positive for CD30

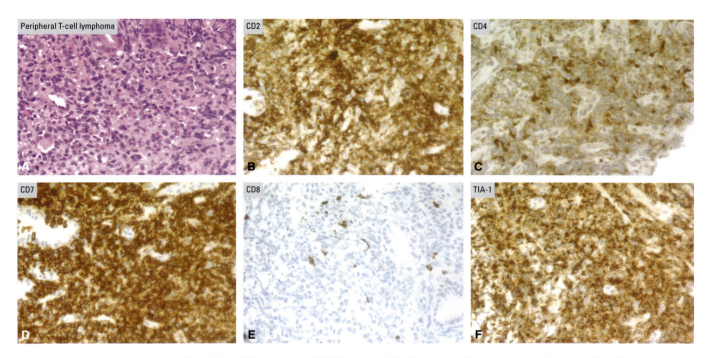

Figure 15.63 Stomach – peripheral T-cell lymphoma. (**A**) Histology. (**B–F**) Immunohistochemistry. Neoplastic cells are positive for CD2 (**B**), CD4 (**C**) and CD7 (**D**), and also show expression of TIA-1 (**F**). CD8 is negative (**E**)

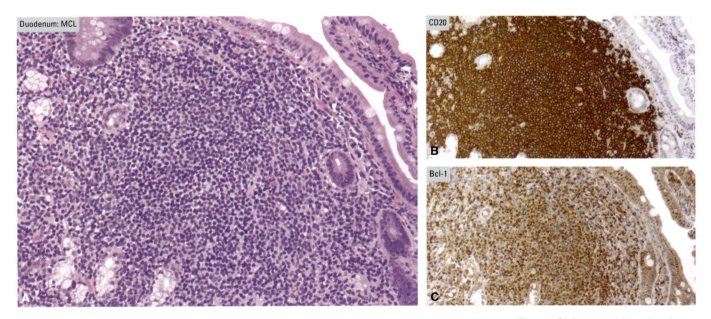

Figure 15.64 Duodenum – mantle cell lymphoma. (**A**) Diffuse small cell lymphoid infiltrate. (**B** and **C**) Immunohistochemistry: lymphomatous cells are positive for CD20 (**B**) and bcl-1 (**C**)

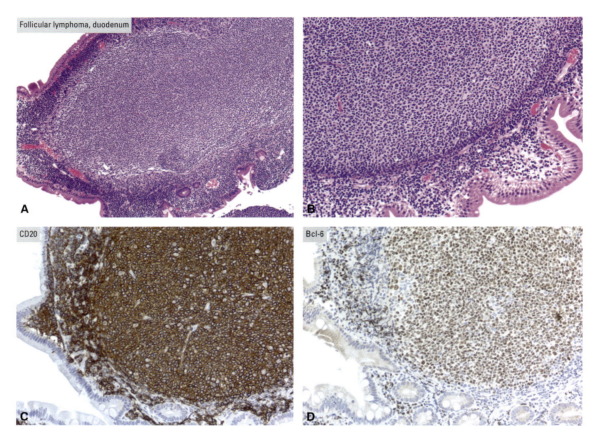

Figure 15.65   Duodenum – follicular lymphoma. (**A** and **B**) Histologic section shows a prominent nodular lymphoid infiltrate. (**C** and **D**) Immunohistochemistry: neoplastic B-cells coexpress CD20 (**C**) and bcl-6 (**D**)

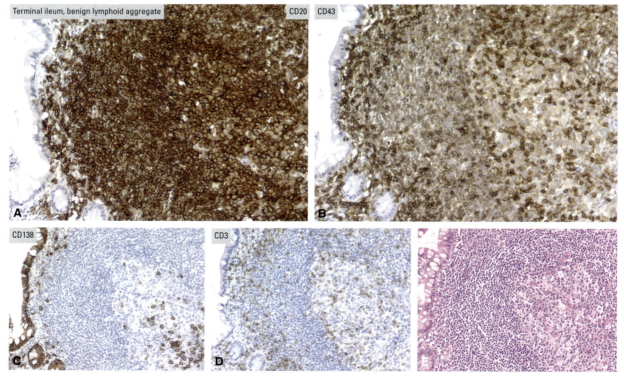

Figure 15.66   Terminal ileum – benign (reactive) lymphoid infiltrate. (**A–D**) Immunohistochemistry. Benign B-cells in the mucosa of terminal ileum are positive for CD20 (**A**) and CD43 (**B**). Aberrant expression of CD43 by B-cells in terminal ileum often is present. Rare scattered CD138+ plasma cells (**C**) and small CD3+ T-cells (**D**) are also positive for CD43. (**E**) Histology showing reactive lymphoid infiltrate with germinal center

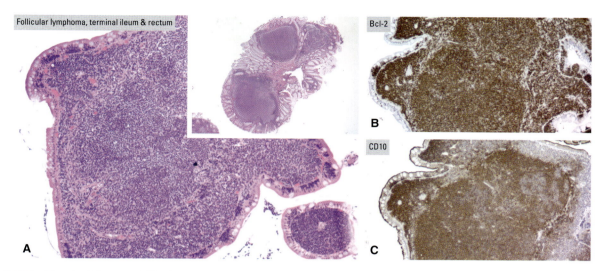

Figure 15.67 Terminal ileum – follicular lymphoma. (**A**) Nodular lymphoid infiltrate. (**B** and **C**) B-cells coexpress bcl-2 (**B**) and CD10 (**C**)

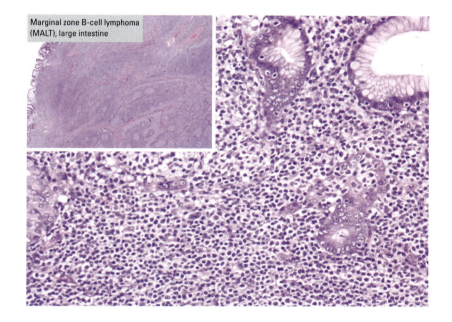

Figure 15.68 Large intestine – marginal zone B-cell lymphoma. Dense lymphoid infiltrate with majority of cells showing clear cytoplasm. Prominent lymphoepithelial lesions are noted

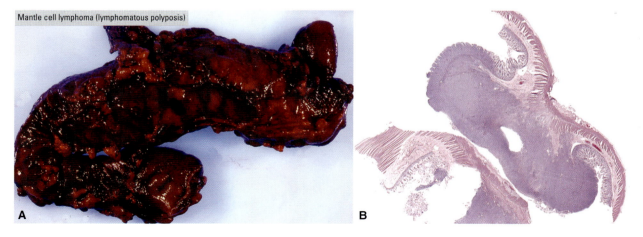

Figure 15.69 Large intestine – mantle cell lymphoma (lymphomatous polyposis). (**A**) Gross picture. Numerous polypoid structures are present. (**B**) Low magnification shows polypoid tumor composed of dense lymphoid infiltrate

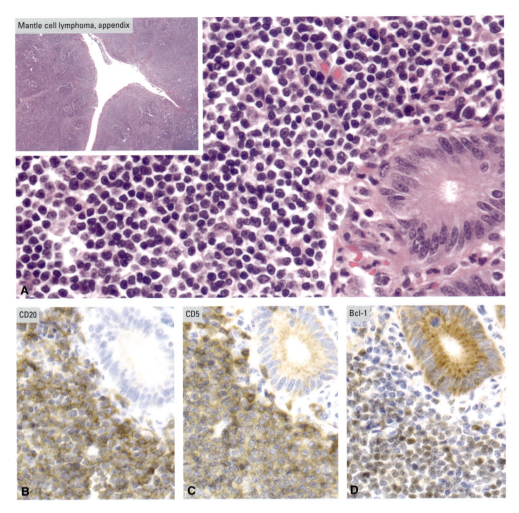

Figure 15.70 Large intestine – mantle cell lymphoma (appendix). (**A**) Dense lymphoid infiltrate of small lymphocytes. (**B–D**) Immunohistochemistry: lymphomatous cells are positive for CD20 (**B**), CD5 (**C**) and bcl-1 (**D**)

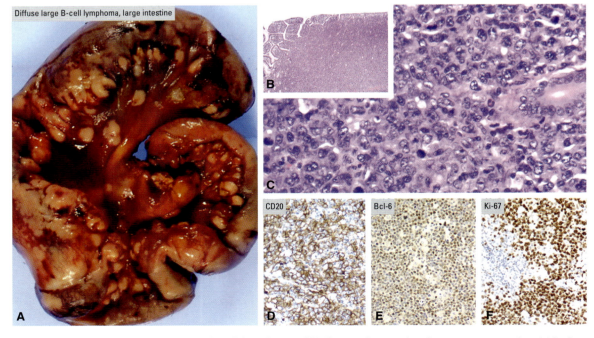

Figure 15.71 Large intestine – diffuse large B-cell lymphoma. (**A**) Gross picture showing numerous polypoid lesions. (**B**) Low magnification with dense lymphoid infiltrate. (**C**) Large lymphoid cells predominate. (**D–F**) Immunohistochemistry: neoplastic B-cells are positive for CD20 (**D**) and bcl-6 (**C**), and show strong expression of Ki-67, approaching 80% (**F**)

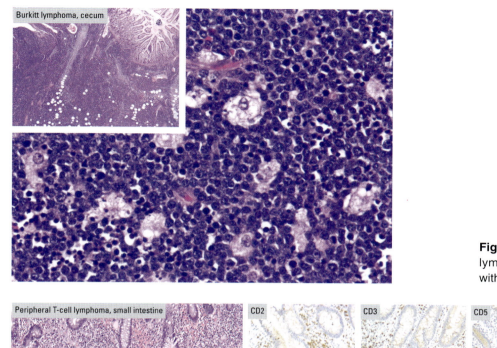

Figure 15.72   Large intestine – Burkitt lymphoma. Dense lymphoid infiltrate with starry-sky pattern

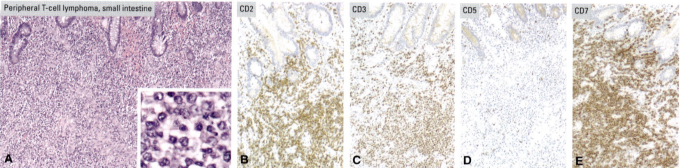

Figure 15.73   Small intestine – peripheral T-cell lymphoma. (**A**) Mucosa and submucosa with numerous atypical lymphoid cells. (**B–E**) Immunohistochemistry: lymphomatous cells are positive for CD2 (**B**), CD3 (**C**) and CD7 (**E**). CD5 is aberrantly absent (**D**)

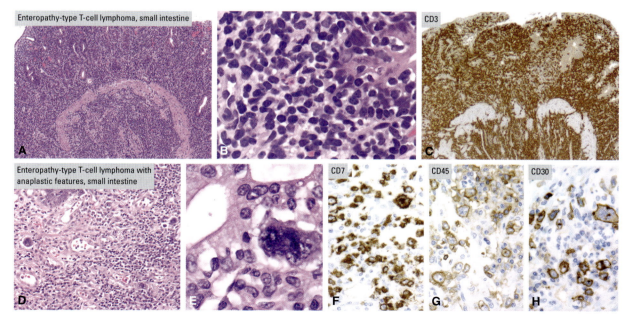

Figure 15.74   Small intestine – enteropathy-type T-cell lymphoma (two cases) (**A–C**) Case no. 1. (**A**) Prominent monotonous lymphoid infiltrate with mucosal ulceration. (**B**) High magnification shows medium-sized lymphocytes with irregular nuclei. (**C**) Neoplastic lymphocytes express CD3. (**D–H**) Case no. 2. (**D**) Small intestinal mucosa with pleomorphic lymphoid infiltrate. (**E**) Scattered large cells resembling Reed–Sternberg cells are present. (**F–H**) Immunohistochemistry: neoplastic cells are positive for CD7 (**F**), CD45 (**G**) and CD30 (**H**)

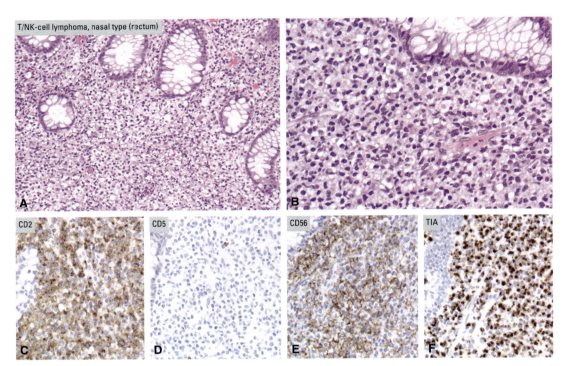

Figure 15.75 Large intestine – extranodal NK/T-cell lymphoma, nasal type. (**A** and **B**) Atypical lymphoid infiltrate. (**C–F**) Immunohistochemistry: tumor cells are positive for CD2 (**C**), CD56 (**E**) and TIA (**F**). CD5 is not expressed (**D**)

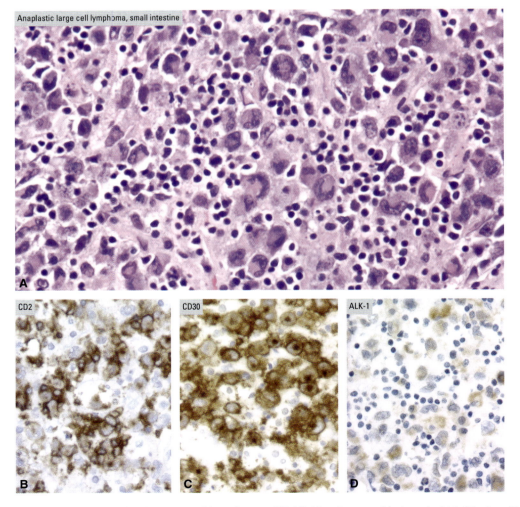

Figure 15.76 Small intestine – anaplastic large cell lymphoma. (**A**) Highly pleomorphic lymphoid infiltrate with characteristic nuclear shapes. (**B–D**) Immunohistochemistry: tumor cells express CD2 (**B**), CD30 (**C**) and ALK-1 (**D**)

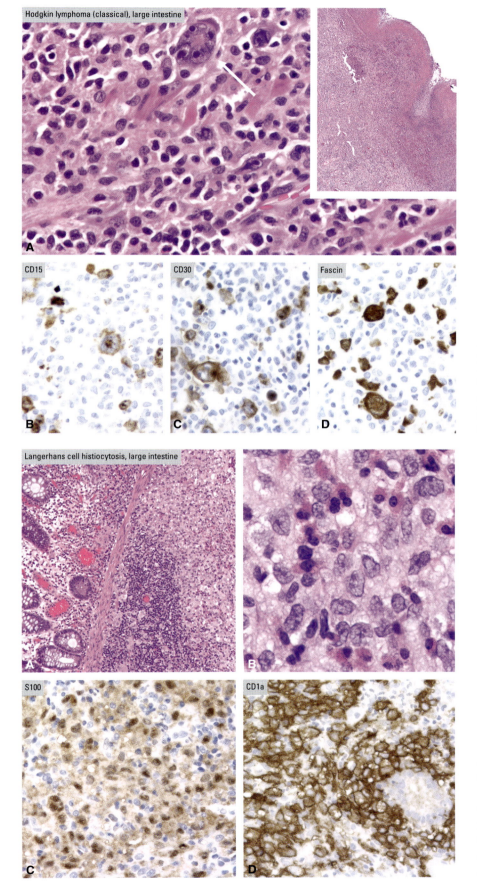

Figure 15.77 Large intestine – classical Hodgkin lymphoma. (**A**) Histology showing typical multinucleated Reed–Sternberg cells (arrow). (**B–D**) Immunohistochemistry: large cells are positive for CD15 (**B**), CD30 (**C**) and fascin (**D**)

Figure 15.78 Large intestine – Langerhans cell histiocytosis. (**A**) Pleomorphic infiltrate with clusters of cells with pale eosinophilic cytoplasm. (**B**) High magnification shows large cells with pale, vacuolated cytoplasm and irregular nuclei. (**C** and **D**) Neoplastic cells are positive for S100 (**C**) and CD1a (**D**)

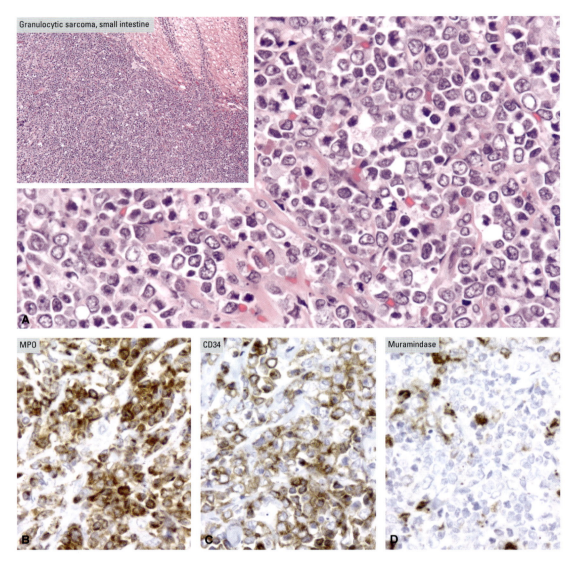

Figure 15.79   Large intestine – extramedullary myeloid tumor (granulocytic sarcoma). (**A**) Large cell mononuclear infiltrate with blastoid morphology. (**B–D**) Immunohistochemistry: large cells express myeloperoxidase (**B**), CD34 (**C**) and, focally, muramidase (**D**)

References

1. Arber DA, Lopategui JR, et al. Chronic lymphoproliferative disorders involving blood and bone marrow. Am J Clin Pathol 1993; 99: 494–503

2. Bartl R, Frisch B. Clinical significance of bone marrow biopsy and plasma cell morphology in MM and MGUS. Pathol Biol (Paris) 1999; 47: 158–68

3. Buhr T, Georgii A, et al. Histologic findings in bone marrow biopsies of patients with thrombocythemic cell counts. Ann Hematol 1992; 64: 286–91

4. Buhr T, Busche G, et al. Evolution of myelofibrosis in chronic idiopathic myelofibrosis as evidenced in sequential bone marrow biopsy specimens. Am J Clin Pathol 2003; 119: 152–8.

5. Burkhardt R, Frisch B, et al. Bone biopsy in haematological disorders. J Clin Pathol 1982; 35: 257–84

6. Florena AM, Iannitto E, et al. Bone marrow biopsy in hemophagocytic syndrome. Virchows Arch 2002; 441: 335–44

7. Foucar K. Bone Marrow Pathology, 2nd edn. ASCP Press, 2001.

8. Georgii A, Vykoupil KF, et al. Chronic myeloproliferative disorders in bone marrow biopsies. Pathol Res Pract 1990; 186: 3–27

9. Lambertenghi-Deliliers G, Pozzoli E, et al. Bone marrow biopsy in chronic myeloid leukemia: significance of some histological parameters. Haematologica 1986; 71: 113–16

10. Lambertenghi-Deliliers G, Annaloro C, et al. Incidence and histological features of bone marrow involvement in malignant lymphomas. Ann Hematol 1992; 65: 61–5

11. Thiele J, Kvasnicka HM. Diagnostic differentiation of essential thrombocythaemia from thrombocythaemias associated with chronic idiopathic myelofibrosis by discriminate analysis of bone marrow features – a clinicopathological study on 272 patients. Histol Histopathol 2003; 18: 93–102

12. Costes V, Duchayne E, et al. Intrasinusoidal bone marrow infiltration: a common growth pattern for different lymphoma subtypes. Br J Haematol 2002; 119: 916–22

13. Schenka AA, Gascoyne RD, et al. Prominent intrasinusoidal infiltration of the bone marrow by mantle cell lymphoma. Hum Pathol 2003; 34: 789–91

14. Borowitz MJ, Guenther KL, et al. Immunophenotyping of acute leukemia by flow cytometric analysis. Use of CD45 and right-angle light scatter to gate on leukemic blasts in three-color analysis. Am J Clin Pathol 1993; 100: 534–40

15. Borowitz MJ, Bray R, et al. U.S.–Canadian Consensus recommendations on the immunophenotypic analysis of hematologic neoplasia by flow cytometry: data analysis and interpretation. Cytometry 1997; 30: 236–44

16. Borowitz MJ. Flow cytometry testing in PNH. How much is enough? Cytometry 2000; 42: 221–2

17. Cabezudo E, Carrara P, et al. Quantitative analysis of CD79b, CD5 and CD19 in mature B-cell lymphoproliferative disorders. Haematologica 1999; 84: 413–18

18. DiGiuseppe JA, Borowitz MJ. Clinical utility of flow cytometry in the chronic lymphoid leukemias. Semin Oncol 1998; 25: 6–10

19. Dunphy CH. Combining morphology and flow cytometric immunophenotyping to evaluate bone marrow specimens for B-cell malignant neoplasms. Am J Clin Pathol 1998; 109: 625–30

20. Gorczyca W, Weisberger J, et al. An approach to diagnosis of T-cell lymphoproliferative disorders by flow cytometry. Cytometry 2002; 50: 177–90

21. Gorczyca W, Tugulea S, et al. Flow cytometry in the diagnosis of mediastinal tumors with emphasis on differentiating thymocytes from precursor T-lymphoblastic lymphoma/leukemia. Leuk Lymphoma 2004; 45: 529–38

22. Gorczyca W. Differential diagnosis of T-cell lymphoproliferative disorders by flow cytometry multicolor immunophenotyping. Correlation with morphology. In: Darzynkiewicz Z, ed. Methods in Cell Biology, Vol. 75. Flow Cytometry, 4th edn. Academic Press, 2004

23. Gorczyca W. Flow cytometry immunophenotypic characteristics of monocytic population in acute monocytic leukemia (AML-M5), acute myelomonocytic leukemia (AML-M4) and chronic myelomonocytic leukemia (CMML). In: Darzynkiewicz Z, ed. Methods in Cell Biology Vol. 75. Flow Cytometry, 4th edn. Academic Press, 2004

24. Ichinohasama R, DeCoteau JF, et al. Three-color flow cytometry in the diagnosis of malignant lymphoma based on the comparative cell morphology of lymphoma cells and reactive lymphocytes. Leukemia 1997; 11: 1891–903

25. Jennings CD, Foon KA. Recent advances in flow cytometry: application to the diagnosis of hematologic malignancy. Blood 1997; 90: 2863–92

26. Khalidi HS, Medeiros LJ, et al. The immunophenotype of adult acute myeloid leukemia: high frequency of lymphoid antigen expression and comparison of immunophenotype, French–American–British classification, and karyotypic abnormalities. Am J Clin Pathol 1998; 109: 211–20

27. Khalidi HS, Chang KL, et al. Acute lymphoblastic leukemia. Survey of immunophenotype, French–American–British classification, frequency of myeloid antigen expression, and karyotypic abnormalities in 210 pediatric and adult cases. Am J Clin Pathol 1999; 111: 467–76

28. Kussick SJ, Wood BL. Using 4-color flow cytometry to identify abnormal myeloid populations. Arch Pathol Lab Med 2003; 127: 1140–7

29. Martinez A, Aymerich M, et al. Routine use of immunophenotype by flow cytometry in tissues with suspected hematological malignancies. Cytometry 2003; 56B: 8–15

30. Orfao A, Ortuno F, et al. Immunophenotyping of acute leukemias and myelodysplastic syndromes. Cytometry 2004; 58A: 62–71

31. Weir EG, Borowitz MJ. Flow cytometry in the diagnosis of acute leukemia. Semin Hematol 2001; 38: 124–38

32. Weisberger J, Wu CD, et al. Differential diagnosis of malignant lymphomas and related disorders by specific pattern of expression of immunophenotypic markers revealed by multiparameter flow cytometry (Review). Int J Oncol 2000; 17: 1165–77

33. Weisberger J, Cornfield D, et al. Down-regulation of pan-T-cell antigens, particularly CD7, in acute infectious mononucleosis. Am J Clin Pathol 2003; 120: 49–55

34. Yamaguchi M, Seto M, et al. De novo CD5+ diffuse large B-cell lymphoma: a clinicopathologic study of 109 patients. Blood 2002; 99: 815–21.

35. Del Poeta G, Maurillo L, et al. Clinical significance of CD38 expression in chronic lymphocytic leukemia. Blood 2001; 98: 2633–9.

36. Wiestner A, Rosenwald A, et al. ZAP-70 expression identifies a chronic lymphocytic leukemia subtype with unmutated immunoglobulin genes, inferior clinical outcome, and distinct gene expression profile. Blood 2003; 101: 4944–51.

37. Barry TS, Jaffe ES, et al. CD5+ follicular lymphoma: a clinicopathologic study of three cases. Am J Clin Pathol 2002; 118: 589–98

38. Hastrup N, Ralfkiaer E, et al. Aberrant phenotypes in peripheral T cell lymphomas. J Clin Pathol 1989; 42: 398–402

39. Li S, Eshleman JR, et al. Lack of surface immunoglobulin light chain expression by flow cytometric immunophenotyping can help diagnose peripheral B-cell lymphoma. Am J Clin Pathol 2002; 118: 229–34

40. Dong H, Gorczyca W, et al. B-cell lymphomas with coexpression of CD5 and CD10. Am J Clin Pathol 2003; 119: 218–30

41. Ginaldi L, Matutes E, et al. Differential expression of CD3 and CD7 in T-cell malignancies: a quantitative study by flow cytometry. Br J Haematol 1996; 93: 921–7

42. Arber DA, Molecular diagnostic approach to non-Hodgkin's lymphoma. J Mol Diagn 2000; 2: 178–90

43. Arber DA, Braziel RM, et al. Evaluation of T cell receptor testing in lymphoid neoplasms: results of a multicenter study of 29 extracted DNA and paraffin-embedded samples. J Mol Diagn 2001; 3: 133–40

44. Ashton-Key M, Diss TC, et al. Molecular analysis of T-cell clonality in ulcerative jejunitis and enteropathy-associated T-cell lymphoma. Am J Pathol 1997; 151: 493–8

45. Bain BJ. Classification of acute leukaemia: the need to incorporate cytogenetic and molecular genetic information. J Clin Pathol 1998; 51: 420–3

46. Bakels V, van Oostveen JW, et al. Immunophenotyping and gene rearrangement analysis provide additional criteria to differentiate between cutaneous T-cell lymphomas and pseudo-T-cell lymphomas. Am J Pathol 1997; 150: 1941–9

47. Bea S, Lopez-Guillermo A, et al. Genetic imbalances in progressed B-cell chronic lymphocytic leukemia and transformed large-cell lymphoma (Richter's syndrome). Am J Pathol 2002; 161: 957–68

48. Bene MC, Bernier M, et al. Acute myeloid leukaemia M0: haematological, immunophenotypic and cytogenetic characteristics and their prognostic significance: an analysis in 241 patients. Br J Haematol 2001; 113: 737–45

49. Boultwood J, Fidler C. Chromosomal deletions in myelodysplasia. Leuk Lymphoma 1995; 17: 71–8

50. Caligiuri MA, Strout MP, et al. Molecular biology of acute myeloid leukemia. Semin Oncol 1997; 24: 32–44

51. Campo E. Genetic and molecular genetic studies in the diagnosis of B-cell lymphomas I: mantle cell lymphoma, follicular lymphoma, and Burkitt's lymphoma. Hum Pathol 2003; 34: 330–5

52. Cortes JE, Talpaz M, et al. Prognostic significance of cytogenetic clonal evolution in patients with chronic myelogenous leukemia on imatinib mesylate therapy. Blood 2003; 101: 3794–800

53. Costello R, Sainty D, et al. Clinical and biological aspects of Philadelphia-negative/BCR-negative chronic myeloid leukemia. Leuk Lymphoma 1997; 25: 225–32

54. Dave BJ, Nelson M, et al. Cytogenetic characterization of diffuse large cell lymphoma using multi-color fluorescence in situ hybridization. Cancer Genet Cytogenet 2002; 132: 125–32

55. Debes-Marun CS, Dewald GW, et al. Chromosome abnormalities clustering and its implications for pathogenesis and prognosis in myeloma. Leukemia 2003; 17: 427–36

56. Delforge M. Understanding the pathogenesis of myelodysplastic syndromes. Hematol J 2003; 4: 303–9

57. Dewald GW, Kyle RA, et al. The clinical significance of cytogenetic studies in 100 patients with multiple myeloma, plasma cell leukemia, or amyloidosis. Blood 1985; 66: 380–90

58. Dohner H, Stilgenbauer S, et al. Genomic aberrations and survival in chronic lymphocytic leukemia. N Engl J Med 2000; 343: 1910–16

59. Falini B. Anaplastic large cell lymphoma: pathological, molecular and clinical features. Br J Haematol 2001; 114: 741–60

60. Fenaux P, Chomienne C, et al. Acute promyelocytic leukemia: biology and treatment. Semin Oncol 1997; 24: 92–102

61. Fend F, Quintanilla-Martinez L, et al. Composite low grade B-cell lymphomas with two immunophenotypically distinct cell populations are true biclonal lymphomas. A molecular analysis using laser capture microdissection. Am J Pathol 1999; 154: 1857–66

62. Frizzera G, Wu CD, et al. The usefulness of immunophenotypic and genotypic studies in the diagnosis and classification of hematopoietic and lymphoid neoplasms. An update. Am J Clin Pathol 1999; 111(1 Suppl 1): S13–39

63. Geddes AA, Bowen DT, Jacobs A. Clonal karyotype abnormalities and clinical progress in the myelodysplastic syndrome. Br J Haematol 1990; 76: 194–202

64. Grimwade D. The clinical significance of cytogenetic abnormalities in acute myeloid leukaemia. Best Pract Res Clin Haematol 2001; 14: 497–529

65. Grimwade D, Walker H, et al. The predictive value of hierarchical cytogenetic classification in older adults with acute myeloid leukemia (AML): analysis of 1065 patients entered into the United Kingdom Medical Research Council AML11 trial. Blood 2001; 98: 1312–20

66. Khoury H, Lestou VS, et al. Multicolor karyotyping and clinicopathological analysis of three intravascular lymphoma cases. Mod Pathol 2003; 16: 716–24

67. Klippel P, Strunk E, et al. Quantification of PRV-1 mRNA distinguishes polycythemia vera from secondary erythrocytosis. Blood 2003; 102: 3569–74

68. Ott G, Katzenberger T, et al. Cytomorphologic, immunohistochemical, and cytogenetic profiles of follicular lymphoma: 2 types of follicular lymphoma grade 3. Blood 2002; 99: 3806–12

69. Rosenwald A, Wright G, et al. Molecular diagnosis of primary mediastinal B cell lymphoma identifies a clinically favorable subgroup of diffuse large B cell lymphoma related to Hodgkin lymphoma. J Exp Med 2003; 198: 851–62

70. Stein H, Hummel M, et al. Molecular biology of Hodgkin's disease. Cancer Surv 1997; 30: 107–23

71. Tefferi A, Mathew P, et al. The 5q- syndrome: a scientific and clinical update. Leuk Lymphoma 1994; 14: 375–8

72. Armitage JO, Weisenburger DD. New approach to classifying non-Hodgkin's lymphomas: clinical features of the major histologic subtypes. Non-Hodgkin's Lymphoma Classification Project. J Clin Oncol 1998; 16: 2780–95

73. Chan JK, Banks PM, et al. A proposal for classification of lymphoid neoplasms (by the International Lymphoma Study Group). Histopathology 1994; 25: 517–36

74. Chan JK, Banks PM, et al. A revised European–American classification of lymphoid neoplasms proposed by the International Lymphoma Study Group. A summary version. Am J Clin Pathol 1995; 103: 543–60

75. Frizzera G. Recent progress in lymphoma classification. Curr Opin Oncol 1997; 9: 392–402

76. Harris NL, Jaffe ES, et al. Lymphoma classification proposal: clarification. Blood 1995; 85: 857–60

77. Harris NL. A practical approach to the pathology of lymphoid neoplasms: a revised European–American classification from the International Lymphoma Study Group. Important Adv Oncol 1995; 111–40

78. Harris NL, Jaffe ES, et al. World Health Organization classification of neoplastic diseases of the hematopoietic and lymphoid tissues: report of the Clinical Advisory Committee meeting – Airlie House, Virginia, November 1997. J Clin Oncol 1999; 17: 3835–49

79. Harris NL, Jaffe ES, et al. The World Health Organization classification of neoplasms of the hematopoietic and lymphoid tissues: report of the Clinical Advisory Committee meeting – Airlie House, Virginia, November, 1997. Hematol J 2000; 1: 53–66

80. Harris NL, Jaffe ES, et al. Lymphoma classification – from controversy to consensus: the R.E.A.L. and WHO Classification of lymphoid neoplasms. Ann Oncol 2000; 11(Suppl 1): 3–10

81. Harris NL, Stein H, et al. New approaches to lymphoma diagnosis. Hematology (Am Soc Hematol Educ Program) 2001; 194–220

82. Hauke RJ, Armitage JO. A new approach to non-Hodgkin's lymphoma. Intern Med 2000; 39: 197–208

83. Isaacson PG. The current status of lymphoma classification. Br J Haematol 2000; 109: 258–66

84. Jaffe ES, Harris NL, et al. World Health Organization Classification of lymphomas: a work in progress. Ann Oncol 1998; 9(Suppl 5): S25–30

85. Jaffe ES, Harris NL, et al. World Health Organization classification of neoplastic diseases of the hematopoietic and lymphoid tissues. A progress report. Am J Clin Pathol 1999; 111(1 Suppl 1): S8–12

86. Knowles DM. Biology of non-Hodgkin's lymphoma. Cancer Treat Res 2001; 104: 149–200

87. Vardiman JW, Harris NL, et al. The World Health Organization (WHO) classification of the myeloid neoplasms. Blood 2002; 100: 2292–302

88. Harris NL, Jaffe ES, et al. The World Health Organization classification of neoplastic diseases of the haematopoietic and lymphoid tissues: Report of the Clinical Advisory Committee Meeting, Airlie House, Virginia, November 1997. Histopathology 2000; 36: 69–86

89. Chadburn A, Narayanan S. Lymphoid malignancies: immunophenotypic analysis. Adv Clin Chem 2003; 37: 293–353

90. de Leval L, Ferry JA, et al. Expression of bcl-6 and CD10 in primary mediastinal large B-cell lymphoma: evidence for derivation from germinal center B cells? Am J Surg Pathol 2001; 25: 1277–82

91. de Leval L, Harris NL, et al. Cutaneous B-cell lymphomas of follicular and marginal zone types: use of Bcl-6, CD10, Bcl-2, and CD21 in differential diagnosis and classification. Am J Surg Pathol 2001; 25: 732–41

92. de Leval L, Harris NL, et al. Variability of immunophenotype in diffuse large B-cell lymphoma and its clinical relevance. Histopathology 2003; 43: 509–28

93. Diebold J, Anderson JR, et al. Diffuse large B-cell lymphoma: a clinicopathologic analysis of 444 cases classified according to the updated Kiel classification. Leuk Lymphoma 2002; 43: 97–104

94. Engelhard M, Brittinger G, et al. Subclassification of diffuse large B-cell lymphomas according to the Kiel classification: distinction of centroblastic and immunoblastic lymphomas is a significant prognostic risk factor. Blood 1997; 89: 2291–7

95. Hans CP, Weisenburger DD, et al. Confirmation of the molecular classification of diffuse large B-cell lymphoma by immunohisto-chemistry using a tissue microarray. Blood 2004; 103: 275–82

96. Nakamura N, Nakamine H, et al. The distinction between Burkitt lymphoma and diffuse large B-cell lymphoma with c-myc rearrangement. Mod Pathol 2002; 15: 771–6

97. Pileri SA, Ceccarelli C, et al. Molecular findings and classification of malignant lymphomas. Acta Haematol 1996; 95: 181–7

98. Pileri SA, Dirnhofer S, et al. Diffuse large B-cell lymphoma: one or more entities? Present controversies and possible tools for its subclassification. Histopathology 2002; 41: 482–509

99. Thieblemont C, Nasser V, et al. Small lymphocytic lymphoma, marginal zone B-cell lymphoma, and mantle cell lymphoma exhibit distinct gene expression profiles allowing molecular diagnosis. Blood 2004; 103: 2727–37

100. Torlakovic E, Torlakovic G, et al. The value of anti-Pax-5 immunostaining in routinely fixed and paraffin-embedded sections. A novel pan-pre-B and B-cell marker. Am J Surg Pathol 2002; 26: 1343–50

101. Ben-Ezra J, Burke JS, et al. Small lymphocytic lymphoma: a clinicopathologic analysis of 268 cases. Blood 1989; 73: 579–87

102. Caligaris-Cappio F, Hamblin TJ. B-cell chronic lymphocytic leukemia: a bird of a different feather. J Clin Oncol 1999; 17: 399–408

103. Caligaris-Cappio F. Biology of chronic lymphocytic leukemia. Rev Clin Exp Hematol 2000; 4: 5–21

104. Criel A, Verhoef G, et al. Further characterization of morpho-logically defined typical and atypical CLL: a clinical, immuno-phenotypic, cytogenetic and prognostic study on 390 cases. Br J Haematol 1997; 97: 383–91

105. Criel A, Michaux L, et al. The concept of typical and atypical chronic lymphocytic leukaemia. Leuk Lymphoma 1999; 33: 33–45

106. Gonzalez H, Maloum K, et al. Cleaved lymphocytes in chronic lymphocytic leukemia: a detailed retrospective analysis of diag-nostic features. Leuk Lymphoma 2002; 43: 555–64

107. Lennert K, Feller AC. Histopathology of Non-Hodgkin Lymphomas, 2nd edn. Springer Verlag, Berlin, 1992

108. Matutes E, Polliack A. Morphological and immunophenotypic features of chronic lymphocytic leukemia. Rev Clin Exp Hematol 2000; 4: 22–47

109. Montesserat E, Villamor N, et al. Bone marrow assessment in B-cell chronic lymphocytic leukemia: aspirate or biopsy? A comparative study. Br J Haematol 1996; 93: 11–16

110. Bonato M, Pittaluga S, et al. Lymph node histology in typical and atypical chronic lymphocytic leukemia. Am J Surg Pathol 1998; 22: 49–56

111. Melo JV, Catovsky D, et al. Chronic lymphocytic leukemia and prolymphocytic leukemia: a clinicopathological reappraisal. Blood Cells 1987; 12: 339–53

112. Melo JV, Catovsky D, et al. The relationship between chronic lymphocytic leukaemia and prolymphocytic leukaemia. IV. Analysis of survival and prognostic features. Br J Haematol 1987; 65: 23–9

113. Ghia P, Guida G, et al. The pattern of CD38 expression defines a distinct subset of chronic lymphocytic leukemia (CLL) patients at risk of disease progression. Blood 2003; 101: 1262–9

114. Hamblin TJ, Orchard JA, et al. CD38 expression and immunoglobulin variable region mutations are independent prognostic variables in chronic lymphocytic leukemia, but CD38 expression may vary during the course of the disease. Blood 2002; 99: 1023–9

115. Dohner H, Stilgenbauer S, et al. Chromosome aberrations in B-cell chronic lymphocytic leukemia: reassessment based on molecular cytogenetic analysis. J Mol Med 1999; 77: 266–81

116. Matutes E. Trisomy 12 in chronic lymphocytic leukaemia. Leuk Res 1996; 20: 375–7

117. Juliusson G, Merup M. Cytogenetics in chronic lymphocytic leukemia. Semin Oncol 1998; 25: 19–26

118. Brecher M, Banks PM. Hodgkin's disease variant of Richter's syn-drome. Report of eight cases. Am J Clin Pathol 1990; 93: 333–9

119. Giles FJ, O'Brien SM, et al. Chronic lymphocytic leukemia in (Richter's) transformation. Semin Oncol 1998; 25: 117–25

120. Matolcsy A, Inghirami G, et al. Molecular genetic demonstration of the diverse evolution of Richter's syndrome (chronic lympho-cytic leukemia and subsequent large cell lymphoma). Blood 1994; 83: 1363–72

121. Matolcsy A, Chadburn A, et al. De novo CD5-positive and Richter's syndrome-associated diffuse large B cell lymphomas are genotypically distinct. Am J Pathol 1995; 147: 207–16

122. Matolcsy A, Casali P, et al. Different clonal origin of B-cell popu-lations of chronic lymphocytic leukemia and large-cell lymphoma in Richter's syndrome. Ann N Y Acad Sci 1995; 764: 496–503

123. Matolcsy A. High-grade transformation of low-grade non-Hodgkin's lymphomas: mechanisms of tumor progression. Leuk Lymphoma 1999; 34: 251–9

124. Matutes E, Brito-Babapulle V, et al. T-cell chronic lymphocytic leukaemia: the spectrum of mature T-cell disorders. Nouv Rev Fr Hematol 1988; 30: 347–51

125. Momose H, Jaffe ES, et al. Chronic lymphocytic leukemia/small lymphocytic lymphoma with Reed–Sternberg-like cells and possible transformation to Hodgkin's disease. Mediation by Epstein-Barr virus. Am J Surg Pathol 1992; 16: 859–67

126. Nakamura N, Kuze T, et al. Richter transformation of a T cell phe-notype with p53 gene mutation. Eur J Haematol 1997; 59: 331–2

127. Nakamura N, Abe M. Richter syndrome in B-cell chronic lymphocytic leukemia. Pathol Int 2003; 53: 195–203

128. Kroft SH, Howard MS, et al. De novo CD5[+] diffuse large B-cell lymphomas. A heterogeneous group containing an unusual form of splenic lymphoma. Am J Clin Pathol 2000; 114: 523–33

129. Matolcsy A. Primary effusion lymphoma: a new non-Hodgkin's lymphoma entity. Pathol Oncol Res 1999; 5: 87–9

130. Matolcsy A, Schattner EJ, et al. Clonal evolution of B cells in transformation from low- to high-grade lymphoma. Eur J Immunol 1999; 29: 1253–64

131. Andriko JA, Aguilera NS, et al. Waldenstrom's macroglobulinemia: a clinicopathologic study of 22 cases. Cancer 1997; 80: 1926–35

132. Desikan KR, Dhodapkar MV, et al. Waldenstrom's macroglobulinemia. Curr Treat Options Oncol 2000; 1: 97–103

133. Dimopoulos MA, Panayiotidis P, et al. Waldenstrom's macroglobulinemia: clinical features, complications, and management. J Clin Oncol 2000; 18: 214–26

134. Kraus MD. Lymphoplasmacytic lymphoma/Waldenstrom macroglobulinemia: one disease or three? Am J Clin Pathol 2001; 116: 799–801

135. Remstein ED, Hanson CA, et al. Despite apparent morphologic and immunophenotypic heterogeneity, Waldenstrom's macroglobulinemia is consistently composed of cells along a morphologic continuum of small lymphocytes, plasmacytoid lymphocytes, and plasma cells. Semin Oncol 2003; 30: 182–6

136. San Miguel JF, Vidriales MB, et al. Immunophenotypic analysis of Waldenstrom's macroglobulinemia. Semin Oncol 2003; 30: 187–95

137. Bhatia JD, Krausz VK, et al. Crystal-storing histiocytosis: a disorder occurring in plasmacytic tumors expressing immunoglobulin kappa light chain. Hum Pathol 1999; 30: 1441–8

138. Lebeau A, Zeindl-Eberhart E, et al. Generalized crystal-storing histiocytosis associated with monoclonal gammopathy: molecular analysis of a disorder with rapid clinical course and review of the literature. Blood 2002; 100: 1817–27

139. Llobet M, Castro P, et al. Massive crystal-storing histiocytosis associated with low-grade malignant B-cell lymphoma of MALT-type of the parotid gland. Diagn Cytopathol 1997; 17: 148–52

140. Andriko JA, Swerdlow SH, et al. Is lymphoplasmacytic lymphoma/immunocytoma a distinct entity? A clinicopathologic study of 20 cases. Am J Surg Pathol 2001; 25: 742–51

141. Berger F, Felman P, et al. Non-MALT marginal zone B-cell lymphomas: a description of clinical presentation and outcome in 124 patients. Blood 2000; 95: 1950–6

142. de Wolf-Peeters C, Pittaluga S, et al. Marginal zone B-cell lymphomas including mucosa-associated lymphoid tissue type lymphoma (MALT), monocytoid B-cell lymphoma and splenic marginal zone cell lymphoma and their relation to the reactive marginal zone. Leuk Lymphoma 1997; 26: 467–78

143. Harris NL. Low-grade B-cell lymphoma of mucosa-associated lymphoid tissue and monocytoid B-cell lymphoma. Related entities that are distinct from other low-grade B-cell lymphomas. Arch Pathol Lab Med 1993; 117: 771–5

144. Camacho FI, Mollejo M, et al. Progression to large B-cell lymphoma in splenic marginal zone lymphoma: a description of a series of 12 cases. Am J Surg Pathol 2001; 25: 1268–76

145. Catovsky D, Matutes E. Splenic lymphoma with circulating villous lymphocytes/splenic marginal-zone lymphoma. Semin Hematol 1999; 36: 148–54

146. Chacon JI, Mollejo M, et al. Splenic marginal zone lymphoma: clinical characteristics and prognostic factors in a series of 60 patients. Blood 2002; 100: 1648–54

147. Dogan A, Isaacson PG. Splenic marginal zone lymphoma. Semin Diagn Pathol 2003; 20: 121–7

148. Franco V, Florena AM, et al. Splenic marginal zone lymphoma. Blood 2003; 101: 2464–72

149. Harris S, Wilkins BS, et al. Splenic marginal zone expansion in B-cell lymphomas of gastrointestinal mucosa-associated lymphoid tissue (MALT) is reactive and does not represent homing of neoplastic lymphocytes. J Pathol 1996; 179: 49–53

150. Iannitto E, Ammatuna E, et al. Prognostic features of splenic lymphoma with villous lymphocytes. Br J Haematol 2003; 123: 370–1

151. Isaacson PG, Matutes E, et al. The histopathology of splenic lymphoma with villous lymphocytes. Blood 1994; 84: 3828–34

152. Isaacson PG. Splenic marginal zone lymphoma. Blood 1996; 88: 751–2

153. Mollejo M, Menarguez J, et al. Splenic marginal zone lymphoma: a distinctive type of low-grade B-cell lymphoma. A clinicopathological study of 13 cases. Am J Surg Pathol 1995; 19: 1146–57

154. Mollejo M, Algara P, et al. Splenic small B-cell lymphoma with predominant red pulp involvement: a diffuse variant of splenic marginal zone lymphoma? Histopathology 2002; 40: 22–30

155. Parry-Jones N, Matutes E, et al. Prognostic features of splenic lymphoma with villous lymphocytes: a report on 129 patients. Br J Haematol 2003; 120: 759–64

156. Piris MA, Mollejo M, et al. A marginal zone pattern may be found in different varieties of non-Hodgkin's lymphoma: the morphology and immunohistology of splenic involvement by B-cell lymphomas simulating splenic marginal zone lymphoma. Histopathology 1998; 33: 230–9

157. Thieblemont C, Berger F, et al. Mucosa-associated lymphoid tissue lymphoma is a disseminated disease in one third of 158 patients analyzed. Blood 2000; 95: 802–6

158. Thieblemont C, Felman P, et al. Splenic marginal-zone lymphoma: a distinct clinical and pathological entity. Lancet Oncol 2003; 4: 95–103

159. Arber DA, Rappaport H, et al. Non-Hodgkin's lymphoproliferative disorders involving the spleen. Mod Pathol 1997; 10: 18–32

160. Arcaini L, Paulli M, et al. Marginal zone-related neoplasms of splenic and nodal origin. Haematologica 2003; 88: 80–93

161. Mollejo M, Algara P, et al. Large B-cell lymphoma presenting in the spleen: identification of different clinicopathologic conditions. Am J Surg Pathol 2003; 27: 895–902

162. Piris MA, Orradre JL, et al. Monocytoid B-cell lymphoma – a MALT tumour? Histopathology 1990; 17: 287–8

163. Camacho FI, Algara P, et al. Nodal marginal zone lymphoma: a heterogeneous tumor: a comprehensive analysis of a series of 27 cases. Am J Surg Pathol 2003; 27: 762–71

164. Campo E, Miquel R, et al. Primary nodal marginal zone lymphomas of splenic and MALT type. Am J Surg Pathol 1999; 23: 59–68

165. Nathwani BN, Anderson JR, et al. Marginal zone B-cell lymphoma: a clinical comparison of nodal and mucosa-associated lymphoid tissue types. Non-Hodgkin's Lymphoma Classification Project. J Clin Oncol 1999; 17: 2486–92

166. Nathwani BN, Drachenberg MR, et al. Nodal monocytoid B-cell lymphoma (nodal marginal-zone B-cell lymphoma). Semin Hematol 1999; 36: 128–38

167. Nathwani BN, Drachenberg MR, et al. Primary nodal marginal zone lymphomas of splenic and MALT type. Am J Surg Pathol 2000; 24: 317–19

168. Zucca E, Conconi A, et al. Nongastric marginal zone B-cell lymphoma of mucosa-associated lymphoid tissue. Blood 2003; 101: 2489–95

169. Bailey EM, Ferry JA, et al. Marginal zone lymphoma (low-grade B-cell lymphoma of mucosa-associated lymphoid tissue type) of skin and subcutaneous tissue: a study of 15 patients. Am J Surg Pathol 1996; 20: 1011–23

170. Baldassano MF, Bailey EM, et al. Cutaneous lymphoid hyperplasia and cutaneous marginal zone lymphoma: comparison of morphologic and immunophenotypic features. Am J Surg Pathol 1999; 23: 88–96

171. Cavalli F, Isaacson PG, et al. MALT lymphomas. Hematology (Am Soc Hematol Educ Program): 2001; 241–58

172. Harris NL. Extranodal lymphoid infiltrates and mucosa-associated lymphoid tissue (MALT). A unifying concept. Am J Surg Pathol 1991; 15: 879–84

173. Isaacson PG, Spencer J. Malignant lymphoma of mucosa-associated lymphoid tissue. Histopathology 1987; 11: 445–62

174. Isaacson PG. Lymphomas of mucosa-associated lymphoid tissue (MALT). Histopathology 1990; 16: 617–19

175. Isaacson PG. Gastrointestinal lymphoma. Hum Pathol 1994; 25: 1020–9

176. Isaacson PG, Banks PM, et al. Primary low-grade hepatic B-cell lymphoma of mucosa-associated lymphoid tissue (MALT)-type. Am J Surg Pathol 1995; 19: 571–5

177. Isaacson PG, Spencer J. The biology of low grade MALT lymphoma. J Clin Pathol 1995; 48: 395–7

178. Ott MM, Rosenwald A, et al. Marginal zone B-cell lymphomas (MZBL) arising at different sites represent different biological entities. Genes Chromosomes Cancer 2000; 28: 380–6

179. Wenzel C, Dieckmann K, et al. CD5 expression in a lymphoma of the mucosa-associated lymphoid tissue (MALT)-type as a marker for early dissemination and aggressive clinical behavior. Leuk Lymphoma 2001; 42: 823–9

180. Wenzel C, Fiebiger W, et al. Extranodal marginal zone B-cell lymphoma of mucosa-associated lymphoid tissue of the head and neck area: high rate of disease recurrence following local therapy. Cancer 2003; 97: 2236–41

181. Zinzani PL, Tani M, et al. Extranodal marginal zone B-cell lymphoma of MALT-type of the lung: single-center experience with 12 patients. Leuk Lymphoma 2003; 44: 821–4

182. Eck M, Schmausser B, et al. MALT-type lymphoma of the stomach is associated with Helicobacter pylori strains expressing the CagA protein. Gastroenterology 1997; 112: 1482–6

183. Eck M, Greiner A, et al. Evaluation of Helicobacter pylori in gastric MALT-type lymphoma: differences between histologic and serologic diagnosis. Mod Pathol 1999; 12: 1148–51

184. Eck M, Schmausser B, et al. Helicobacter pylori in gastric mucosa-associated lymphoid tissue type lymphoma. Recent Results Cancer Res 2000; 156: 9–18

185. Isaacson PG. Gastric lymphoma and Helicobacter pylori. N Engl J Med 1994; 330: 1310–11

186. Isaacson PG, Spencer J. Gastric lymphoma and Helicobacter pylori. Important Adv Oncol 1996; 111–21

187. Isaacson PG, Diss TC, et al. Long-term follow-up of gastric MALT lymphoma treated by eradication of H. pylori with antibodies. Gastroenterology 1999; 117: 750–1

188. Isaacson PG. Gastric MALT lymphoma: from concept to cure. Ann Oncol 1999; 10: 637–45

189. Nakamura S, Aoyagi K, et al. B-cell monoclonality precedes the development of gastric MALT lymphoma in Helicobacter pylori-associated chronic gastritis. Am J Pathol 1998; 152: 1271–9

190. Ye H, Liu H, et al. High incidence of t(11; 18)(q21; q21) in Helicobacter pylori-negative gastric MALT lymphoma. Blood 2003; 101: 2547–50

191. Chuang SS, Lee C, et al. High frequency of t(11; 18) in gastric mucosa-associated lymphoid tissue lymphomas in Taiwan, including one patient with high-grade transformation. Br J Haematol 2003; 120: 97–100

192. Ott G, Katzenberger T, et al. The t(11; 18)(q21; q21) chromosome translocation is a frequent and specific aberration in low-grade but not high-grade malignant non-Hodgkin's lymphomas of the mucosa-associated lymphoid tissue (MALT-) type. Cancer Res 1997; 57: 3944–8

193. Starostik P, Patzner J, et al. Gastric marginal zone B-cell lymphomas of MALT type develop along 2 distinct pathogenetic pathways. Blood 2002; 99: 3–9

194. Fischbach W, Dragosics B, et al. Primary gastric B-cell lymphoma: results of a prospective multicenter study. The German–Austrian Gastrointestinal Lymphoma Study Group. Gastroenterology 2000; 119: 1191–202

195. Isaacson PG, Spencer J, et al. Primary B-cell gastric lymphoma. Hum Pathol 1986; 17: 72–82

196. Nakamura S, Tsuneyoshi M. Primary gastric T-cell lymphoma with and without human T-lymphotropic virus type 1. Cancer 1998; 82: 998–1000

197. McCullough JE, Kim CH, et al. Mantle zone lymphoma of the colon simulating diffuse inflammatory bowel disease. Role of immunohistochemistry in establishing the diagnosis. Dig Dis Sci 1992; 37: 934–8

198. Bouroncle BA. Thirty-five years in the progress of hairy cell leukemia. Leuk Lymphoma 1994; 14(Suppl 1): 1–12

199. Frassoldati A, Lamparelli T, et al. Hairy cell leukemia: a clinical review based on 725 cases of the Italian Cooperative Group (ICGHCL). Italian Cooperative Group for Hairy Cell Leukemia. Leuk Lymphoma 1994; 13: 307–16

200. Hounieu H, Chittal SM, et al. Hairy cell leukemia. Diagnosis of bone marrow involvement in paraffin-embedded sections with monoclonal antibody DBA.44. Am J Clin Pathol 1992; 98: 26–33

201. Matutes E, Wotherspoon A, et al. The natural history and clinico-pathological features of the variant form of hairy cell leukemia. Leukemia 2001; 15: 184–6

202. Pittaluga S, Tierens A, et al. How reliable is histologic examination of bone marrow trephine biopsy specimens for the staging of non-Hodgkin lymphoma? A study of hairy cell leukemia and mantle cell lymphoma involvement of the bone marrow trephine specimen by histologic, immunohistochemical, and polymerase chain reaction techniques. Am J Clin Pathol 1999; 111: 179–84

203. Sun T, Dittmar K, et al. Relationship between hairy cell leukemia variant and splenic lymphoma with villous lymphocytes: presentation of a new concept. Am J Hematol 1996; 51: 282–8

204. Mercieca J, Matutes E, et al. Massive abdominal lymphadenopathy in hairy cell leukaemia: a report of 12 cases. Br J Haematol 1992; 82: 547–54

205. Matutes E, Wotherspoon A, et al. The variant form of hairy-cell leukaemia. Best Pract Res Clin Haematol 2003; 16: 41–56

206. Sainati L, Matutes E, et al. A variant of hairy cell leukemia resistant to alpha-interferon: clinical and phenotypic characteristics of 17 patients. Blood 1990; 76: 157–62

207. Barlogie B, Epstein J, et al. Plasma cell myeloma – new biological insights and advances in therapy. Blood 1989; 73: 865–79

208. Barlogie B. Advances in therapy of multiple myeloma: lessons from acute leukemia. Clin Cancer Res 1997; 3(12 Pt 2): 2605–13

209. Bartl R, Frisch B, et al. Bone marrow histology in myeloma: its importance in diagnosis, prognosis, classification and staging. Br J Haematol 1982; 51: 361–75

210. Bartl R, Frisch B, et al. Histologic classification and staging of multiple myeloma. A retrospective and prospective study of 674 cases. Am J Clin Pathol 1987; 87: 342–55

211. Bartl R. Histologic classification and staging of multiple myeloma. Hematol Oncol 1988; 6: 107–13

212. Ho PJ, Campbell LJ, et al. The biology and cytogenetics of multiple myeloma. Rev Clin Exp Hematol 2002; 6: 276–300

213. Fonseca R, Coignet LJ, et al. Cytogenetic abnormalities in multiple myeloma. Hematol Oncol Clin North Am 1999; 13: 1169–80, viii

214. Fonseca R, Oken MM, et al. Deletions of chromosome 13 in multiple myeloma identified by interphase FISH usually denote large deletions of the q arm or monosomy. Leukemia 2001; 15: 981–6

215. Fonseca R, Bailey RJ, et al. Genomic abnormalities in monoclonal gammopathy of undetermined significance. Blood 2002; 100: 1417–24

216. Fonseca R, Blood EA, et al. Myeloma and the t(11; 14)(q13; q32); evidence for a biologically defined unique subset of patients. Blood 2002; 99: 3735–41

217. Fonseca R, Blood E, et al. Clinical and biologic implications of recurrent genomic aberrations in myeloma. Blood 2003; 101: 4569–75

218. Hoechtlen-Vollmar W, Menzel G, et al. Amplification of cyclin D1 gene in multiple myeloma: clinical and prognostic relevance. Br J Haematol 2000; 109: 30–8

219. Zhan F, Barlogie B, et al. Toward the identification of distinct molecular and clinical entities of multiple myeloma using global gene expression profiling. Semin Hematol 2003; 40: 308–20

220. Durie BG. Multiple myeloma: what's new. CA Cancer J Clin 2001; 51: 271–2, 263

221. Garcia-Sanz R, Orfao A, et al. Primary plasma cell leukemia: clinical, immunophenotypic, DNA ploidy, and cytogenetic characteristics. Blood 1999; 93: 1032–7

222. Kyle RA. Benign monoclonal gammopathy – after 20–35 years of follow-up. Mayo Clin Proc 1993; 68: 26–36

223. Alexiou C, Kau RJ, et al. Extramedullary plasmacytoma: tumor occurrence and therapeutic concepts. Cancer 1999; 85: 2305–14

224. Lee CK, Ma ES, et al. Plasmablastic transformation of multiple myeloma. Hum Pathol 2003; 34: 710–14

225. Hollowood K, Goodlad JR. Follicular lymphomas. Histopathology 1996; 29: 195

226. Isaacson PG. Malignant lymphomas with a follicular growth pattern. Histopathology 1996; 28: 487–95

227. Lai R, Weiss LM, et al. Frequency of CD43 expression in non-Hodgkin lymphoma. A survey of 742 cases and further characterization of rare CD43+ follicular lymphomas. Am J Clin Pathol 1999; 111: 488–94

228. Jardin F, Gaulard P, et al. Follicular lymphoma without t(14; 18) and with BCL-6 rearrangement: a lymphoma subtype with distinct pathological, molecular and clinical characteristics. Leukemia 2002; 16: 2309–17

229. Skinnider BF, Horsman DE, et al. Bcl-6 and Bcl-2 protein expression in diffuse large B-cell lymphoma and follicular lymphoma: correlation with 3q27 and 18q21 chromosomal abnormalities. Hum Pathol 1999; 30: 803–8

230. Horsman DE, Okamoto I, et al. Follicular lymphoma lacking the t(14; 18)(q32; q21): identification of two disease subtypes. Br J Haematol 2003; 120: 424–33

231. Hans CP, Weisenburger DD, et al. A significant diffuse component predicts for inferior survival in grade 3 follicular lymphoma, but cytologic subtypes do not predict survival. Blood 2003; 101: 2363–7

232. Natkunam Y, Warnke RA, et al. Blastic/blastoid transformation of follicular lymphoma. Immunohistologic and molecular analyses of five cases. Am J Surg Pathol 2002; 24: 525–34

233. Franco R, Fernandez-Vazquez A, et al. Cutaneous presentation of follicular lymphomas. Mod Pathol 2001; 14: 913–19

234. Hashimoto Y, Nakamura N, et al. Multiple lymphomatous polyposis of the gastrointestinal tract is a heterogeneous group

that includes mantle cell lymphoma and follicular lymphoma: analysis of somatic mutation of immunoglobulin heavy chain gene variable region. Hum Pathol 1999; 30: 581–7

235. Melo JV, Robinson DS, et al. Morphology and immunology of circulating cells in leukaemic phase of follicular lymphoma. J Clin Pathol 1988; 41: 951–9

236. Mirza I, Macpherson N, et al. Primary cutaneous follicular lymphoma: an assessment of clinical, histopathologic, immunophenotypic, and molecular features. J Clin Oncol 2002; 20: 647–55

237. Nadal E, Martinez A, et al. Primary follicular lymphoma arising in the ampulla of Vater. Ann Hematol 2002; 81: 228–31

238. Yoshino T, Miyake K, et al. Increased incidence of follicular lymphoma in the duodenum. Am J Surg Pathol 2000; 24: 688–93

239. Willemze R, Kerl H, et al. EORTC classification for primary cutaneous lymphomas: a proposal from the Cutaneous Lymphoma Study Group. Blood 1997; 90: 354–71

240. Argatoff LH, Connors JM, et al. Mantle cell lymphoma: a clinicopathologic study of 80 cases. Blood 1997; 89: 2067–78

241. Banks PM, Chan J, et al. Mantle cell lymphoma. A proposal for unification of morphologic, immunologic, and molecular data. Am J Surg Pathol 1992; 16: 637–40

242. Bosch F, Lopez-Guillermo A, et al. Mantle cell lymphoma: presenting features, response to therapy, and prognostic factors. Cancer 1998; 82: 567–75

243. de Boer CJ, van Krieken JH, et al. Cyclin D1 messenger RNA overexpression as a marker for mantle cell lymphoma. Oncogene 1995; 10: 1833–40

244. de Boer CJ, Schuuring E, et al. Cyclin D1 protein analysis in the diagnosis of mantle cell lymphoma. Blood 1995; 86: 2715–23

245. Harris NL. Mantle cell lymphoma. J Clin Oncol 1994; 12: 876–7

246. Harris AW, Bodrug SE, et al. Cyclin D1 as the putative bcl-1 oncogene. Curr Top Microbiol Immunol 1995; 194: 347–53

247. Lai R, Medeiros LJ. Pathologic diagnosis of mantle cell lymphoma. Clin Lymphoma 2000; 1: 197–206; discussion 207–8

248. Leitch HA, Gascoyne RD, et al. Limited-stage mantle-cell lymphoma. Ann Oncol 2003; 14: 1555–61

249. Majlis A, Pugh WC, et al. Mantle cell lymphoma: correlation of clinical outcome and biologic features with three histologic variants. J Clin Oncol 1997; 15: 1664–71

250. Swerdlow SH, Zukerberg LR, et al. The morphologic spectrum of non-Hodgkin's lymphomas with BCL1/cyclin D1 gene rearrangements. Am J Surg Pathol 1996; 20: 627–40

251. Weisenburger DD, Vose JM, et al. Mantle cell lymphoma. A clinicopathologic study of 68 cases from the Nebraska Lymphoma Study Group. Am J Hematol 2000; 64: 190–6

252. Campo E, Raffeld M, et al. Mantle-cell lymphoma. Semin Hematol 1999; 36: 115–27

253. Kumar S, Krenacs L, et al. bc1-1 rearrangement and cyclin D1 protein expression in multiple lymphomatous polyposis. Am J Clin Pathol 1996; 105: 737–43

254. Pittaluga S, Verhoef G, et al. 'Small' B-cell non-Hodgkin's lymphomas with splenomegaly at presentation are either mantle cell lymphoma or marginal zone cell lymphoma. A study based on histology, cytology, immunohistochemistry, and cytogenetic analysis. Am J Surg Pathol 1996; 20: 211–23

255. Liu Z, Dong HY, et al. CD5- mantle cell lymphoma. Am J Clin Pathol 2002; 118: 216–24

256. Bea S, Ribas M, et al. Increased number of chromosomal imbalances and high-level DNA amplifications in mantle cell lymphoma are associated with blastoid variants. Blood 1999; 93: 4365–74

257. Laszlo T, Matolcsy A. Blastic transformation of mantle cell lymphoma: genetic evidence for a clonal link between the two stages of the tumour. Histopathology 1999; 35: 355–9

258. Ott G, Kalla J, et al. The cytomorphological spectrum of mantle cell lymphoma is reflected by distinct biological features. Leuk Lymphoma 1998; 32: 55–63

259. Pittaluga S, Tierens A, et al. Blastic variant of mantle cell lymphoma shows a heterogeneous pattern of somatic mutations of the rearranged immunoglobulin heavy chain variable genes. Br J Haematol 1998; 102: 1301–6

260. Soslow RA, Zukerberg LR, et al. BCL-1 (PRAD-1/cyclin D-1) overexpression distinguishes the blastoid variant of mantle cell lymphoma from B-lineage lymphoblastic lymphoma. Mod Pathol 1997; 10: 810–17

261. Chikatsu N, Kojima H, et al. ALK+, CD30-, CD20- large B-cell lymphoma containing anaplastic lymphoma kinase (ALK) fused to clathrin heavy chain gene (CLTC). Mod Pathol 2003; 16: 828–32

262. de Leval L, Braaten KM, et al. Diffuse large B-cell lymphoma of bone: an analysis of differentiation-associated antigens with clinical correlation. Am J Surg Pathol 2003; 27: 1269–77

263. Gascoyne RD, Lamant L, et al. ALK-positive diffuse large B-cell lymphoma is associated with Clathrin-ALK rearrangements: report of 6 cases. Blood 2003; 102: 2568–73

264. Haralambieva E, Pulford KA, et al. Anaplastic large-cell lymphomas of B-cell phenotype are anaplastic lymphoma kinase (ALK) negative and belong to the spectrum of diffuse large B-cell lymphomas. Br J Haematol 2000; 109: 584–91

265. Jaffe ES. Hematopathology: integration of morphologic features and biologic markers for diagnosis. Mod Pathol 1999; 12: 109–15

266. Maes B, Anastasopoulou A, et al. Among diffuse large B-cell lymphomas, T-cell-rich/histiocyte-rich BCL and CD30+ anaplastic B-cell subtypes exhibit distinct clinical features. Ann Oncol 2001; 12: 853–8

267. Pileri S, Falini B, et al. Lymphohistiocytic T-cell lymphoma (anaplastic large cell lymphoma CD30+/Ki-1+ with a high content of reactive histiocytes). Histopathology 1990; 16: 383–91

268. Pileri SA, Zinzani PL, et al. Diffuse large B-cell lymphoma with primary retroperitoneal presentation: clinico-pathologic study of nine cases. Ann Oncol 2001; 12: 1445–53

269. Felgar RE, Steward KR, et al. T-cell-rich large-B-cell lymphomas contain non-activated CD8+ cytolytic T cells, show increased

tumor cell apoptosis, and have lower Bcl-2 expression than diffuse large-B-cell lymphomas. Am J Pathol 1998; 153: 1707–15

270. Dogan A, Burke JS, et al. Micronodular T-cell/histiocyte-rich large B-cell lymphoma of the spleen: histology, immunophenotype, and differential diagnosis. Am J Surg Pathol 2003; 27: 903–11

271. Fraga M, Sanchez-Verde L, et al. T-cell/histiocyte-rich large B-cell lymphoma is a disseminated aggressive neoplasm: differential diagnosis from Hodgkin's lymphoma. Histopathology 2002; 41: 216–29

272. Jaffe ES, Gonzalez CL, et al. T-cell-rich B-cell lymphomas. Am J Surg Pathol 1991; 15: 491–2

273. Li S, Griffin CA, et al. Primary cutaneous T-cell-rich B-cell lymphoma: clinically distinct from its nodal counterpart? Mod Pathol 2001; 14: 10–13

274. Lim MS, Beaty M, et al. T-cell/histiocyte-rich large B-cell lymphoma: a heterogeneous entity with derivation from germinal center B cells. Am J Surg Pathol 2002; 26: 1458–66

275. Pileri SA, Ascani S, et al. Diffuse large B-cell lymphoma (DLBCL), anaplastic variant. Report on a problematic case primarily arising in the stomach. Haematologica 2002; 87: ECR40

276. Lai R, Medeiros LJ, et al. Sinusoidal CD30-positive large B-cell lymphoma: a morphologic mimic of anaplastic large cell lymphoma. Mod Pathol 2000; 13: 223–8

277. Brown RS, Campbell C, et al. Plasmablastic lymphoma: a new subcategory of human immunodeficiency virus-related non-Hodgkin's lymphoma. Clin Oncol (R Coll Radiol) 1998; 10: 327–9

278. Delecluse HJ, Anagnostopoulos I, et al. Plasmablastic lymphomas of the oral cavity: a new entity associated with the human immunodeficiency virus infection. Blood 1997; 89: 1413–20

279. Dupin N, Diss TL, et al. HHV-8 is associated with a plasmablastic variant of Castleman disease that is linked to HHV-8-positive plasmablastic lymphoma. Blood 2000; 95: 1406–12

280. Gaidano G, Cerri M, et al. Molecular histogenesis of plasmablastic lymphoma of the oral cavity. Br J Haematol 2002; 119: 622–8

281. Nguyen DD, Loo BW Jr, et al. Plasmablastic lymphoma presenting in a human immunodeficiency virus-negative patient: a case report. Ann Hematol 2003; 82: 521–5

282. Delsol G, Lamant L, et al. A new subtype of large B-cell lymphoma expressing the ALK kinase and lacking the 2; 5 translocation. Blood 1997; 89: 1483–90

283. Chittal SM, Brousset P, et al. Large B-cell lymphoma rich in T-cells and simulating Hodgkin's disease. Histopathology 1991; 19: 211–20

284. Elgin J, Phillips G, et al. Hodgkin's and non-Hodgkin's lymphoma: spectrum of morphologic and immunophenotypic overlap. Ann Diagn Pathol 1999; 3: 263–75

285. Harris NL. The relationship between Hodgkin's disease and non-Hodgkin's lymphoma. Semin Diagn Pathol 1992; 9: 304–10

286. Harris NL. Differential diagnosis between Hodgkin's disease and non-Hodgkin's lymphoma. Int Rev Exp Pathol 1992; 33: 1–25

287. Harris NL. The many faces of Hodgkin's disease around the world: what have we learned from its pathology? Ann Oncol 1998; 9(Suppl 5): S45–56

288. Harris NL. Hodgkin's disease: classification and differential diagnosis. Mod Pathol 1999; 12: 159–75

289. Nguyen DT, Diamond LW, et al. Differential diagnosis of L26-positive, CD15-negative Hodgkin's disease and large B-cell lymphoma with a high content of reactive T-cells: a morphologic and immunohistochemical study. Hematopathol Mol Hematol 1996; 10: 135–50

290. Piris M, Brown DC, et al. CD30 expression in non-Hodgkin's lymphoma. Histopathology 1990; 17: 211–18

291. Savage KJ, Monti S, et al. The molecular signature of mediastinal large B-cell lymphoma differs from that of other diffuse large B-cell lymphomas and shares features with classical Hodgkin's lymphoma. Blood 2003; 102: 3871–9

292. Chang KL, Kamel OW, et al. Pathologic features of nodular lymphocyte predominance Hodgkin's disease in extranodal sites. Am J Surg Pathol 1995; 19: 1313–24

293. Falini B, Bigerna B, et al. Distinctive expression pattern of the BCL-6 protein in nodular lymphocyte predominance Hodgkin's disease. Blood 1996; 87: 465–71

294. Kraus MD, Haley J. Lymphocyte predominance Hodgkin's disease. The use of bcl-6 and CD57 in diagnosis and differential diagnosis. Am J Surg Pathol 2000; 24: 1068–78

295. Allory Y, Challine D, et al. Bone marrow involvement in lymphomas with hemophagocytic syndrome at presentation: a clinicopathologic study of 11 patients in a Western institution. Am J Surg Pathol 2001; 25: 865–74

296. Abou-Elella AA, Weisenburger DD, et al. Primary mediastinal large B-cell lymphoma: a clinicopathologic study of 43 patients from the Nebraska Lymphoma Study Group. J Clin Oncol 1999; 17: 784–90

297. Barth TF, Leithauser F, et al. Mediastinal B-cell lymphoma, a lymphoma type with several characteristics unique among diffuse large B-cell lymphomas. Ann Hematol 2001; 80(Suppl 3): B49–53

298. Barth TF, Leithauser F, et al. Mediastinal (thymic) large B-cell lymphoma: where do we stand? Lancet Oncol 2002; 3: 229–34

299. Cazals-Hatem D, Lepage E, et al. Primary mediastinal large B-cell lymphoma. A clinicopathologic study of 141 cases compared with 916 nonmediastinal large B-cell lymphomas, a GELA ('Groupe d'Etude des Lymphomes de l'Adulte') study. Am J Surg Pathol 1996; 20: 877–88

300. Davis RE, Dorfman RF, et al. Primary large-cell lymphoma of the thymus: a diffuse B-cell neoplasm presenting as primary mediastinal lymphoma. Hum Pathol 1990; 21: 1262–8

301. Paulli M, Strater J, et al. Mediastinal B-cell lymphoma: a study of its histomorphologic spectrum based on 109 cases. Hum Pathol 1999; 30: 178–87

302. Kirn D, Mauch P, et al. Large-cell and immunoblastic lymphoma of the mediastinum: prognostic features and treatment outcome in 57 patients. J Clin Oncol 1993; 11: 1336–43

303. Pileri SA, Gaidano G, et al. Primary mediastinal B-cell lymphoma: high frequency of BCL-6 mutations and consistent expression of the transcription factors OCT-2, BOB.1, and PU.1 in the absence of immunoglobulins. Am J Pathol 2003; 162: 243–53

304. Sander CA, Jaffe ES, et al. Mediastinal lymphoblastic lymphoma with an immature B-cell B-cell immunophenotype. Am J Surg Pathol 1992; 16: 300–5

305. Suster S. Primary large-cell lymphomas of the mediastinum. Semin Diagn Pathol 1999; 16: 51–64

306. Tsang P, Cesarman E, et al. Molecular characterization of primary mediastinal B cell lymphoma. Am J Pathol 1996; 148: 2017–25

307. Zinzani PL, Martelli M, et al. Primary mediastinal large B-cell lymphoma with sclerosis: a clinical study of 89 patients treated with MACOP-B chemotherapy and radiation therapy. Haematologica 2001; 86: 187–91

308. Higgins JP, Warnke RA. CD30 expression is common in mediastinal large B-cell lymphoma. Am J Clin Pathol 1999; 112: 241–7

309. Ferry JA, Harris NL, et al. Intravascular lymphomatosis (malignant angioendotheliomatosis). A B-cell neoplasm expressing surface homing receptors. Mod Pathol 1988; 1: 444–52

310. Ascoli V, Signoretti S, et al. Primary effusion lymphoma in HIV-infected patients with multicentric Castleman's disease. J Pathol 2001; 193: 200–9

311. Cobo F, Hernandez S, et al. Expression of potentially oncogenic HHV-8 genes in an EBV-negative primary effusion lymphoma occurring in an HIV-seronegative patient. J Pathol 1999; 189: 288–93

312. Gaidano G, Carbone A. Primary effusion lymphoma: a liquid phase lymphoma of fluid-filled body cavities. Adv Cancer Res 2001; 80: 115–46

313. Jaffe ES. Primary body cavity-based AIDS-related lymphomas. Evolution of a new disease entity. Am J Clin Pathol 1996; 105: 141–3

314. Klein U, Gloghini A, et al. Gene expression profile analysis of AIDS-related primary effusion lymphoma (PEL) suggests a plasmablastic derivation and identifies PEL-specific transcripts. Blood 2003; 101: 4115–21

315. Nador RG, Cesarman E, et al. Primary effusion lymphoma: a distinct clinicopathologic entity associated with the Kaposi's sarcoma-associated herpes virus. Blood 1996; 88: 645–56

316. Nakamura Y, Tajima F, et al. Primary effusion lymphoma of the left scrotum. Intern Med 2003; 42: 351–3

317. Simonelli C, Spina M, et al. Clinical features and outcome of primary effusion lymphoma in HIV-infected patients: a single-institution study. J Clin Oncol 2003; 21: 3948–54

318. Wilson KS, McKenna RW, et al. Primary effusion lymphomas exhibit complex and recurrent cytogenetic abnormalities. Br J Haematol 2002; 116: 113–21

319. Chan AC, Chan JK, et al. Anaplastic large cell lymphoma presenting as a pleural effusion and mimicking primary effusion lymphoma. A report of 2 cases. Acta Cytol 2003; 47: 809–16

320. Lai R, Medeiros LJ, et al. Sinusoidal CD30-positive large B-cell lymphoma: a morphologic mimic of anaplastic large cell lymphoma. Mod Pathol 2000; 13: 223–8

321. Carbone A, Canzonieri V, et al. Burkitt's lymphoma: historical background and recent insights into classification and pathogenesis. Ann Otol Rhinol Laryngol 2000; 109: 693–702

322. Harris E, Paneesha S, et al. Burkitt's lymphoma: single-centre experience with modified BFM protocol. Clin Lab Haematol 2002; 24: 111–14

323. Jaffe ES, Diebold J, et al. Burkitt's lymphoma: a single disease with multiple variants. The World Health Organization classification of neoplastic diseases of the hematopoietic and lymphoid tissues. Blood 1999; 93: 1124

324. Takada K. Role of Epstein-Barr virus in Burkitt's lymphoma. Curr Top Microbiol Immunol 2001; 258: 141–51

325. Braziel RM, Arber DA, et al. The Burkitt-like lymphomas: a Southwest Oncology Group study delineating phenotypic, and clinical features. Blood 2001; 97: 3713–20

326. Davi F, Delecluse HJ, et al. Burkitt-like lymphomas in AIDS patients: characterization within a series of 103 human immunodeficiency virus-associated non-Hodgkin's lymphomas. Burkitt's Lymphoma Study Group. J Clin Oncol 1998; 16: 3788–95

327. Fenaux P, Bourhis JH, et al. Burkitt's acute lymphocytic leukemia (L3ALL) in adults. Hematol Oncol Clin North Am 2001; 15: 37–50

328. Lin P, Jones D, et al. Precursor B-cell lymphoblastic lymphoma: a predominantly extranodal tumor with low propensity for leukemic involvement. Am J Surg Pathol 2000; 24: 1480–90

329. Maitra A, McKenna RW, et al. Precursor B-cell lymphoblastic lymphoma. A study of nine cases lacking blood and bone marrow involvement and review of the literature. Am J Clin Pathol 2001; 115: 868–75

330. Onciu M, Lai R, et al. Precursor T-cell acute lymphoblastic leukemia in adults. Age-related immunophenotypic, cytogenetic, and molecular subsets. Am J Clin Pathol 2002; 117: 252–8

331. Guinee D Jr, Jaffe E, et al. Pulmonary lymphomatoid granulomatosis. Evidence for a proliferation of Epstein-Barr virus infected B-lymphocytes with a prominent T-cell component and vasculitis. Am J Surg Pathol 1994; 18: 753–64

332. Jaffe ES, Wilson WH. Lymphomatoid granulomatosis: pathogenesis, pathology and clinical implications. Cancer Surv 1997; 30: 233–48

333. Katzenstein AL, Peiper SC. Detection of Epstein-Barr virus genomes in lymphomatoid granulomatosis: analysis of 29 cases by the polymerase chain reaction technique. Mod Pathol 1990; 3: 435–41

334. Myers JL, Kurtin PJ, et al. Lymphomatoid granulomatosis. Evidence of immunophenotypic diversity and relationship to Epstein-Barr virus infection. Am J Surg Pathol 1995; 19: 1300–12

335. Nicholson AG, Wotherspoon AC, et al. Lymphomatoid granulomatosis: evidence that some cases represent Epstein-Barr virus-associated B-cell lymphoma. Histopathology 1996; 29: 317–24

336. Beaty MW, Toro J, et al. Cutaneous lymphomatoid granulomatosis: correlation of clinical and biologic features. Am J Surg Pathol 2001; 25: 1111–20

337. Tong T, Cooke B, Barnetson RS. Lymphomatoid granulomatosis. J Am Acad Dermatol 1992; 27(5 Pt 2): 872–6

338. Arrowsmith ER, Macon WR, et al. Peripheral T-cell lymphomas: clinical features and prognostic factors of 92 cases defined by the revised European American lymphoma classification. Leuk Lymphoma 2003; 44: 241–9

339. Ascani S, Zinzani PL, et al. Peripheral T-cell lymphomas. Clinicopathologic study of 168 cases diagnosed according to the R.E.A.L. Classification. Ann Oncol 1997; 8: 583–92

340. Campo E, Gaulard P, et al. Report of the European Task Force on Lymphomas: workshop on peripheral T-cell lymphomas. Ann Oncol 1998; 9: 835–43

341. Chan JK. Peripheral T-cell and NK-cell neoplasms: an integrated approach to diagnosis. Mod Pathol 1999; 12: 177–99

342. Hastrup N, Hamilton-Dutoit S, et al. Peripheral T-cell lymphomas: an evaluation of reproducibility of the updated Kiel classification. Histopathology 1991; 18: 99–105

343. Jaffe ES, Krenacs L, et al. Extranodal peripheral T-cell and NK-cell neoplasms. Am J Clin Pathol 1999; 111(1 Suppl 1): S46–55

344. Jaffe ES, Krenacs L, et al. Classification of cytotoxic T-cell and natural killer cell lymphomas. Semin Hematol 2003; 40: 175–84

345. Loughran TP Jr. Clonal diseases of large granular lymphocytes. Blood 1993; 82: 1–14

346. Matutes E, Catovsky D. Classification of mature T-cell leukemias. Leukemia 2003; 17: 1682–3; author reply 1683

347. Mioduszewska O. T-cell lymphomas. Arch Geschwulstforsch 1979; 49: 685–93

348. Mioduszewska O, Porwit-Ksiazek A. Significance of immunological, cytochemical and immunohistochemical methods in the diagnosis of malignant lymphomas. Mater Med Pol 1984; 16: 44–9

349. Mioduszewska O. T cell leukemia/lymphoma: histogenesis and etiology. Patol Pol 1985; 36: 121–9

350. Mioduszewska O, Kulczycka E. Immunopathological characteristics and course of various peripheral T-cell lymphomas. Nowotwory 1988; 38: 39–53

351. Pileri SA, Ascani S, et al. Peripheral T-cell lymphoma: a developing concept. Ann Oncol 1998; 9: 797–801

352. Pinkus GS, O'Hara CJ, et al. Peripheral/post-thymic T-cell lymphomas: a spectrum of disease. Clinical, pathologic, and immunologic features of 78 cases. Cancer 1990; 65: 971–98

353. Reiser M, Josting A, et al. T-cell non-Hodgkin's lymphoma in adults: clinicopathological characteristics, response to treatment and prognostic factors. Leuk Lymphoma 2002; 43: 805–11

354. Rudiger T, Weisenburger DD, et al. Peripheral T-cell lymphoma (excluding anaplastic large-cell lymphoma): results from the Non-Hodgkin's Lymphoma Classification Project. Ann Oncol 2002; 13: 140–9

355. Chiang AK, Chan AC, et al. Nasal T/natural killer (NK)-cell lymphomas are derived from Epstein-Barr virus-infected cytotoxic lymphocytes of both NK- and T-cell lineage. Int J Cancer 1997; 73: 332–8

356. Guitart J. HIV-1 and an HTLV-II-associated cutaneous T-cell lymphoma. N Engl J Med 2000; 343: 303–4

357. Jaffe ES, Burg G. Report of the symposium on Cutaneous Lymphomas: Sixth International Conference on Malignant Lymphoma. Ann Oncol 1997; (8 Suppl 1): 83–4

358. Loughran TP. HTLV infection and hematologic malignancies. Leuk Res 1996; 20: 457–8

359. Quintanilla-Martinez L, Fend F, et al. Peripheral T-cell lymphoma with Reed–Sternberg-like cells of B-cell phenotype and genotype associated with Epstein-Barr virus infection. Am J Surg Pathol 1999; 23: 1233–40

360. de Bruin PC, Kummer JA, et al. Granzyme B-expressing peripheral T-cell lymphomas: neoplastic equivalents of activated cytotoxic T-cells with preference for mucosa-associated lymphoid tissue localization. Blood 1994; 84: 3785–91

361. Knowles DM. Immunophenotypic and immunogenotypic approaches useful in distinguishing benign and malignant lymphoid proliferations. Semin Oncol 1993; 20: 583–610

362. Matutes E, Coelho E, et al. Expression of TIA-1 and TIA-2 in T cell malignancies and T cell lymphocytosis. J Clin Pathol 1996; 49: 154–8

363. Bartlett NL, Longo DL. T-small lymphocyte disorders. Semin Hematol 1999; 36: 164–70

364. Brito-Babapulle V, Maljaie SH, et al. Relationship of T leukaemias with cerebriform nuclei to T-prolymphocytic leukaemia: a cytogenetic analysis with in situ hybridization. Br J Haematol 1997; 96: 724–32

365. Catovsky D, Matutes E, et al. Is T-cell CLL a disease entity? Br J Haematol 1996; 94: 580

366. Matutes E. T-cell prolymphocytic leukemia. Cancer Control 1998; 5: 19–24

367. Matutes E. Chronic T-cell lymphoproliferative disorders. Rev Clin Exp Hematol 2002; 6: 401–20; discussion 449–50

368. Mallett RB, Matutes E, et al. Cutaneous infiltration in T-cell prolymphocytic leukaemia. Br J Dermatol 1995; 132: 263–6

369. Pawson R, Catovsky D, et al. Lack of evidence of HHV-8 in mature T-cell lymphoproliferative disorders. Lancet 1996; 348: 1450–1

370. Pawson R, Schulz TF, et al. The human T-cell lymphotropic viruses types I/II are not involved in T prolymphocytic leukemia and large granular lymphocytic leukemia. Leukemia 1997; 11: 1305–11

371. Pawson R, Schulz T, et al. Absence of HTLV-I/II in T-prolymphocytic leukaemia. Br J Haematol 1998; 102: 872–3

372. Chan WC, Link S, et al. Heterogeneity of large granular lymphocyte proliferations: delineation of two major subtypes. Blood 1986; 68: 1142–53

373. Chan WC, Gu LB, et al. Large granular lymphocyte proliferation with the natural killer-cell phenotype. Am J Clin Pathol 1992; 97: 353–8

374. Kwong YL, Chan AC, et al. CD56+ NK lymphomas: clinico-pathological features and prognosis. Br J Haematol 1997; 97: 821–9

375. Kwong YL, Wong KF. Association of pure red cell aplasia with T large granular lymphocyte leukaemia. J Clin Pathol 1998; 51: 672–5

376. Lamy T, Loughran TP. Large granular lymphocyte leukemia. Cancer Control 1998; 5: 25–33

377. Lamy T, Loughran TP Jr. Current concepts: large granular lymphocyte leukemia. Blood Rev 1999; 13: 230–40

378. Lamy T, Loughran TP Jr. Clinical features of large granular lymphocyte leukemia. Semin Hematol 2003; 40: 185–95

379. Loughran TP Jr, Kadin ME, et al. Leukemia of large granular lymphocytes: association with clonal chromosomal abnormalities and autoimmune neutropenia, thrombocytopenia, and hemolytic anemia. Ann Intern Med 1985; 102: 169–75

380. Loughran TP Jr, Starkebaum G. Large granular lymphocyte leukemia. Report of 38 cases and review of the literature. Medicine (Baltimore) 1987; 66: 397–405

381. Loughran TP Jr, Starkebaum G. Clinical features in large granular lymphocytic leukemia. Blood 1987; 69: 1786

382. Loughran TP Jr, Abbott L, et al. Absence of human herpes virus 8 DNA sequences in large granular lymphocyte (LGL) leukemia. Leuk Lymphoma 1997; 26: 177–80

383. Loughran TP Jr. Chronic T-cell leukemia/lymphoma. Cancer Control 1998; 5: 8–9

384. Macon WR, Williams ME, et al. Natural killer-like T-cell lymphomas: aggressive lymphomas of T-large granular lympho-cytes. Blood 1996; 87: 1474–83

385. Oshimi K. Leukemia and lymphoma of natural killer lineage cells. Int J Hematol 2003; 78: 18–23

386. Sokol L, Loughran TP Jr. Large granular lymphocyte leukemia and natural killer cell leukemia/lymphomas. Curr Treat Options Oncol 2003; 4: 289–96

387. Matutes E, Wotherspoon AC, et al. Transformation of T-cell large granular lymphocyte leukaemia into a high-grade large T-cell lymphoma. Br J Haematol 2001; 115: 801–6

388. Jaffe ES, Clark J, et al. Lymph node pathology of HTLV and HTLV-associated neoplasms. Cancer Res 1985; 45(9 Suppl): 4662s–4s

389. Levine PH, Cleghorn F, et al. Adult T-cell leukemia/lymphoma: a working point-score classification for epidemiological studies. Int J Cancer 1994; 59: 491–3

390. Pawson R, Richardson DS, et al. Adult T-cell leukemia/lymphoma in London: clinical experience of 21 cases. Leuk Lymphoma 1998; 31: 177–85

391. Pawson R. Malignancy: human T-cell lymphotropic virus type I and adult T-cell leukaemia/lymphoma. Hematology 1999; 4: 11–27

392. Chan JK, Ng CS, et al. Most nasal/nasopharyngeal lymphomas are peripheral T-cell neoplasms. Am J Surg Pathol 1987; 11: 418–29

393. Chan JK, Tsang WY, et al. Classification of natural killer cell neoplasms. Am J Surg Pathol 1994; 18: 1177–9

394. Chan JK. Natural killer cell neoplasms. Anat Pathol 1998; 3: 77–145

395. Cheung MM, Chan JK, et al. Natural killer cell neoplasms: a distinctive group of highly aggressive lymphomas/leukemias. Semin Hematol 2003; 40: 221–32

396. Cuadra-Garcia I, Proulx GM, et al. Sinonasal lymphoma: a clinicopathologic analysis of 58 cases from the Massachusetts General Hospital. Am J Surg Pathol 1999; 23: 1356–69

397. Gaal K, Sun NC, et al. Sinonasal NK/T-cell lymphomas in the United States. Am J Surg Pathol 2000; 24: 1511–17

398. Jaffe ES. Nasal and nasal-type T/NK cell lymphoma: a unique form of lymphoma associated with the Epstein-Barr virus. Histopathology 1995; 27: 581–3

399. Jaffe ES, Chan JK, et al. Report of the Workshop on Nasal and Related Extranodal Angiocentric T/Natural Killer Cell Lymphomas. Definitions, differential diagnosis, and epidemi-ology. Am J Surg Pathol 1996; 20: 103–11

400. Jaffe ES. Classification of natural killer (NK) cell and NK-like T-cell malignancies. Blood 1996; 87: 1207–10

401. Natkunam Y, Smoller BR, et al. Aggressive cutaneous NK and NK-like T-cell lymphomas: clinicopathologic, immunohisto-chemical, and molecular analyses of 12 cases. Am J Surg Pathol 1999; 23: 571–81

402. Natkunam Y, Warnke RA, et al. Aggressive natural killer-like T-cell malignancy with leukemic presentation following solid organ transplantation. Am J Clin Pathol 1999; 111: 663–71

403. Oshimi K. NK cell lymphoma. Int J Hematol 2002; 76(Suppl 2): 118–21

404. Ratech H, Burke JS, et al. A clinicopathologic study of malig-nant lymphomas of the nose, paranasal sinuses, and hard palate, including cases of lethal midline granuloma. Cancer 1989; 64: 2525–31

405. Siu LL, Chan JK, et al. Natural killer cell malignancies: clinico-pathologic and molecular features. Histol Histopathol 2002; 17: 539–54

406. Weiss LM, Arber DA, et al. Nasal T-cell lymphoma. Ann Oncol 1994; 5(Suppl 1): 39–42

407. Chan JK, Ng CS, et al. S-100 protein-positive sinusoidal large cell lymphoma. Hum Pathol 1987; 18: 756–9

408. Martin AR, Chan WC, et al. Aggressive natural killer cell lymphoma of the small intestine. Mod Pathol 1995; 8: 467–72

409. Chan JK, Ng CS. Malignant lymphoma, natural killer cells and hemophagocytic syndrome. Pathology 1989; 21: 154–5

410. Chen SH, Wu CS, et al. Primary sinonasal non-Hodgkin's lymphoma masquerading as chronic rhinosinusitis: an issue of routine histopathological examination. J Laryngol Otol 2003; 117: 404–7

411. Cheung MM, Chan JK, et al. Primary non-Hodgkin's lymphoma of the nose and nasopharynx: clinical features, tumor immuno-phenotype, and treatment outcome in 113 patients. J Clin Oncol 1998; 16: 70–7

412. Ferry JA, Sklar J, et al. Nasal lymphoma. A clinicopathologic study with immunophenotypic and genotypic analysis. Am J Surg Pathol 1991; 15: 268–79

413. Liu Q, Ohshima K, et al. Nasal CD56 positive small round cell tumors. Differential diagnosis of hematological, neurogenic, and myogenic neoplasms. Virchows Arch 2001; 438: 271–9

414. Baumgartner AK, Zettl A, et al. High frequency of genetic aberrations in enteropathy-type T-cell lymphoma. Lab Invest 2003; 83: 1509–16

415. de Bruin PC, Connolly CE, et al. Enteropathy-associated T-cell lymphomas have a cytotoxic T-cell phenotype. Histopathology 1997; 31: 313–17

416. Isaacson PG. Intestinal lymphoma and enteropathy. J Pathol 1995; 177: 111–13

417. Isaacson PG. Relation between cryptic intestinal lymphoma and refractory sprue. Lancet 2000; 356: 178–9

418. Murray A, Cuevas EC, et al. Study of the immunohisto-chemistry and T cell clonality of enteropathy-associated T cell lymphoma. Am J Pathol 1995; 146: 509–19

419. Pricolo VE, Mangi AA, et al. Gastrointestinal malignancies in patients with celiac sprue. Am J Surg 1998; 176: 344–7

420. Chott A, Haedicke W, et al. Most CD56$^+$ intestinal lymphomas are CD8$^+$CD5$^-$ T-cell lymphomas of monomorphic small to medium size histology. Am J Pathol 1998; 153: 1483–90

421. Chott A, Vesely M, et al. Classification of intestinal T-cell neoplasms and their differential diagnosis. Am J Clin Pathol 1999; 111(1 Suppl 1): S68–74

422. Foss HD, Stein H. Pathology of intestinal lymphomas. Recent Results Cancer Res 2000; 156: 33–41

423. Isaacson PG. Gastrointestinal lymphomas of T- and B-cell types. Mod Pathol 1999; 12: 151–8

424. Pulte D, Murray J. Celiac disease and diffuse T-cell lymphoma of the colon. Gastrointest Endosc 2001; 53: 379–81

425. Alonsozana EL, Stamberg J, et al. Isochromosome 7q: the primary cytogenetic abnormality in hepatosplenic gamma delta T cell lymphoma. Leukemia 1997; 11: 1367–72

426. Belhadj K, Reyes F, et al. Hepatosplenic gamma delta T-cell lymphoma is a rare clinicopathologic entity with poor outcome: report on a series of 21 cases. Blood 2003; 10: 4261–92

427. Chang KL, Arber DA. Hepatosplenic gamma delta T-cell lymphoma – not just alphabet soup. Adv Anat Pathol 1998; 5: 21–9

428. Cooke CB, Krenacs L, et al. Hepatosplenic T-cell lymphoma: a distinct clinicopathologic entity of cytotoxic gamma delta T-cell origin. Blood 1996; 88: 4265–74

429. Farcet JP, Gaulard P, et al. Hepatosplenic T-cell lymphoma: sinusal/sinusoidal localization of malignant cells expressing the T-cell receptor gamma delta. Blood 1990; 75: 2213–19

430. Kumar S, Lawlor C, et al. Hepatosplenic T-cell lymphoma of alphabeta lineage. Am J Surg Pathol 2001; 25: 970–1

431. Przybylski GK, Wu H, et al. Hepatosplenic and subcutaneous panniculitis-like gamma/delta T cell lymphomas are derived from different Vdelta subsets of gamma/delta T lymphocytes. J Mol Diagn 2000; 2: 11–19

432. Suarez F, Wlodarska I, et al. Hepatosplenic alphabeta T-cell lymphoma: an unusual case with clinical, histologic, and cyto-genetic features of gammadelta hepatosplenic T-cell lymphoma. Am J Surg Pathol 2000; 24: 1027–32

433. Wong KF, Chan JK, et al. Hepatosplenic gamma delta T-cell lymphoma. A distinctive aggressive lymphoma type. Am J Surg Pathol 1995; 19: 718–26

434. Lai R, Larratt LM, et al. Hepatosplenic T-cell lymphoma of alphabeta lineage in a 16-year-old boy presenting with hemolytic anemia and thrombocytopenia. Am J Surg Pathol 2000; 24: 459–63

435. Macon WR, Levy NB, et al. Hepatosplenic alphabeta T-cell lymphomas: a report of 14 cases and comparison with hepatosplenic gammadelta T-cell lymphomas. Am J Surg Pathol 2001; 25: 285–96

436. Chan JK. Splenic involvement by peripheral T-cell and NK-cell neoplasms. Semin Diagn Pathol 2003; 20: 105–20

437. Jaffe ES. Malignant lymphomas: pathology of hepatic involvement. Semin Liver Dis 1987; 7: 257–68

438. Rueffer U, Sieber M, et al. Spleen involvement in Hodgkin's lymphoma: assessment and risk profile. Ann Hematol 2003; 82: 390–6

439. Hoque SR, Child FJ, et al. Subcutaneous panniculitis-like T-cell lymphoma: a clinicopathological, immunophenotypic and mol-ecular analysis of six patients. Br J Dermatol 2003; 148: 516–25

440. Jaffe ES, Sander CA, et al. Cutaneous lymphomas: a proposal for a unified approach to classification using the R.E.A.L./WHO Classification. Ann Oncol 2000; 11(Suppl 1): 17–21

441. Kumar S, Krenacs L, et al. Subcutaneous panniculitic T-cell lymphoma is a tumor of cytotoxic T lymphocytes. Hum Pathol 1998; 29: 397–403

442. Papenfuss JS, Aoun P, et al. Subcutaneous panniculitis-like T-cell lymphoma: presentation of 2 cases and observations. Clin Lymphoma 2002; 3: 175–80

443. Salhany KE, Macon WR, et al. Subcutaneous panniculitis-like T-cell lymphoma: clinicopathologic, immunophenotypic, and genotypic analysis of alpha/beta and gamma/delta subtypes. Am J Surg Pathol 1998; 22: 881–93

444. Kummer JA, Vermeer MH, et al. Most primary cutaneous CD30-positive lymphoproliferative disorders have a CD4-positive cytotoxic T-cell phenotype. J Invest Dermatol 1997; 109: 636–40

445. Greer JP, Kinney MC, et al. T cell and NK cell lymphoprolifer-ative disorders. Hematology (Am Soc Hematol Educ Program) 2001; 259–81

446. Boulland ML, Wechsler J, et al. Primary CD30-positive cutaneous T-cell lymphomas and lymphomatoid papulosis frequently express cytotoxic proteins. Histopathology 2000; 36: 136–44

447. Chang SE, Choi HJ, et al. A case of primary cutaneous CD56+, TdT+, CD4+, blastic NK-cell lymphoma in a 19-year-old woman. Am J Dermatopathol 2002; 24: 72–5

448. Fernandez-Vazquez A, Rodriguez-Peralto JL, et al. Primary cutaneous large B-cell lymphoma: the relation between morphology, clinical presentation, immunohistochemical markers, and survival. Am J Surg Pathol 2001; 25: 307–15

449. Gonzalez CL, Medeiros LJ, et al. T-cell lymphoma involving subcutaneous tissue. A clinicopathologic entity commonly associated with hemophagocytic syndrome. Am J Surg Pathol 1991; 15: 17–27

450. Herrera E, Gallardo M, et al. Primary cutaneous CD30 (Ki-1)-positive non-anaplastic B-cell lymphoma. J Cutan Pathol 2002; 29: 181–4

451. Bakels V, Van Oostveen JW, et al. Diagnostic and prognostic significance of clonal T-cell receptor beta gene rearrangements in lymph nodes of patients with mycosis fungoides. J Pathol 1993; 170: 249–55

452. Delfau-Larue MH, Petrella T, et al. Value of clonality studies of cutaneous T lymphocytes in the diagnosis and follow-up of patients with mycosis fungoides. J Pathol 1998; 184: 185–90

453. Diamandidou E, Cohen PR, et al. Mycosis fungoides and Sezary syndrome. Blood 1996; 88: 2385–409

454. Diamandidou E, Colome-Grimmer M, et al. Transformation of mycosis fungoides/Sezary syndrome: clinical characteristics and prognosis. Blood 1998; 92: 1150–9

455. Diamandidou E, Colome M, et al. Prognostic factor analysis in mycosis fungoides/Sezary syndrome. J Am Acad Dermatol 1999; 40(6 Pt 1): 914–24

456. Falini B, Pileri S, et al. Peripheral T-cell lymphoma associated with hemophagocytic syndrome. Blood 1990; 75: 434–44

457. Kim YH, Hoppe RT. Mycosis fungoides and the Sezary syndrome. Semin Oncol 1999; 26: 276–89

458. Kim YH, Liu HL, et al. Long-term outcome of 525 patients with mycosis fungoides and Sezary syndrome: clinical prognostic factors and risk for disease progression. Arch Dermatol 2003; 139: 857–66

459. Smoller BR, Detwiler SP, et al. Role of histology in providing prognostic information in mycosis fungoides. J Cutan Pathol 1998; 25: 311–15

460. Vermeer MH, Geelen FA, et al. Expression of cytotoxic proteins by neoplastic T cells in mycosis fungoides increases with progression from plaque stage to tumor stage disease. Am J Pathol 1999; 154: 1203–10

461. Vergier B, de Muret A, et al. Transformation of mycosis fungoides: clinicopathological and prognostic features of 45 cases. French Study Group of Cutaneous Lymphomas. Blood 2000; 95: 2212–18

462. Pawson R, Matutes E, et al. Sezary cell leukaemia: a distinct T cell disorder or a variant form of T prolymphocytic leukaemia? Leukemia 1997; 11: 1009–13

463. Perez-Ordonez B, Rosai J. Follicular dendritic cell tumor: review of the entity. Semin Diagn Pathol 1998; 15: 144–54

464. Guitart J, Kennedy J, et al. Histologic criteria for the diagnosis of mycosis fungoides: proposal for a grading system to standardize pathology reporting. J Cutan Pathol 2001; 28: 174–83

465. Santucci M, Pimpinelli N, et al. Cytotoxic/natural killer cell cutaneous lymphomas. Report of EORTC Cutaneous Lymphoma Task Force Workshop. Cancer 2003; 97: 610–27

466. Bekkenk MW, Geelen FA, et al. Primary and secondary cutaneous CD30(+) lymphoproliferative disorders: a report from the Dutch Cutaneous Lymphoma Group on the long-term follow-up data of 219 patients and guidelines for diagnosis and treatment. Blood 2000; 95: 3653–61

467. Bekkenk MW, Vermeer MH, et al. Peripheral T-cell lymphomas unspecified presenting in the skin: analysis of prognostic factors in a group of 82 patients. Blood 2003; 102: 2213–19

468. Chan JK, Ng CS, et al. Angiocentric T-cell lymphoma of the skin. An aggressive lymphoma distinct from mycosis fungoides. Am J Surg Pathol 1988; 12: 861–76

469. Connors JM, Hsi ED, et al. Lymphoma of the skin. Hematology (Am Soc Hematol Educ Program): 2002; 263–82

470. Franco R, Fernandez-Vazquez A, et al. Cutaneous follicular B-cell lymphoma: description of a series of 18 cases. Am J Surg Pathol 2001; 25: 875–83

471. Kadin ME, Carpenter C. Systemic and primary cutaneous anaplastic large cell lymphomas. Semin Hematol 2003; 40: 244–56

472. Toro JR, Liewehr DJ, et al. Gamma-delta T-cell phenotype is associated with significantly decreased survival in cutaneous T-cell lymphoma. Blood 2003; 101: 3407–12

473. DeCoteau JF, Butmarc JR, et al. The t(2; 5) chromosomal translocation is not a common feature of primary cutaneous CD30+ lymphoproliferative disorders: comparison with anaplastic large-cell lymphoma of nodal origin. Blood 1996; 87: 3437–41

474. Bekkenk MW, Kluin PM, et al. Lymphomatoid papulosis with a natural killer-cell phenotype. Br J Dermatol 2001; 145: 318–22

475. Carbone A, Gloghini A, et al. BCL-6 protein expression in human peripheral T-cell neoplasms is restricted to CD30+ anaplastic large-cell lymphomas. Blood 1997; 90: 2445–50

476. Gaulard P, Bourquelot P, et al. Expression of the alpha/beta and gamma/delta T-cell receptors in 57 cases of peripheral T-cell lymphomas. Identification of a subset of gamma/delta T-cell lymphomas. Am J Pathol 1990; 137: 617–28

477. Gaulard P, Kanavaros P, et al. Bone marrow histologic and immunohistochemical findings in peripheral. T-cell lymphoma: a study of 38 cases. Hum Pathol 1991; 22: 331–8

478. Nakamura N, Suzuki S, et al. Peripheral T-cell lymphoma other than angioimmunoblastic T-cell lymphoma (AILD), with follicular dendritic cells proliferation and infection of B immunoblasts with Epstein-Barr virus. Fukushima J Med Sci 1999; 45: 45–51

479. O'Shea JJ, Jaffe ES, et al. Peripheral T cell lymphoma presenting as hypereosinophilia with vasculitis. Clinical, pathologic, and immunologic features. Am J Med 1987; 82: 539–45

480. Sun T, Susin M, et al. T-cell lymphoma associated with natural killer-like T-cell reaction. Am J Hematol 1998; 57: 331–7

481. Gorczyca W, Tsang P, et al. CD30-positive T-cell lymphomas co-expressing CD15: an immunohistochemical analysis. Int J Oncol 2003; 22: 319–24

482. Felgar RE, Furth EE, et al. Histiocytic necrotizing lymphadenitis (Kikuchi's disease): in situ end-labeling, immunohistochemical, and serologic evidence supporting cytotoxic lymphocyte-mediated apoptotic cell death. Mod Pathol 1997; 10: 231–41

483. Menasce LP, Banerjee SS, et al. Histiocytic necrotizing lymphadenitis (Kikuchi–Fujimoto disease): continuing diagnostic difficulties. Histopathology 1998; 33: 248–54

484. Attygalle A, Al-Jehani R, et al. Neoplastic T cells in angioimmunoblastic T-cell lymphoma express CD10. Blood 2002; 99: 627–33

485. Ferry JA. Angioimmunoblastic T-cell lymphoma. Adv Anat Pathol 2002; 9: 273–9

486. Frizzera G, Kaneko Y, et al. Angioimmunoblastic lymphadenopathy and related disorders: a retrospective look in search of definitions. Leukemia 1989; 3: 1–5

487. Jaffe ES. Angioimmunoblastic T-cell lymphoma: new insights, but the clinical challenge remains. Ann Oncol 1995; 6: 631–2

488. Lome-Maldonado C, Canioni D, et al. Angio-immunoblastic T cell lymphoma (AILD-TL) rich in large B cells and associated with Epstein-Barr virus infection. A different subtype of AILD-TL? Leukemia 2002; 16: 2134–41

489. Nakamura S, Sasajima Y, et al. Angioimmunoblastic T-cell lymphoma (angioimmunoblastic lymphadenopathy with dysproteinemia [AILD]-type T-cell lymphoma) followed by Hodgkin's disease associated with Epstein-Barr virus. Pathol Int 1995; 45: 958–64

490. Dogan A, Attygalle AD, et al. Angioimmunoblastic T-cell lymphoma. A review. Br J Haematol 2003; 121: 681–91

491. Benharroch D, Meguerian-Bedoyan Z, et al. ALK-positive lymphoma: a single disease with a broad spectrum of morphology. Blood 1998; 91: 2076–84

492. Chadburn A, Cesarman E, et al. CD30 (Ki-1) positive anaplastic large cell lymphomas in individuals infected with the human immunodeficiency virus. Cancer 1993; 72: 3078–90

493. Chan JK, Ng CS, et al. Anaplastic large cell Ki-1 lymphoma. Delineation of two morphological types. Histopathology 1989; 15: 11–34

494. Chan JK. Anaplastic large cell lymphoma: redefining its morphologic spectrum and importance of recognition of the ALK-positive subset. Adv Anat Pathol 1998; 5: 281–313

495. Delsol G, Mason D. 'Hallmark' cells in nodal cytotoxic lymphomas. Am J Surg Pathol 2000; 24: 1309–10

496. Gascoyne RD, Aoun P, et al. Prognostic significance of anaplastic lymphoma kinase (ALK) protein expression in adults with anaplastic large cell lymphoma. Blood 1999; 93: 3913–21

497. Falcao RP, Garcia AB, et al. Blastic CD4 NK cell leukemia/lymphoma: a distinct clinical entity. Leuk Res 2002; 26: 803–7

498. Jaffe ES. Anaplastic large cell lymphoma: the shifting sands of diagnostic hematopathology. Mod Pathol 2001; 14: 219–28

499. Kinney MC, Kadin ME. The pathologic and clinical spectrum of anaplastic large cell lymphoma and correlation with ALK gene dysregulation. Am J Clin Pathol 1999; 111(1 Suppl 1): S56–67

500. Morris SW, Xue L, et al. ALK⁺ CD30⁺ lymphomas: a distinct molecular genetic subtype of non-Hodgkin's lymphoma. Br J Haematol 2001; 113: 275–95

501. Nakamura S, Shiota M, et al. Anaplastic large cell lymphoma: a distinct molecular pathologic entity: a reappraisal with special reference to p80(NPM/ALK) expression. Am J Surg Pathol 1997; 21: 1420–32

502. Ott G, Bastian BC, et al. A lymphohistocytic variant of anaplastic large cell lymphoma with demonstration of the t(2; 5)(p23; q35) chromosome translocation. Br J Haematol 1998; 100: 187–90

503. Paulli M, Vallisa D, et al. ALK positive lymphohistocytic variant of anaplastic large cell lymphoma in an adult. Haematologica 2001; 86: 260–5

504. Pileri SA, Piccaluga A, et al. Anaplastic large cell lymphoma: update of findings. Leuk Lymphoma 1995; 18: 17–25

505. Pileri SA, Milani M, et al. Anaplastic large cell lymphoma: a concept reviewed. Adv Clin Pathol 1998; 2: 285–96

506. Pittaluga S, Wlodarska I, et al. The monoclonal antibody ALK1 identifies a distinct morphological subtype of anaplastic large cell lymphoma associated with 2p23/ALK rearrangements. Am J Pathol 1997; 151: 343–51

507. Stein H, Foss HD, et al. CD30(+) anaplastic large cell lymphoma: a review of its histopathologic, genetic, and clinical features. Blood 2000; 96: 3681–95

508. Szomor A, Zenou P, et al. Genotypic analysis in primary systemic anaplastic large cell lymphoma. Pathol Oncol Res 2003; 9: 104–6

509. ten Berge RL, Oudejans JJ, et al. ALK expression in extranodal anaplastic large cell lymphoma favors systemic disease with (primary) nodal involvement and a good prognosis and occurs before dissemination. J Clin Pathol 2000; 53: 445–50

510. Tilly H, Gaulard P, et al. Primary anaplastic large-cell lymphoma in adults: clinical presentation, immunophenotype, and outcome. Blood 1997; 90: 3727–34

511. Weisenburger DD, Anderson JR, et al. Systemic anaplastic large-cell lymphoma: results from the non-Hodgkin's lymphoma classification project. Am J Hematol 2001; 67: 172–8

512. Zinzani PL, Bendandi M, et al. Anaplastic large-cell lymphoma: clinical and prognostic evaluation of 90 adult patients. J Clin Oncol 1996; 14: 955–62

513. Bayle C, Charpentier A, et al. Leukaemic presentation of small cell variant anaplastic large cell lymphoma: report of four cases. Br J Haematol 1999; 104: 680–8

514. Fraga M, Brousset P, et al. Bone marrow involvement in anaplastic large cell lymphoma. Immunohistochemical detection of minimal disease and its prognostic significance. Am J Clin Pathol 1995; 103: 82–9

515. Greer JP, Kinney MC, et al. Clinical features of 31 patients with Ki-1 anaplastic large-cell lymphoma. J Clin Oncol 1991; 9: 539–47

516. Onciu M, Behm FG, et al. ALK-positive anaplastic large cell lymphoma with leukemic peripheral blood involvement is a clinicopathologic entity with an unfavorable prognosis. Am J Clin Pathol 2003; 120: 617–25

517. ten Berge RL, de Bruin PC, et al. ALK-negative anaplastic large cell lymphoma demonstrates similar poor prognosis to peripheral T-cell lymphoma, unspecified. Histopathology 2003; 43: 462–9

518. Kinney MC, Collins RD, et al. A small-cell-predominant variant of primary Ki-1 (CD30)+ T-cell lymphoma. Am J Surg Pathol 1993; 17: 859–68

519. Falini B, Bigerna B, et al. ALK expression defines a distinct group of T/null lymphomas ('ALK lymphomas') with a wide morphological spectrum. Am J Pathol 1998; 153: 875–86

520. Falini B, Pulford K, et al. Lymphomas expressing ALK fusion protein(s) other than NPM-ALK. Blood 1999; 94: 3509–15

521. Falini B, Pileri S, et al. ALK+ lymphoma: clinico-pathological findings and outcome. Blood 1999; 93: 2697–706

522. Brousset P, Rochaix P, et al. High incidence of Epstein-Barr virus detection in Hodgkin's disease and absence of detection in anaplastic large-cell lymphoma in children. Histopathology 1993; 23: 189–91

523. Chittal SM, Delsol G. The interface of Hodgkin's disease and anaplastic large cell lymphoma. Cancer Surv 1997; 30: 87–105

524. Weisenburger DD, Gordon BG, et al. Occurrence of the t(2; 5)(p23; q35) in non-Hodgkin's lymphoma. Blood 1996; 87: 3860–8

525. Harvell J, Vaseghi M, et al. Large atypical cells of lymphomatoid papulosis are CD56-negative: a study of 18 cases. J Cutan Pathol 2002; 29: 88–92

526. Anagnostopoulos I, Hansmann ML, et al. European Task Force on Lymphoma project on lymphocyte predominance Hodgkin disease: histologic and immunohistologic analysis of submitted cases reveals 2 types of Hodgkin disease with a nodular growth pattern and abundant lymphocytes. Blood 2000; 96: 1889–99

527. Ashton-Key M, Isaacson PG. CD45 immunostaining in T-cell-rich B-cell lymphoma and lymphocyte predominance Hodgkin's disease. J Pathol 1997; 181: 462–3

528. Boudova L, Torlakovic E, et al. Nodular lymphocyte-predominant Hodgkin lymphoma with nodules resembling T-cell/histiocyte-rich B-cell lymphoma: differential diagnosis between nodular lymphocyte-predominant Hodgkin lymphoma and T-cell/histiocyte-rich B-cell lymphoma. Blood 2003; 102: 3753–8

529. Chandi L, Kumar L, et al. Hodgkin's disease: a retrospective analysis of 15 years experience at a large referral centre. Natl Med J India 1998; 11: 212–17

530. Chittal SM, Caveriviere P, et al. Monoclonal antibodies in the diagnosis of Hodgkin's disease. The search for a rational panel. Am J Surg Pathol 1988; 12: 9–21

531. Diehl V, Josting A. Hodgkin's disease. Cancer J 2000; 6(Suppl 2): S150–8

532. Ferry JA, Harris NL. The pathology of hodgkin's disease: what's new? Semin Radiat Oncol 1996; 6: 121–30

533. Isaacson PG, Ashton–Key M. Phenotype of Hodgkin and Reed–Sternberg cells. Lancet 1996; 347: 481

534. Kuppers R, Rajewsky K, et al. L&H cells in lymphocyte-predominant Hodgkin's disease. N Engl J Med 1998; 338: 763–4; author reply 764–5

535. Mason DY, Banks PM, et al. Nodular lymphocyte predominance Hodgkin's disease. A distinct clinicopathological entity. Am J Surg Pathol 1994; 18: 526–30

536. Pileri SA, Ascani S, et al. Hodgkin's lymphoma: the pathologist's viewpoint. J Clin Pathol 2002; 55: 162–76

537. Pileri SA, Sabattini E, et al. How do we define Hodgkin's disease? The authors' reply. J Clin Pathol 2003; 56: 159

538. Stein H, Marafioti T, et al. Down-regulation of BOB.1/OBF.1 and Oct2 in classical Hodgkin disease but not in lymphocyte predominant Hodgkin disease correlates with immunoglobulin transcription. Blood 2001; 97: 496–501

539. Uherova P, Valdez R, et al. Nodular lymphocyte predominant Hodgkin lymphoma. An immunophenotypic reappraisal on a single-institution experience. Am J Clin Pathol 2003; 119: 192–8

540. Zukerberg LR, Collins AB, et al. Coexpression of CD15 and CD20 by Reed–Sternberg cells in Hodgkin's disease. Am J Pathol 1991; 139: 475–83

541. Nguyen PL, Ferry JA, et al. Progressive transformation of germinal centers and nodular lymphocyte predominance Hodgkin's disease: a comparative immunohistochemical study. Am J Surg Pathol 1999; 23: 27–33

542. Ferry JA, Zukerberg LR, et al. Florid progressive transformation of germinal centers. A syndrome affecting young men, without early progression to nodular lymphocyte predominance Hodgkin's disease. Am J Surg Pathol 1992; 16: 252–8

543. McBride JA, Rodriguez J, et al. T-cell-rich B large-cell lymphoma simulating lymphocyte-rich Hodgkin's disease. Am J Surg Pathol 1996; 20: 193–201

544. Rudiger T, Gascoyne RD, et al. Workshop on the relationship between nodular lymphocyte predominant Hodgkin's lymphoma and T cell/histiocyte-rich B cell lymphoma. Ann Oncol 2002; 13(Suppl): 44–51

545. MacLennan KA, Bennett MH, et al. Relationship of histopathologic features to survival and relapse in nodular sclerosing Hodgkin's disease. A study of 1659 patients. Cancer 1989; 64: 1686–93

546. von Wasilewski S, Franklin J, et al. Nodular sclerosing Hodgkin disease: new grading predicts prognosis in intermediate and advanced stages. Blood 2003; 101: 4063–9

547. Camilleri-Broet S, Audouin J, et al. ALK is not expressed in Hodgkin disease. Blood 2001; 97: 1901–2

548. Chadburn A, Frizzera G. Mediastinal large B-cell lymphoma vs classic Hodgkin lymphoma. Am J Clin Pathol 1999; 112: 155–8

549. Barosi G. Myelofibrosis with myeloid metaplasia: diagnostic definition and prognostic classification for clinical studies and treatment guidelines. J Clin Oncol 1999; 17: 2954–70

550. Bilgrami S, Greenberg BR. Polycythemia rubra vera. Semin Oncol 1995; 22: 307–26

551. Buhr T, Georgii A, et al. Myelofibrosis in chronic myeloproliferative disorders. Incidence among subtypes according to the Hannover Classification. Pathol Res Pract 1993; 189: 121–32

552. Cervantes F, Pereira A, et al. The changing profile of idiopathic myelofibrosis: a comparison of the presenting features of patients diagnosed in two different decades. Eur J Haematol 1998; 60: 101–5

553. Cervantes F, Alvarez-Larran A, et al. Myelofibrosis with myeloid metaplasia following essential thrombocythaemia: actuarial probability, presenting characteristics and evolution in a series of 195 patients. Br J Haematol 2002; 118: 786–90

554. Dickstein JI, Vardiman JW. Hematopathologic findings in the myeloproliferative disorders. Semin Oncol 1995; 22: 355–73

555. Georgii A, Buhr T, et al. Classification and staging of Ph-negative myeloproliferative disorders by histopathology from bone marrow biopsies. Leuk Lymphoma 1996; 22(Suppl 1): 15–29

556. Goldman JM, Melo JV. Chronic myeloid leukemia – advances in biology and new approaches to treatment. N Engl J Med 2003; 349: 1451–64

557. Georgii A, Buesche G, et al. The histopathology of chronic myeloproliferative diseases. Baillieres Clin Haematol 1998; 11: 721–49

558. Iland HJ, Laszlo J, et al. Differentiation between essential thrombocythemia and polycythemia vera with marked thrombocytosis. Am J Hematol 1987; 25: 191–201

559. Jantunen R, Juvonen E, et al. Essential thrombocythemia at diagnosis: causes of diagnostic evaluation and presence of positive diagnostic findings. Ann Hematol 1998; 77: 101–6

560. Kreft A, Weiss M, et al. Chronic idiopathic myelofibrosis: prognostic impact of myelofibrosis and clinical parameters on event-free survival in 122 patients who presented in prefibrotic and fibrotic stages. A retrospective study identifying subgroups of different prognoses by using the RECPAM method. Ann Hematol 2003; 82: 605–11

561. Lorand-Metze I, Vassallo J, et al. Histological and cytological heterogeneity of bone marrow in Philadelphia-positive chronic myelogenous leukaemia at diagnosis. Br J Haematol 1987; 67: 45–9

562. Lorand-Metze I. Bone marrow morphology at diagnosis as a prognostic parameter in Philadelphia-positive chronic myelogenous leukaemia (CML). Br J Haematol 1989; 71: 163

563. Michiels JJ, Kutti J, et al. Diagnosis, pathogenesis and treatment of the myeloproliferative disorders essential thrombocythemia, polycythemia vera and essential megakaryocytic granulocytic metaplasia and myelofibrosis. Neth J Med 1999; 54: 46–62

564. Murphy S. Polycythemia vera. Dis Mon 1992; 38: 153–212

565. Najean Y, Arrago JP, et al. The 'spent' phase of polycythemia vera: hypersplenism in the absence of myelofibrosis. Br J Haematol 1984; 56: 163–70

566. Schmitt-Graeff A, Thiele J, et al. Essential thrombocythemia with ringed sideroblasts: a heterogeneous spectrum of diseases, but not a distinct entity. Haematologica 2000; 87: 392–9

567. Spivak JL, Barosi G, et al. Chronic myeloproliferative disorders. Hematology (Am Soc Hematol Educ Program) 2003; 200–24

568. Spivak JL. Diagnosis of the myeloproliferative disorders: resolving phenotypic mimicry. Semin Hematol 2003; 40(1 Suppl): 1–5

569. Thiele J, Kvasnicka HM. Chronic myeloproliferative disorders with thrombocythemia: a comparative study of two classification systems (PVSG, WHO) on 839 patients. Ann Hematol 2003; 82: 148–52

570. Bock O, Serinsoz E, et al. The polycythemia rubra vera-1 gene is constitutively expressed by bone marrow cells and does not discriminate polycythemia vera from reactive and other chronic myeloproliferative disorders. Br J Haematol 2003; 123: 472–4

571. Buhr T, Choritz H, et al. The impact of megakaryocyte proliferation of the evolution of myelofibrosis. Histological follow-up study in 186 patients with chronic myeloid leukaemia. Virchows Arch A Pathol Anat Histopathol 1992; 420: 473–8

572. Cervantes F, Colomer D, et al. Chronic myeloid leukemia of thrombocythemic onset: a CML subtype with distinct hematological and molecular features? Leukemia 1996; 10: 1241–3

573. Harrison CN, Gale RE, et al. A large proportion of patients with a diagnosis of essential thrombocythemia do not have a clonal disorder and may be at lower risk of thrombotic complications. Blood 1999; 93: 417–24

574. Koike T, Uesugi Y, et al. 5q-syndrome presenting as essential thrombocythemia: myelodysplastic syndrome or chronic myeloproliferative disorders? Leukemia 1995; 9: 517–18

575. Kralovics R, Buser AS, et al. Comparison of molecular markers in a cohort of patients with chronic myeloproliferative disorders. Blood 2003; 102: 1869–71

576. Murphy S, Peterson P, et al. Experience of the Polycythemia Vera Study Group with essential thrombocythemia: a final report on diagnostic criteria, survival, and leukemic transition by treatment. Semin Hematol 1997; 34: 29–39

577. Murphy S. Diagnostic criteria and prognosis in polycythemia vera and essential thrombocythemia. Semin Hematol 1999; 36(1 Suppl 2): 9–13

578. Barosi G, Viarengo G, et al. Diagnostic and clinical relevance of the number of circulating CD34(+) cells in myelofibrosis with myeloid metaplasia. Blood 2001; 98: 3249–55

579. Barosi G. Myelofibrosis with myeloid metaplasia. Hematol Oncol Clin North Am 2003; 17: 1211–26

580. Harrison CN. Current trends in essential thrombocythaemia. Br J Haematol 2002; 117: 796–808

581. Harrison CN, Donohoe S, et al. Patients with essential thrombocythaemia have an increased prevalence of antiphospholipid antibodies which may be associated with thrombosis. Thromb Haemost 2002; 87: 802–7

582. Harrison CN, Green AR. Essential thrombocythemia. Hematol Oncol Clin North Am 2003; 17: 1175–90, vii

583. Gale RE. Pathogenic markers in essential thrombocythemia. Curr Hematol Rep 2003; 2: 242–7

584. Klippel P, Strunk E, et al. Biochemical characterization of PRV-1, a novel hematopoietic cell surface receptor, which is overexpressed in polycythemia rubra vera. Blood 2002; 100: 2441–8

585. Teofili L, Martini M, et al. Overexpression of the polycythemia rubra vera-1 gene in essential thrombocythemia. J Clin Oncol 2002; 15: 4249–52

586. Cervantes F, Lopez-Guillermo A, et al. An assessment of the clinicohematological criteria for the accelerated phase of chronic myeloid leukemia. Eur J Haematol 1996; 57: 286–91

587. Cervantes F, Hernandez-Boluda JC, et al. Imatinib mesylate therapy of chronic phase chronic myeloid leukemia resistant or intolerant to interferon: results and prognostic factors for response and progression-free survival in 150 patients. Haematologica 2003; 88: 1117–22

588. Cortes J, Talpaz M, et al. Effects of age on prognosis with imatinib mesylate therapy for patients with Philadelphia chromosome-positive chronic myelogenous leukemia. Cancer 2003; 98: 1105–13

589. Druker BJ, O'Brien SG, et al. Chronic myelogenous leukemia. Hematology (Am Soc Hematol Educ Program): 2002; 111–35

590. Faderl S, Talpaz M, et al. Chronic myelogenous leukemia: biology and therapy. Ann Intern Med 1999; 131: 207–19

591. Feldman E, Najfeld V, et al. The emergence of Ph⁻, trisomy-8⁺ cells in patients with chronic myeloid leukemia treated with imatinib mesylate. Exp Hematol 2003; 31: 702–7

592. Garcia-Manero G, Faderl S, et al. Chronic myelogenous leukemia: a review and update of therapeutic strategies. Cancer 2003; 98: 437–57

593. Gotlib V, Darji J, et al. Eosinophilic variant of chronic myeloid leukemia with vascular complications. Leuk Lymphoma 2003; 44: 1609–13

594. Hernandez-Boluda JC, Cervantes F, et al. Blast crisis of Ph-positive chronic myeloid leukemia with isochromosome 17q: report of 12 cases and review of the literature. Leuk Lymphoma 2000; 38: 83–90

595. Khalidi HS, Brynes RK, Medeiros LJ, et al. The immunophenotype of blast transformation of chronic myelogenous leukemia: a high frequency of mixed lineage phenotype in 'lymphoid' blasts and a comparison of morphologic, immunophenotypic, and molecular findings. Mod Pathol 1998; 11: 1211–21

596. Lowenberg B. Minimal residual disease in chronic myeloid leukemia. N Engl J Med 2003; 349: 1399–401

597. Nadal E, Cervantes F, et al. Hypercalcemia as the presenting feature of t-cell lymphoid blast crisis of ph-positive chronic myeloid leukemia. Leuk Lymphoma 2001; 41: 203–6

598. Nair C, Chopra H, et al. Immunophenotype and ultrastructural studies in blast crisis of chronic myeloid leukemia. Leuk Lymphoma 1995; 19: 309–13

599. Sawyers CL. Chronic myeloid leukemia. N Engl J Med 1999; 340: 1330–8

600. Anderson JE, Appelbaum FR. Myelodysplasia and myeloproliferative disorders. Curr Opin Hematol 1997; 4: 261–7

601. Lin CC, Manshourin T, et al. Proliferation and apoptosis in acute and chronic leukemias and myelodysplastic syndrome. Leuk Res 2002; 26: 551–9

602. Anastasi J, Feng J, et al. The relationship between secondary chromosomal abnormalities and blast transformation in chronic myelogenous leukemia. Leukemia 1995; 9: 628–33

603. Anastasi J, Feng J, et al. Lineage involvement by BCR/ABL in Ph⁺ lymphoblastic leukemias: chronic myelogenous leukemia presenting in lymphoid blast vs Ph⁺ acute lymphoblastic leukemia. Leukemia 1996; 10: 795–802

604. Cortes JE, Talpaz M, et al. Chronic myelogenous leukemia: a review. Am J Med 1996; 100: 555–70

605. Derderian PM, Kantarjian HM, et al. Chronic myelogenous leukemia in the lymphoid blastic phase: characteristics, treatment response, and prognosis. Am J Med 1993; 94: 69–74

606. Urbano-Ispizua A, Cervantes F, et al. Immunophenotypic characteristics of blast crisis of chronic myeloid leukaemia: correlations with clinico-biological features and survival. Leukemia 1993; 7: 1349–54

607. Bain BJ. Cytogenetic and molecular genetic aspects of eosinophilic leukaemias. Br J Haematol 2003; 122: 173–9

608. Brito-Babapulle F. Clonal eosinophilic disorders and the hypereosinophilic syndrome. Blood Rev 1997; 11: 129–45

609. Brito-Babapulle F. The eosinophilias, including the idiopathic hypereosinophilic syndrome. Br J Haematol 2003; 121: 203–23

610. Granjo E, Lima M, et al. Chronic eosinophilic leukaemia presenting with erythroderma, mild eosinophilia and hyper-IgE: clinical, immunological and cytogenetic features and therapeutic approach. A case report. Acta Haematol 2002; 107: 108–12

611. Guitart J. Idiopathic eosinophilia. N Engl J Med 2000; 342: 659–60; author reply 660–1

612. Kueck BD, Smith RE, et al. Eosinophilic leukemia: a myeloproliferative disorder distinct from the hypereosinophilic syndrome. Hematol Pathol 1991; 5: 195–205

613. Messinezy M, Westwood NB, et al. Serum erythropoietin values in erythrocytoses and in primary thrombocythaemia. Br J Haematol 2002; 117: 47–53

614. Najean Y, Deschamps A, et al. Acute leukemia and myelodysplasia in polycythemia vera. A clinical study with long-term follow-up. Cancer 1988; 61: 89–95

615. Pearson TC. The risk of thrombosis in essential thrombocythemia and polycythemia vera. Semin Oncol 2002; 29 (3 Suppl 10): 16–21

616. Pearson TC. Primary thrombocythaemia: diagnosis and management. Br J Haematol 1991; 78: 145–8

617. Cervantes F, Barosi G, et al. Myelofibrosis with myeloid metaplasia in adult individuals 30 years old or younger: presenting features, evolution and survival. Eur J Haematol 2001; 66: 324–7

618. Guardiola P, Anderson JE, et al. Myelofibrosis with myeloid metaplasia. N Engl J Med 2000; 343: 659; author reply 659–60

619. Hehlmann R, Jahn M, et al. Essential thrombocythemia. Clinical characteristics and course of 61 cases. Cancer 1988; 61: 2487–96

620. Murphy S, Iland H, et al. Essential thrombocythemia: an interim report from the Polycythemia Vera Study Group. Semin Hematol 1986; 23: 177–82

621. Sterkers Y, Preudhomme C, et al. Acute myeloid leukemia and myelodysplastic syndromes following essential thrombocythemia treated with hydroxyurea: high proportion of cases with 17p deletion. Blood 1998; 91: 616–22

622. George TI, Arber DA. Pathology of the myeloproliferative diseases. Hematol Oncol Clin North Am 2003; 17: 1101–27

623. Bain BJ. The relationship between the myelodysplastic syndromes and the myeloproliferative disorders. Leuk Lymphoma 1999; 34: 443–9

624. Cambier N, Baruchel A, et al. Chronic myelomonocytic leukemia: from biology to therapy. Hematol Cell Ther 1997; 39: 41–8

625. Cortes J. CMML: a biologically distinct myeloproliferative disease. Curr Hematol Rep 2003; 2: 202–8

626. Germing U, Gattermann N, et al. Problems in the classification of CMML – dysplastic versus proliferative type. Leuk Res 1998; 22: 871–8

627. Kouides PA, Bennett JM. Transformation of chronic myelomonocytic leukemia to acute lymphoblastic leukemia: case report and review of the literature of lymphoblastic transformation of myelodysplastic syndrome. Am J Hematol 1995; 49: 157–62

628. Michaux JL, Martiat P. Chronic myelomonocytic leukaemia (CMML) – a myelodysplastic or myeloproliferative syndrome? Leuk Lymphoma 1993; 9: 35–41

629. Neuwirtova R, Mocikova K, et al. Mixed myelodysplastic and myeloproliferative syndromes. Leuk Res 1996; 20: 717–26

630. Voglova J, Chrobak L, et al. Myelodysplastic and myeloproliferative type of chronic myelomonocytic leukemia – distinct subgroups or two stages of the same disease? Leuk Res 2001; 25: 493–9

631. Fenaux P, Beuscart R, et al. Prognostic factors in adult chronic myelomonocytic leukemia: an analysis of 107 cases. J Clin Oncol 1988; 6: 1417–24

632. Germing U, Gattermann N, et al. Validation of the WHO proposals for a new classification of primary myelodysplastic syndromes: a retrospective analysis of 1600 patients. Leuk Res 2000; 24: 983–92

633. Germing U, Gattermann N, et al. Two types of acquired idiopathic sideroblastic anaemia (AISA): a time-tested distinction. Br J Haematol 2000; 108: 724–8

634. Germing U, Strupp C, et al. New prognostic parameters for chronic myelomonocytic leukemia. Blood 2002; 100: 731–2; author reply 732–3

635. Carroll AJ, Poon MC, et al. Sideroblastic anemia associated with thrombocytosis and a chromosome 3 abnormality. Cancer Genet Cytogenet 1986; 22: 183–7

636. Perez Sanchez I, Perez Corrala A, et al. Sideroblastic anaemia with reactive thrombocytosis versus myelodysplastic/myeloproliferative disease. Leuk Lymphoma 2003; 44: 557–9

637. Albitar M, Manshouri T, et al. Myelodysplastic syndrome is not merely 'preleukemia'. Blood 2002; 100: 791–8

638. Aul C, Bowen DT, et al. Pathogenesis, etiology and epidemiology of myelodysplastic syndromes. Haematologica 1998; 83: 71–86

639. Bennett JM, Kouides PA, et al. The myelodysplastic syndromes: morphology, risk assessment, and clinical management (2002). Int J Hematol 2002; 76(Suppl 2): 228–38

640. Bowen D, Culligan D, et al. Guidelines for the diagnosis and therapy of adult myelodysplastic syndromes. Br J Haematol 2003; 120: 187–200

641. Foucar K, Langdon RM 2nd, et al. Myelodysplastic syndromes. A clinical and pathologic analysis of 109 cases. Cancer 1985; 56: 553–61

642. Greenberg P, Cox C, et al. International scoring system for evaluating prognosis in myelodysplastic syndromes. Blood 1997; 89: 2079–88

643. Greenberg PL. Risk factors and their relationship to prognosis in myelodysplastic syndromes. Leuk Res 1998; 22(Suppl 1): S3–6

644. Greenberg PL, Sanz GF, et al. Prognostic scoring systems for risk assessment in myelodysplastic syndromes. Forum (Genova) 1999; 9: 17–31

645. Greenberg P, Anderson J, et al. Problematic WHO reclassification of myelodysplastic syndromes. Members of the International MDS Study Group. J Clin Oncol 2000; 18: 3447–52

646. Greenberg PL, Young NS, et al. Myelodysplastic syndromes. Hematology (Am Soc Hematol Educ Program) 2002; 136–61

647. Heaney ML, Golde DW. Myelodysplasia. N Engl J Med 1999; 340: 1649–60

648. Kouides PA, Bennett JM. Morphology and classification of the myelodysplastic syndromes and their pathologic variants. Semin Hematol 1996; 33: 95–110

649. Kouides PA, Bennett JM. Understanding the myelodysplastic Syndromes. Oncologist 1997; 2: 389–401

650. Greenberg PL. Apoptosis and its role in the myelodysplastic syndromes: implications for disease natural history and treatment. Leuk Res 1998; 22: 1123–36

651. Huh YO, Jilani I, et al. More cell death in refractory anemia with excess blasts in transformation than in acute myeloid leukemia. Leukemia 2002; 16: 2249–52

652. Armitage JO, Carbone PP, et al. Treatment-related myelodysplasia and acute leukemia in non-Hodgkin's lymphoma patients. J Clin Oncol 2003; 21: 897–906

653. Aul C, Gattermann N, et al. Primary myelodysplastic syndromes: analysis of prognostic factors in 235 patients and proposals for an improved scoring system. Leukemia 1992; 6: 52–9

654. Haase D, Binder C, et al. Increased risk for therapy-associated hematologic malignancies in patients with carcinoma of the breast and combined homozygous gene deletions of glutathione transferases M1 and T1. Leuk Res 2002; 26: 249–54

655. Latagliata R, Petti MC, et al. Therapy-related myelodysplastic syndrome–acute myelogenous leukemia in patients treated for acute promyelocytic leukemia: an emerging problem. Blood 2002; 99: 822–4

656. Laughlin MJ, McGaughey DS, et al. Secondary myelodysplasia and acute leukemia in breast cancer patients after autologous bone marrow transplant. J Clin Oncol 1998; 16: 1008–12

657. Misgeld E, Germing U, et al. Secondary myelodysplastic syndrome – after fludarabine therapy of a low-grade non Hodgkin's lymphoma. Leuk Res 2001; 25: 95–8

658. Orazi A, Cattoretti G, et al. Therapy-related myelodysplastic syndromes: FAB classification, bone marrow histology, and immunohistology in the prognostic assessment. Leukemia 1993; 7: 838–47

659. Wattel E, Lai JL, et al. De novo myelodysplastic syndrome (MDS) with deletion of the long arm of chromosome 20: a subtype of MDS with distinct hematological and prognostic features? Leuk Res 1993; 17: 921–6

660. Bram S, Swolin B, et al. Is monosomy 5 an uncommon aberration? Fluorescence in situ hybridization reveals translocations and deletions in myelodysplastic syndromes or acute myelocytic leukemia. Cancer Genet Cytogenet 2003; 142: 107–14

661. Cermak J, Michalova K, et al. A prognostic impact of separation of refractory cytopenia with multilineage dysplasia and 5q-syndrome from refractory anemia in primary myelodysplastic syndrome. Leuk Res 2003; 27: 221–9

662. Chang CC, Cleveland RP. Decreased CD10-positive mature granulocytes in bone marrow from patients with myelodysplastic syndrome. Arch Pathol Lab Med 2000; 124: 1152–6

663. Cherry AM, Brockman SR, et al. Comparison of interphase FISH and metaphase cytogenetics to study myelodysplastic syndrome: an Eastern Cooperative Oncology Group (ECOG) study. Leuk Res 2003; 27: 1085–90

664. Dunkley SM, Manoharan A, et al. Myelodysplastic syndromes: prognostic significance of multilineage dysplasia in patients with refractory anemia or refractory anemia with ringed sideroblasts. Blood 2002; 99: 3870–1; author reply 3871

665. Giagounidis AA, Germing U, et al. Clinical, morphological, cytogenetic, and prognostic features of patients with myelodysplastic syndromes and del(5q) including band q31. Leukemia 2004; 18: 113–19

666. Haase D, Feuring-Buske M, et al. Cytogenetic analysis of CD34+ subpopulations in AML and MDS characterized by the expression of CD38 and CD117. Leukemia 1997; 11: 674–9

667. Lambertenghi Deliliers G, Annaloro C, et al. The diagnostic and prognostic value of bone marrow immunostaining in myelodysplastic syndromes. Leuk Lymphoma 1998; 28: 231–9

668. Oriani A, Annaloro C, et al. Bone marrow histology and CD34 immunostaining in the prognostic evaluation of primary myelodysplastic syndromes. Br J Haematol 1996; 92: 360–4

669. Soligo DA, Oriani A, et al. CD34 immunohistochemistry of bone marrow biopsies: prognostic significance in primary myelodysplastic syndromes. Am J Hematol 1994; 46: 9–17

670. Stetler-Stevenson M, Arthur DC, et al. Diagnostic utility of flow cytometric immunophenotyping in myelodysplastic syndrome. Blood 2001; 98: 979–87

671. Vallespi T, Imbert M, et al. Diagnosis, classification, and cytogenetics of myelodysplastic syndromes. Haematologica 1998; 83: 258–75

672. Strupp C, Gattermann N, et al. Refractory anemia with excess of blasts in transformation: analysis of reclassification according to the WHO proposals. Leuk Res 2003; 27: 397–404

673. Lambertenghi-Deliliers G, Orazi A, et al. Myelodysplastic syndrome with increased marrow fibrosis: a distinct clinico-pathological entity. Br J Haematol 1991; 78: 161–6

674. Lambertenghi-Deliliers G, Annaloro C, et al. Myelodysplastic syndrome associated with bone marrow fibrosis. Leuk Lymphoma 1992; 8: 51–5

675. Maschek H, Georgii A, et al. Myelofibrosis in primary myelodysplastic syndromes: a retrospective study of 352 patients. Eur J Haematol 1992; 48: 208–14

676. Bain BJ, Moorman AV, et al. Myelodysplastic syndromes associated with 11q23 abnormalities. European 11q23 Workshop participants. Leukemia 1998; 12: 834–9

677. Boultwood J, Wainscoat JS. Clonality in the myelodysplastic syndromes. Int J Hematol 2001; 73: 411–15

678. Haase D, Fonatsch C, et al. Cytogenetic findings in 179 patients with myelodysplastic syndromes. Ann Hematol 1995; 70: 171–87

679. Lewis S, Oscier D, et al. Hematological features of patients with myelodysplastic syndromes associated with a chromosome 5q deletion. Am J Hematol 1995; 49: 194–200

680. Rosati S, Mick R, et al. Refractory cytopenia with multilineage dysplasia: further characterization of an 'unclassifiable' myelodysplastic syndrome. Leukemia 1996; 10: 20–6

681. Boultwood J, Lewis S, et al. The 5q-syndrome. Blood 1994; 84: 3253–60

682. Mathew P, Tefferi A, et al. The 5q- syndrome: a single-institution study of 43 consecutive patients. Blood 1993; 81: 1040–5

683. Washington LT, Doherty D, et al. Myeloid disorders with deletion of 5q as the sole karyotypic abnormality: the clinical and pathologic spectrum. Leuk Lymphoma 2002; 43: 761–5

684. Arber DA, Carter NH, et al. Value of combined morphologic, cytochemical, and immunophenotypic features in predicting recurrent cytogenetic abnormalities in acute myeloid leukemia. Hum Pathol 2003; 34: 479–83

685. Arber DA, Stein AS, et al. Prognostic impact of acute myeloid leukemia classification. Importance of detection of recurring cytogenetic abnormalities and multilineage dysplasia on survival. Am J Clin Pathol 2003; 119: 672–80

686. Brunning RD. Classification of acute leukemias. Semin Diagn Pathol 2003; 20: 142–53

687. Gahn B, Haase D, et al. De novo AML with dysplastic hematopoiesis: cytogenetic and prognostic significance. Leukemia 1996; 10: 946–51

688. Grimwade D, Lo Coco F. Acute promyelocytic leukemia: a model for the role of molecular diagnosis and residual disease monitoring in directing treatment approach in acute myeloid leukemia. Leukemia 2002; 16: 1959–73

689. Heaney ML, Golde DW. Critical evaluation of the World Health Organization classification of myelodysplasia and acute myeloid leukemia. Curr Oncol Rep 2000; 2: 140–3

690. Szczepanski T, Orfao A, et al. Minimal residual disease in leukaemia patients. Lancet Oncol 2001; 2: 409–17

691. Arber DA, Glackin C, et al. Presence of t(8; 21)(q22; q22) in myeloperoxidase-positive, myeloid surface antigen-negative acute myeloid leukemia. Am J Clin Pathol 1997; 107: 68–73

692. Delaunay J, Vey N, et al. Prognosis of inv(16)/t(16; 16) acute myeloid leukemia (AML): a survey of 110 cases from the French AML Intergroup. Blood 2003; 102: 462–9

693. Nishii K, Usui E, et al. Characteristics of t(8; 21) acute myeloid leukemia (AML) with additional chromosomal abnormality: concomitant trisomy 4 may constitute a distinctive subtype of t(8; 21) AML. Leukemia 2003; 17: 731–7

694. Arber DA, Jenkins KA, et al. CD79 alpha expression in acute myeloid leukemia. High frequency of expression in acute promyelocytic leukemia. Am J Pathol 1996; 149: 1105–10

695. Baer MR, Stewart CC, et al. Acute myeloid leukemia with 11q23 translocations: myelomonocytic immunophenotype by multiparameter flow cytometry. Leukemia 1998; 12: 317–25

696. Basso G, Lanza F, et al. Flow cytometric immunophenotyping of acute lymphoblastic leukemia: is the time ready for consensus the guidelines? J Biol Regul Homeost Agents 2002; 16: 257–8

697. Delgado J, Morado M, et al. CD56 expression in myeloperoxidase-negative FAB M5 acute myeloid leukemia. Am J Hematol 2002; 69: 28–30

698. Escribano L, Ocqueteau M, et al. Expression of the c-kit (CD117) molecule in normal and malignant hematopoiesis. Leuk Lymphoma 1998; 30: 459–66

699. Garcia Vela JA, Martin M, et al. Acute myeloid leukemia M2 and t(8; 21)(q22; q22) with an unusual phenotype: myeloperoxidase (+), CD13 (–), CD14 (–), and CD33(–). Ann Hematol 1999; 78: 237–40

700. Grimwade D, Walker H, et al. The importance of diagnostic cytogenetics on outcome in AML: analysis of 1,612 patients entered into the MRC AML 10 trial. The Medical Research Council Adult and Children's Leukaemia Working Parties. Blood 1998; 92: 2322–33

701. Hans CP, Finn WG, et al. Usefulness of anti-CD117 in the flow cytometric analysis of acute leukemia. Am J Clin Pathol 2002; 117: 301–5

702. Kotylo PK, Seo I, et al. Flow cytometric immunophenotypic characterization of pediatric and adult minimally differentiated acute myeloid leukemia (AML-M0). Am J Clin Pathol 2000; 113: 193–200

703. Legrand O, Perrot JY, et al. The immunophenotype of 177 adults with acute myeloid leukemia: proposal of a prognostic score. Blood 2000; 96: 870–7

704. Peffault de Latour R, Legrand O, et al. Comparison of flow cytometry and enzyme cytochemistry for the detection of myeloperoxidase in acute myeloid leukaemia: interests of a new positivity threshold. Br J Haematol 2003; 122: 211–16

705. Rizzatti EG, Garcia AB, et al. Expression of CD117 and CD11b in bone marrow can differentiate acute promyelocytic leukemia from recovering benign myeloid proliferation. Am J Clin Pathol 2002; 118: 31–7

706. Thalhammer-Scherrer R, Mitterbauer G, et al. The immunophenotype of 325 adult acute leukemias. Am J Clin Pathol 2002; 117: 380–9

707. Chevallier N, Corcoran CM, et al. The ETO protein of t(8; 21) AML is a corepressor for the Bcl-6 B-cell lymphoma oncoprotein. Blood 2004; 103: 1454–63

708. Ferrara F, Di Noto R, et al. Immunophenotypic analysis enables the correct prediction of t(8; 21) in acute myeloid leukaemia. Br J Haematol 1998; 102: 444–8

709. Hurwitz CA, Raimondi SC, et al. Distinctive immunophenotypic features of t(8; 21)(q22; q22) acute myeloblastic leukemia in children. Blood 1992; 80: 3182–8

710. Yamamoto K, Nagata K, et al. CD7$^+$ near-tetraploid acute myeloblastic leukemia M2 with double t(8; 21)(q22; q22) translocations and Aml1/ETO rearrangements detected by fluorescence in situ hybridization analysis. Int J Hematol 2001; 74: 316–21

711. Fenaux P, Degos L. Differentiation therapy for acute promyelocytic leukemia. N Engl J Med 1997; 337: 1076–7

712. Fenaux P, Chomienne C, et al. Treatment of acute promyelocytic leukaemia. Best Pract Res Clin Haematol 2001; 14: 153–74

713. Fenaux P, Chevret S, et al. Treatment of older adults with acute promyelocytic leukaemia. Best Pract Res Clin Haematol 2003; 16: 495–501

714. Grimwade D, Biondi A, et al. Characterization of acute promyelocytic leukemia cases lacking the classic t(15; 17): results of the European Working Party. Blood 2000; 96: 1297–308

715. Arber DA, Jenkins KA. Paraffin section immunophenotyping of acute leukemias in bone marrow specimens. Am J Clin Pathol 1996; 106: 462–8

716. Nagendra S, Meyerson H, et al. Leukemias resembling acute promyelocytic leukemia, microgranular variant. Am J Clin Pathol 2002; 117: 651–7

717. Fenaux P, Vanhaesbroucke C, et al. Acute monocytic leukaemia in adults: treatment and prognosis in 99 cases. Br J Haematol 1990; 75: 41–8

718. Gil-Mateo MP, Miquel FJ, et al. Aleukemic 'leukemia cutis' of monocytic lineage. J Am Acad Dermatol 1997; 36(5 Pt 2): 837–40

719. Killick S, Matutes E, et al. Acute erythroid leukemia (M6): outcome of bone marrow transplantation. Leuk Lymphoma 1999; 35: 99–107

720. Peterson LC, Parkin JL, et al. Acute basophilic leukemia. A clinical, morphologic, and cytogenetic study of eight cases. Am J Clin Pathol 1991; 96: 160–70

721. Horny HP, Kaiserling E, et al. Bone marrow mastocytosis associated with an undifferentiated extramedullary tumor of hemopoietic origin. Arch Pathol Lab Med 1997; 121: 423–6

722. Traweek ST, Arber DA, et al. Extramedullary myeloid cell tumors. An immunohistochemical and morphologic study of 28 cases. Am J Surg Pathol 1993; 17: 1011–19

723. Carbonell F, Swansbury J, et al. Cytogenetic findings in acute biphenotypic leukaemia. Leukemia 1996; 10: 1283–7

724. Hanson CA, Abaza M, et al. Acute biphenotypic leukaemia: immunophenotypic and cytogenetic analysis. Br J Haematol 1993; 84: 49–60

725. Killick S, Matutes E, et al. Outcome of biphenotypic acute leukemia. Haematologica 1999; 84: 699–706

726. Legrand O, Perrot JY, et al. Adult biphenotypic acute leukaemia: an entity with poor prognosis which is related to unfavorable cytogenetics and P-glycoprotein over-expression. Br J Haematol 1998; 100: 147–55

727. Matutes E, Morilla R, et al. Definition of acute biphenotypic leukemia. Haematologica 1997; 82: 64–6

728. De Zen L, Orfao A, et al. Quantitative multiparametric immunophenotyping in acute lymphoblastic leukemia: correlation with specific genotype. I. ETV6/AML1 ALLs identification. Leukemia 2000; 14: 1225–31

729. Khalidi HS, O'Donnell MR, et al. Adult precursor-B acute lymphoblastic leukemia with translocations involving chromosome band 19p13 is associated with poor prognosis. Cancer Genet Cytogenet 1999; 109: 58–65

730. Lukas DR, Bentley G, et al. Ewing sarcoma vs lymphoblastic lymphoma. A comparative immunohistochemical study. Am J Clin Pathol 2001; 115: 11–17

731. Navid F, Mosijczuk AD, et al. Acute lymphoblastic leukemia with the (8; 14)(q24; q32) translocation and FAB L3 morphology associated with a B-precursor immunophenotype: the Pediatric Oncology Group experience. Leukemia 1999; 13: 135–41

732. Pui CH, Rivera GK, et al. Clinical significance of CD10 expression in childhood acute lymphoblastic leukemia. Leukemia 1993; 7: 35–40

733. Tabernero MD, Bortoluci AM, et al. Adult precursor B-ALL with BCR/ABL gene rearrangements displays a unique immunophenotype based on the pattern of CD10, CD34, CD13 and CD38 expression. Leukemia 2001; 15: 406–14

734. Vasef MA, Brynes RK, et al. Surface immunoglobulin light chain-positive acute lymphoblastic leukemia of FAB L1 or L2 type: a report of 6 cases in adults. Am J Clin Pathol 1998; 110: 143–9

735. Kita K, Nakase K, et al. Phenotypical characteristics of acute myelocytic leukemia associated with the t(8; 21)(q22; q22) chromosomal abnormality: frequent expression of immature B-cell antigen CD19 together with stem cell antigen CD34. Blood 1992; 80: 470–7

736. Rimsha LM, Larson RS, et al. Benign hematogone-rich lymphoid proliferations can be distinguished from B-lineage acute lymphoblastic leukemia by integration of morphology, immunophenotype, adhesion molecule expression, and architectural features. Am J Clin Pathol 2000; 114: 66–75

737. Nakamura S, Koshikawa T, et al. Lymphoblastic lymphoma expressing CD56 and TdT. Am J Surg Pathol 1998; 22: 135–7

738. Bayerl MG, Rakozy CK, et al. Blastic natural killer cell lymphoma/leukemia: a report of seven cases. Am J Clin Pathol 2002; 117: 41–50

739. DiGiuseppe JA, Louie DC, et al. Blastic natural killer cell leukemia/lymphoma: a clinicopathologic study. Am J Surg Pathol 1997; 21: 1223–30

740. Feuillard J, Jacob MC, et al. Clinical and biologic features of CD4$^+$CD56$^+$ malignancies. Blood 2002; 99: 1556–63

741. Khoury JD, Medeiros LJ, et al. CD56(+) TdT(+) blastic natural killer cell tumor of the skin: a primitive systemic malignancy related to myelomonocytic leukemia. Cancer 2002; 94: 2401–8

742. Leroux D, Mugneret F, et al. CD4$^+$, CD56$^+$ DC2 acute leukemia is characterized by recurrent clonal chromosomal changes affecting 6 major targets: a study of 21 cases by the Groupe Français de Cytogénétique Hématologique. Blood 2002; 99: 4154–9

743. Petrella T, Dalac S, et al. CD4$^+$ CD56$^+$ cutaneous neoplasms: a distinct hematological entity? Groupe Français d'Etude des Lymphomes Cutanés (GFELC). Am J Surg Pathol 1999; 23: 137–46

744. Petrella T, Comeau MR, et al. 'Agranular CD4$^+$ CD56$^+$ hematodermic neoplasm' (blastic NK-cell lymphoma) originates from a population of CD56$^+$ precursor cells related to plasmacytoid monocytes. Am J Surg Pathol 2002; 26: 852–62

745. Copie-Bergman C, Wotherspoon AC, et al. True histiocytic lymphoma: a morphologic, immunohistochemical, and molecular genetic study of 13 cases. Am J Surg Pathol 1998; 22: 1386–92

746. Hanson CA, Jaszcz W, et al. True histiocytic lymphoma: histopathologic, immunophenotypic and genotypic analysis. Br J Haematol 1989; 73: 187–98

747. Isaacson PG. Histiocytic malignancy. Histopathology 1985; 9: 1007–11

748. Kamel OW, Gocke CD, et al. True histiocytic lymphoma: a study of 12 cases based on current definition. Leuk Lymphoma 1995; 18: 81–6

749. Miettinen M, Fletcher CD, et al. True histiocytic lymphoma of small intestine. Analysis of two S-100 protein-positive cases with features of interdigitating reticulum cell sarcoma. Am J Clin Pathol 1993; 100: 285–92

750. Milchgrub S, Kamel OW, et al. Malignant histiocytic neoplasms of the small intestine. Am J Surg Pathol 1992; 16: 11–20

751. Pileri SA, Grogan TM, et al. Tumours of histiocytes and accessory dendritic cells: an immunohistochemical approach to classification from the International Lymphoma Study Group based on 61 cases. Histopathology 2002; 41: 1–29

752. Soria C, Orradre JL, et al. True histiocytic lymphoma (monocytic sarcoma). Am J Dermatopathol 1992; 14: 511–17

753. Soslow RA, Davis RE, et al. True histiocytic lymphoma following therapy for lymphoblastic neoplasms. Blood 1996; 87: 5207–12

754. Gonzalez CL, Jaffe ES. The histiocytoses: clinical presentation and differential diagnosis. Oncology (Huntingt) 1990; 4: 47–60; discussion 60, 62

755. Hage C, Willman CL, et al. Langerhans' cell histiocytosis (histiocytosis X): immunophenotype and growth fraction. Hum Pathol 1993; 24: 840–5

756. Howarth DM, Gilchrist GS, et al. Langerhans cell histiocytosis. Diagnosis, natural history, management, and outcome. Cancer 1999; 85: 2278–90

757. Lieberman PH, Jones CR, et al. Langerhans cell (eosinophilic) granulomatosis. A clinicopathologic study encompassing 50 years. Am J Surg Pathol 1996; 20: 519–52

758. Nezelof C, Basset F. Langerhans cell histiocytosis research. Past, present, and future. Hematol Oncol Clin North Am 1998; 12: 385–406

759. Rosai J, Dorfman RF. Sinus histiocytosis with massive lymphadenopathy. A newly recognized benign clinicopathological entity. Arch Pathol 1969; 87: 63–70

760. Jaffe ES, Costa J, et al. Malignant lymphoma and erythrophagocytosis simulating malignant histiocytosis. Am J Med 1983; 75: 741–9

761. Chan JK, Tsang WY, et al. Follicular dendritic cell tumors of the oral cavity. Am J Surg Pathol 1994; 18: 148–57

762. Chan JK, Fletcher CD, et al. Follicular dendritic cell sarcoma. Clinicopathologic analysis of 17 cases suggesting a malignant potential higher than currently recognized. Cancer 1997; 79: 294–313

763. Choi PC, To KF, et al. Follicular dendritic cell sarcoma of the neck: report of two cases complicated by pulmonary metastases. Cancer 2000; 89: 664–72

764. Hollowood K, Stamp G, et al. Extranodal follicular dendritic cell sarcoma of the gastrointestinal tract. Morphologic, immunohistochemical and ultrastructural analysis of two cases. Am J Clin Pathol 1995; 103: 90–7

765. Perez-Ordonez B, Erlandson RA, et al. Follicular dendritic cell tumor: report of 13 additional cases of a distinctive entity. Am J Surg Pathol 1996; 20: 944–55

766. Austen KF. Systemic mastocytosis. N Engl J Med 1992; 326: 639–40

767. Bain BJ. Systemic mastocytosis and other mast cell neoplasms. Br J Haematol 1999; 106: 9–17

768. Gupta R, Bain BJ, et al. Cytogenetic and molecular genetic abnormalities in systemic mastocytosis. Acta Haematol 2002; 107: 123–8

769. Horan RF, Austen KF. Systemic mastocytosis: retrospective review of a decade's clinical experience at the Brigham and Women's Hospital. J Invest Dermatol 1991; 96: 5S-13S; discussion 13S-14S

770. Horny HP, Parwaresch MR, et al. Bone marrow findings in systemic mastocytosis. Hum Pathol 1985; 16: 808–14

771. Horny HP, Kaiserling E, et al. Lymph node findings in generalized mastocytosis. Histopathology 1992; 21: 439–46

772. Horny HP, Ruck P, et al. Systemic mast cell disease (mastocytosis). General aspects and histopathological diagnosis. Histol Histopathol 1997; 12: 1081–9

773. Horny HP, Sillaber C, et al. Diagnostic value of immunostaining for tryptase in patients with mastocytosis. Am J Surg Pathol 1998; 22: 1132–40

774. Horny HP, Valent P. Diagnosis of mastocytosis: general histopathological aspects, morphological criteria, and immunohistochemical findings. Leuk Res 2001; 25: 543–51

775. Horny HP, Valent P. Histopathological and immunohistochemical aspects of mastocytosis. Int Arch Allergy Immunol 2002; 127: 115–17

776. Jordan JH, Walchshofer S, et al. Immunohistochemical properties of bone marrow mast cells in systemic mastocytosis: evidence for expression of CD2, CD117/Kit, and bcl-x(L). Hum Pathol 2001; 32: 545–52

777. Li CY. Diagnosis of mastocytosis: value of cytochemistry and immunohistochemistry. Leuk Res 2001; 25: 537–41

778. Longley J, Duffy TP, et al. The mast cell and mast cell disease. J Am Acad Dermatol 1995; 32: 545–61; quiz 562–4

779. Longley BJ, Metcalfe DD. A proposed classification of mastocytosis incorporating molecular genetics. Hematol Oncol Clin North Am 2000; 14: 697–701, viii

780. Metcalfe DD, Akin C. Mastocytosis: molecular mechanisms and clinical disease heterogeneity. Leuk Res 2001; 25: 577–82

781. Natkunam Y, Rouse RV. Utility of paraffin section immunohistochemistry for C-KIT (CD117) in the differential diagnosis of systemic mast cell disease involving the bone marrow. Am J Surg Pathol 2000; 24: 81–91

782. Valent P, Horny HP, et al. Diagnostic criteria and classification of mastocytosis: a consensus proposal. Leuk Res 2001; 25: 603–25

783. Valent P, Akin C, et al. Mast cell proliferative disorders: current view on variants recognized by the World Health Organization. Hematol Oncol Clin North Am 2003; 17: 1227–41

784. Valent P, Akin C, et al. Diagnosis and treatment of systemic mastocytosis: state of the art. Br J Haematol 2003; 122: 695–717

785. Valent P, Akin C, et al. Aggressive systemic mastocytosis and related mast cell disorders: current treatment options and proposed response criteria. Leuk Res 2003; 27: 635–41

786. Wilkins BS, Bain BJ. Normal and neoplastic mast cells. Br J Haematol 1999; 106: 1

787. Gine E, Bosch F, et al. Simultaneous diagnosis of hairy cell leukemia and chronic lymphocytic leukemia/small lymphocytic lymphoma: a frequent association? Leukemia 2002; 16: 1454–9

788. Kim H. Composite lymphoma and related disorders. Am J Clin Pathol 1993; 99: 445–51

789. Kuppers R, Sousa AB, et al. Common germinal-center B-cell origin of the malignant cells in two composite lymphomas, involving classical Hodgkin's disease and either follicular lymphoma or B-CLL. Mol Med 2001; 7: 285–92

790. Siebert JD, Mulvaney DA, et al. Utility of flow cytometry in subtyping composite and sequential lymphoma. J Clin Lab Anal 1999; 13: 199–204

Abbreviations

AILD	angioimmunoblastic T-cell lymphoma	DLBCL	diffuse large B-cell lymphoma
ALCL	anaplastic large cell lymphoma	EBV	Epstein–Barr virus
ALIP	abnormal localization of immature precursors	EMA	epithelial membrane antigen
		EMT	extramedullary myeloid tumors
ALK	anaplastic lymphoma kinase	ET	essential thrombocythemia
ALL	acute lymphoblastic leukemia	FC	flow cytometry
AML	acute myeloid leukemia	FDC	follicular dendritic cell
AML1/ETO	AML with t(8;21)	FISH	fluorescence *in situ* hybridization
AML-M0	acute myeloid leukemia, minimally differentiated	FL	hollicular lymphoma
		FS	forward scatter
AML-M1	acute myeloid leukemia without maturation	FSC	forward scatter
		GCC	germinal center cells
AML-M2	acute myeloid leukemia with maturation	GIST	gastrointestinal stromal tumors
AML-M3	acute promyelocytic leukemia	GPHA	glycophorin A
AML-M4	acute myelomonocytic leukemia	HCL	hairy cell leukemia
AML-M4Eo	acute myelomonocytic leukemia with eosinophilia	HHV-8	human herpes virus 8
		HL	(classical) Hodgkin lymphoma
AML-M5	acute monoblastic leukemia	HTLV-I/II	human T-cell lymphotropic viruses
AML-M6	acute erythroid leukemia	IDC	interdigitating reticulum cells
AML-M7	acute megakaryoblastic leukemia	IHC	immunohistochemical
APL	acute promyelocytic leukemia	KS	Kaposi sarcoma
ATLL	adult T-cell leukemia/lymphoma	LBL	lymphoblastic lymphoma
B-ALL/LBL	precursor B-lymphoblastic leukemia/ lymphoma	LCA	leukocyte common antigen
		LGL	large granular lymphocyte
B-CLL	B-chronic lymphocytic leukemia	L&H	lymphocyte and histiocyte cell (-popcorn cell)
B-CLL/SLL	chronic lymphocytic leukemia/small lymphocytic lymphoma	M:E	myeloid to erythroid ratio
		MALT	mucosa-associated lymphoid tissue
BM	bone marrow	MCL	mantle cell lymphoma
B-PLL	B-cell prolymphocytic leukemia	MDS	myelodysplastic syndrome
CIMF	chronic idiopathic myelofibrosis	MF/SS	mycosis fungoides/Sezary syndrome
CML	chronic myelogenous leukemia	MGUS	monoclonal gammapathy of undetermined significance
CMML	chronic myelomonocytic leukemia		
CMPD	chronic myeloproliferative disorders	MM	plasma cell myeloma
CMV	cytomegalovirus	MPO	myeloperoxidase
DC2	blastic NK-cell leukemia/lymphoma	MZL	marginal zone B-cell lymphoma

NHL	non-Hodgkin lymphoma	RCMD	refractory cytopenia with multilineage dysplasia
NK	natural killer		
NLPHL	nodular lymphocyte-predominant Hodgkin lymphoma	RCMD-RS	refractory cytopenia with multilineage dysplasia and ringed sideroblasts
NOS	not otherwise specified	RES	reactive erythrophagocytic syndrome
NS	nodular sclerosis	R–S	Reed–Sternberg
NSE	alpha naphthyl butyrate esterase	SLL	small lymphocytic lymphoma
NSE	non-specific esterase	SLVL	splenic lymphoma with villous lymphocytes
PCR	polymerase chain reaction		
PEL	primary effusion lymphoma	SMZL	splenic marginal zone lymphoma
PAS	periodic acid-Schiff	SS	Sezary syndrome
PTGC	progressive transformation of germinal centers	SSC	side scatter
		T-ALL/LBL	precursor T lymphoblastic leukemia/ lymphoma
PLL	prolymphocytic leukemia		
PV	polycythemia vera	TCR	T-cell antigen receptors
RA	refractory anemia	TCRLBCL	T-cell/histiocyte-rich, large B-cell lymphoma
RA	rheumatoid arthritis		
RAEB	refractory anemia with excess blasts	T-LGL	T-cell large granular lymphocytic leukemia
RARS	refractory anemia with ringed sideroblasts		
		T-PLL	T-cell prolymphocytic leukemia

Index